Encyclopedia of Endoscopy

Encyclopedia of Endoscopy

Edited by **Steven Notley**

hayle medical

New York

Published by Hayle Medical,
30 West, 37th Street, Suite 612,
New York, NY 10018, USA
www.haylemedical.com

Encyclopedia of Endoscopy
Edited by Steven Notley

International Standard Book Number: 978-1-63241-164-8 (Hardback)

Printed in China.

Contents

Preface

Over the recent decade, advancements and applications have progressed exponentially. This has led to the increased interest in this field and projects are being conducted to enhance knowledge. The main objective of this book is to present some of the critical challenges and provide insights into possible solutions. This book will answer the varied questions that arise in the field and also provide an increased scope for furthering studies.

Encyclopedic information regarding the procedure of endoscopy has been illuminated in this book. Endoscopy has played a vital role in the development of modern medicine and other medical specialties. The field of endoscopic procedure has evolved over the last decade. By using varied information, it has provided a better understanding regarding pathogenic mechanisms, description of new entities and applications for early detection, diagnostic procedures and therapeutic procedures. The benefits of various technical advances and modern endoscopic equipment have led to a dynamic evolution of endoscopy. Consequently, endoscopy has outweighed its function as just an examination tool and it has become a rapid and efficient therapeutic tool for various organs including gastrointestinal tract, head and neck, respiratory tract and others. This book is an evidence of the efficacy and usefulness of endoscopy.

I hope that this book, with its visionary approach, will be a valuable addition and will promote interest among readers. Each of the authors has provided their extraordinary competence in their specific fields by providing different perspectives as they come from diverse nations and regions. I thank them for their contributions.

Editor

Section 1

General Aspects

Chapter 1

Endoscopy and Histopathology

Karel Geboes, Karen Geboes and
Anne Jouret-Mourin

Additional information is available at the end of the chapter

1. Introduction

Endoscopy and histopathology are two morphological diagnostic procedures which allow direct examination of organs with optical methods. They can detect abnormalities of the normal anatomy and histology and provide a precise diagnosis. Based on the information derived from these investigations an adequate treatment, either medical or surgical can be proposed. The optical resolution of both methods is different. Classical endoscopy is using essentially the naked eye observation of the tissue which allows a diagnosis of an ulcer or a raised lesion for instance, while histopathology is reaching the cellular and sub-cellular level. The new endoscopic techniques however do increase the optical resolution. The major contributions of histopathology to endoscopy are situated in inflammatory and neoplastic diseases. Histopathology allows a more precise diagnosis of the type of inflammation and a better classification of tumours. This has again an impact upon treatment. For the diagnosis, histopathology can be an essential element, as illustrated by gluten sensitive enteropathy (although serology is also an essential element) or by identification of specific pathogens such as Giardia lamblia, Mycobacterium avium, cryptosporidia.... Histopathology can further be important for the confirmation of a diagnosis but very often it will provide a more precise diagnosis by determining the aetiology of inflammation as illustrated by autoimmune gastritis, or by typing a tumour (adenocarcinoma or lymphoma). In addition, histopathology can provide essential elements for further therapy strategy by demonstrating the presence or absence of risk factors for residual tumour in polypectomy or endoscopic mucosal resection. Indirectly, it offers the possibility of using additional techniques such as biomarkers for dysplasia and cancer or the demonstration of mutations such as KRAS in colorectal cancer or HER2 amplification in oesophageal and gastric cancer.[1, 2].These applications can have important therapeutic consequences. It has been shown for instance that activating mutations of the KRAS gene are associated with poor response to anti-EGFR therapies and that patients with tumors that had high levels of HER2 protein expression derived the greatest benefit from treatment with trastuzumab..

2. What is the influence of endoscopy on the diagnostic yield of histopathology?

2.1. General requirements for the endoscopist and the pathologist

A close collaboration between the endoscopist and the pathologist is essential for an accurate diagnosis. This imposes on each of the partners some constraints.

Overall the endoscopist should provide the pathologists with a copy of the endoscopy report mentioning the sites of the biopsies, a macroscopic description of the lesions if present and the adjacent mucosa and essential clinical information such as the age of the patient, the immune status of the patient, duration of symptoms and treatment if any.

The pathologist should provide information of the quality of the biopsies (number and size and depth of the samples) in order to avoid false conclusions, a degree of probability of his initial diagnosis and if needed suggest particular conditions for further sampling or ancillary techniques such as immune histochemistry. Contentious cases should be selected for clinic pathological discussion.[3]

2.2. Sampling of biopsies

The diagnostic yield of histopathology depends upon the experience of the pathologist but also upon the quality of the biopsy samples and sampling error. The quality of the samples is influenced by a variety of elements such as the size and shape of the biopsy forceps, the nature and location of the disease, the experience of the endoscopist and the number of samples. During endoscopy samples can be obtained by way of different techniques. These include pinch biopsy, suction biopsy with a multipurpose tube (which provides larger samples), brush cytology, endoscopic fine needle aspiration (offering material from deep areas in the lesion) and snare excision or strip biopsy.

Pinch biopsy is the most common technique. Several types of biopsy forceps are available. A distinction can be made between those with elliptical and those with round cups. Generally the samples obtained with elliptical cups are larger. A forceps with round cups may be more appropriate for children in order to avoid complications. The size of the biopsy forceps determines partly the size (surface and depth) of the samples. The small forceps has a width of 1.8 mm when opened. The average forceps has a 2.4 mm diameter and allows to obtain samples containing the muscularis mucosae (and upper submucosa) in 60% of the cases. The larger Jumbo forceps has a 3.4 mm diameter. Samples obtained with this forceps are larger, but, they usually contain not more submucosa and the risk of complications (perforation and bleeding) may be more important, whereas it is minimal with the smaller forceps (if the patient has normal coagulation). A forceps can have a central spike so that it stays in position in the mucosa, during the procedure. The spike can induce artefacts which should not be confused with erosions.

The anatomic location or certain types of lesions may be the reason why samples are of less good quality or superficial in nature. This is often so in areas immediately distal to a stricture, and at the papilla of Vater in the duodenum. The extrahepatic bile ducts and the pancreatic duct are other areas where biopsies are more difficult to obtain and hence usually smaller. If the biopsies of the papilla are taken following sphincterotomy, coagulation artefacts are likely to be present.

In order to obtain samples of appropriate depth air insufflation during the endoscopic examination should be limited. When over-insufflation occurs the mucosa is stretched and pushed towards the underlying submucosa and the samples are likely to be more superficial.

The samples obtained with a forceps are usually limited to the mucosa. Normally they are not suitable for the assessment of submucosal or deeper lesions. This means that they are not good for instance for a diagnosis of "vasculitis", except for small vessel disease. By the use of a "burrowing technique" whereby several biopsies are taken in the same area information of deeply situated lesions can eventually be obtained. An alternative are samples obtained with endoscopic ultrasound guided fine needle aspiration. They are usually smaller but they permit both morphologic and cytologic analysis of lesions within or adjacent to the gastrointestinal (GI) tract. They can be used for the assessment of neoplastic lesions, but because of the small size, they are not good for conditions such as vasculitis.[4]

2.3. Larger samples

Larger samples are obtained with endoscopic mucosal resection (EMR) or endoscopical submucosal resection (ESD) and snare polypectomy. These samples must be handled adequately by the endoscopist or/and in the pathology lab. The histopathological interpretation of these samples provides important information for subsequent management and assessment of the risk for residual cancer. A correct diagnostic process involves, tumour differentiation, precise determination of deep infiltration, lymphatic permeation and adequate determination of the section margin. Identification of this area is easy if the lesion is adequately oriented. In the case of polypectomy, the endoscopist could identify the section margin with India ink or with a pin if the lesion is removed in one piece. The specimen will be cut along the marker. (Fig. 1) In the case of EMR /ESD, ideally, the specimen should be oriented, pinned and stretched on card board in the endoscopy unit.(Fig 2) If the specimen is not removed in one piece, reconstruction of the specimens should be attempted. Painting of the base and margins is useful, as tumour extension to the deep margin implies surgery and remnants of the neoplastic epithelium at the lateral margins indicate re-excision or postoperative destruction.[5, 6] Good communication between the pathologist and the clinicians is important for the assessment of the efficacy of the treatment and for the design of the strategy of the additional treatment which is based upon the depth of invasion of the lesion. If the resection has been performed in piecemeal fashion and the specimen is received in two or more fragments, it may be impossible to determine the true margin of resection, if the endoscopist did not attempt to identify the true margin or placed the true margin in a separate container.[7]

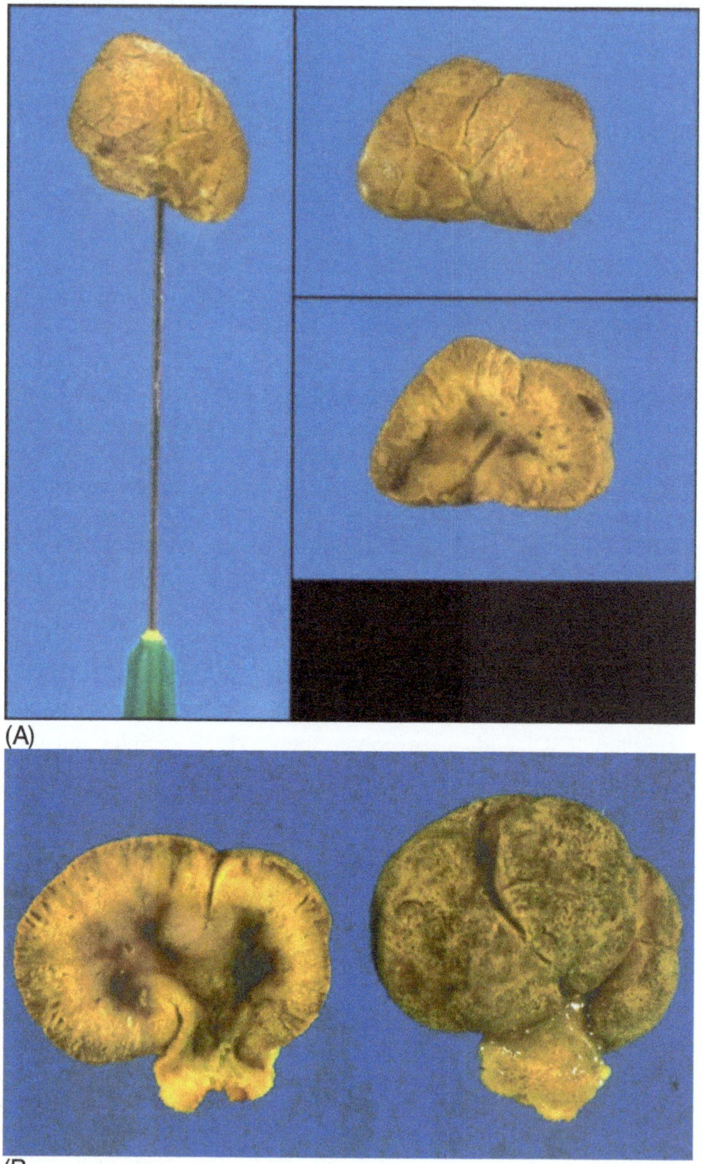

Figure 1. Polypectomy specimen correctly oriented using a needle showing the top (upper right) and the base (lower right) (A) and cut along the orientation (B)

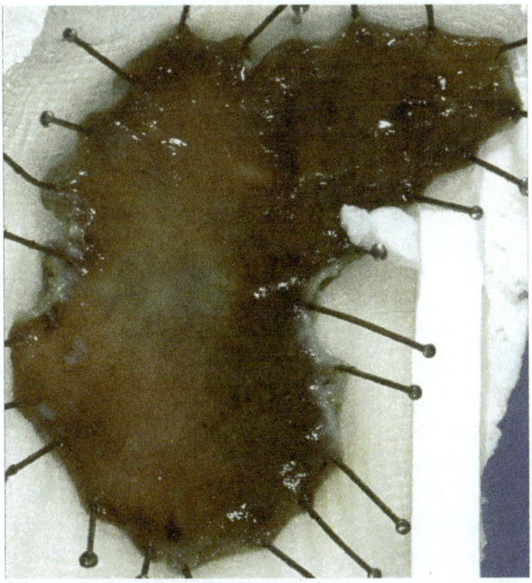

(A)

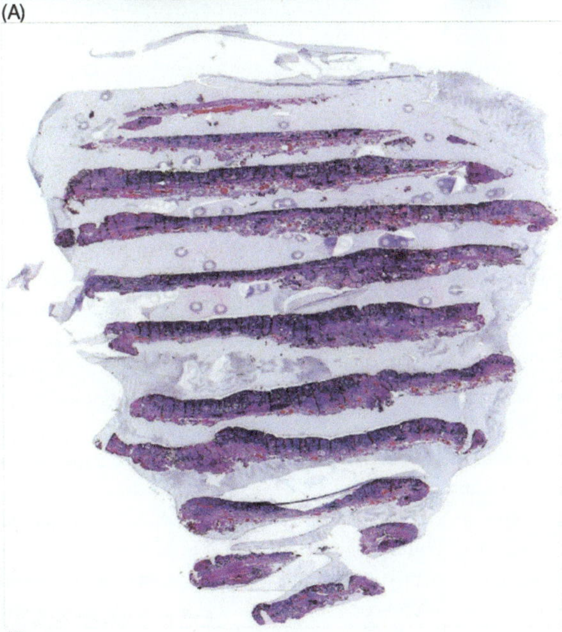

(B

Figure 2. Specimen from endoscopic mucosal resection pinned out and stretched (A) and cut at all levels (B)

2.4. Endoscopic ultrasound-guided fine-needle aspiration biopsy

Endoscopic ultrasound guided fine needle aspiration has become the most accurate modality for characterization of pancreatic cystic and solid lesions, differential diagnosis of indeterminate masses and locoregional staging of some digestive cancers (gastric, oesophagus, pancreas, biliary tract…). It should be performed in the primary mass but also in distant lymph nodes, or metastatic locations. EUS-FNA has a high sensitivity, specificity, positive predictive value and accuracy in the assessment of biliopancreatic tumours. The performance of this technique is dependent on the endoscopist and cytopathologist experience. It is well known that accuracy of FNA increases when the technique is performed by an experienced clinician and when the slides are reviewed by an experienced cytopathologist the collaboration between these two physicians is also very important.[8]

2.5. Number of samples

Several studies have shown that the diagnostic yield of histopathology is increased and sampling error is decreased by increasing the number of biopsies. This has been demonstrated for inflammatory diseases such as chronic idiopathic inflammatory bowel diseases (IBD) and for neoplastic diseases.[9] Therefore different guidelines for endoscopic sampling in various diseases have been developed.[10-12] ECCO guidelines propose to obtain "multiple" biopsies from five sites around the colon (including the rectum) and the ileum for a reliable diagnosis of Crohn's disease. Multiple biopsies imply a minimum of two samples from each site (Table) This is also true for a diagnosis of collagenous or lymphocytic colitis. Thickening of the subepithelial collagen table in collagenous colitis is indeed not homogeneous. Such guidelines are very important in clinical practice. They limit sampling error and compensate for the small size of the samples. However, the introduction of new technologies and modern endoscopes including zoom endoscopy, high magnification endoscopy and more sophisticated techniques such as laser-scanning confocal endoscopy and endo-cytoscopy (microscope incorporated in the endoscope) will change practice in the future by offering the possibility of targeted biopsies. In a recent study at our institute, chromo endoscopy (CE) and narrow band imaging (NBI) were used to detect dysplasia in ulcerative colitis. A total of 268 raised lesions were detected in 83 patients (156 lesions in 45 patients with CE and 112 lesions in 38 patients with NBI). On histology, 44 were shown to be neoplastic (26 lesions in 10 patients with CE and 18 lesions in 12 patients with NBI): 1 adenocarcinoma, 1 high grade dysplasia, 2 dysplasia associated lesion or mass, and 17 adenoma like mass. The new endoscopic techniques are also narrowing the gap between endoscopy and pathology. Laser scanning endoscopy provides a microscopy-level image without obtaining a biopsy specimen. Endo-cytoscopy is based on the technology of light contact microscopy. The tip of an endoscope is placed in direct contact with a dye-stained surface and then the surface is scanned with condensed normal white light, producing cellular-level imaging. Laser endoscopy increases the real time diagnostic yield and can be used to confirm dysplasia with high accuracy. Bio-endoscopy is another technique under consideration. It involves the use of monoclonal antibodies labelled with a fluorescent tag of reporter probes (molecules that enter cells) or fluorescent DNA probes for FISH in order to detect in situ molecular changes or chromosomal instability.[13-16]

Organ	Disease	Location	Area for biopsies	Evidence
Oesophagus	GERD/NERD	Distal esophagus	Z-line 2 cm above Z-line Cardia Stomach (antrum) Hp	?
	Eosinophilic oesophagitis	Entire oesophagus	Proximal, mid Distal esophagus	+
	Barrett's oesophagus	Distal oesophagus	Four quadrant biopsy Every 1cm (short) Every 2 cm (long) (Seattle protocol)	++
Stomach	Gastritis	Entire stomach	Corpus : 2 Antrum 2 Angulus 1 (Sydney protocol) + duodenum	++
Small intestine	Coeliac disease	Descending duodenum	Multiple (4)	++
Colon	Colitis Crohn's disease Ulcerative colitis Microscopic colitis	Ileum Entire colon	Multiple	+
Pouch	Pouchitis	5 cm from Ileoanal anastomosis Anterior and posterior wall		+

Table 1. Recommendations for biopsy strategies in inflammatory conditions of the gastrointestinal tract

While these new techniques can offer real time images and diagnosis, the interpretation of the images still depends on the morphological features of the lesions, as observed with microscopy and some lesions like sessile serrated adenomas are still beyond the reach of real time diagnosis. The endoscopist must therefore have a thorough knowledge of pathology.

3. Specimen handling

Specimen handling should be done carefully in order to allow optimal diagnostic work up. It implies proper identification of the patient, including the age, specification of the site of origin, fixation and in some instances, orientation. Adequate fixation by an appropriate fixative is central to any histological preparation. Tissue that is inadequately fixed will lead to difficulties for cutting, staining and performing ancillary tests. These problems are not correctable in a later stage. Unfortunately there is no "all purpose" fixative. The choice of the appropriate fixative is based on the type of tissue being fixed and on projected needs for ancillary tests, such as special stains, immune histochemistry, in situ hybridization, and electron microscopy. Routine Haematoxylin and eosin staining of multiple sections is adequate in most cases but insufficient in particular situations such as a diagnosis of Hirschsprung's disease or metabolic storage disorders.(Fig 3) For such indications freshly frozen tissue for enzyme histochemistry for the demonstration of acetylcholinesterase activity in nerves, or the identification of fat are needed or tissue fixed in glutaraldehyde for transmission electron microscopy. If possible, the endoscopist should be aware of the clinical indication for the biopsy, and, if necessary contact the pathology laboratory in order to know whether a special fixation is needed. In general formalin (10% neutral buffered formalin, i.e. a 10% v/v solution of 40% formaldehyde gas in water) allows good fixation and application of immune histochemistry as well as molecular analyses. Bouin fixation should therefore be "proscribed". Furthermore it is important to control the duration of fixation. Samples need to be immersed in the fixative immediately and the duration of fixation can have an impact on the quality of the results of ancillary techniques such as immune histochemistry. A minimum of 6 hours and no longer than 48 hours is recommended for adequate molecular biology procedures such as for HER2 immune histochemistry in gastric cancer.[17] Frozen sections will allow application of most ancillary techniques. Freezing must be done properly (by immersion in liquid nitrogen for instance) and quickly in order to avoid the formation of ice cristals. Rapid adequate freezing and prevention of tissue degeneration is equally essential when molecular techniques based on DNA analysis are considered.

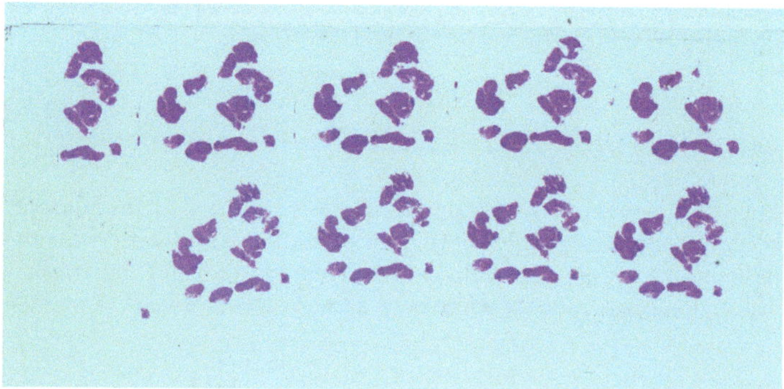

Figure 3. Multiple sections from multiple endoscopic biopsies allow a more complete microscopic analysis

Proper orientation of the tissue samples is important for a correct diagnosis of malabsorptive states such as celiac disease, where the ratio villous height – crypt depth must be assessed and for specimens from endoscopic resections of polyps or early neoplastic lesions.

4. Immune histochemistry and other ancillary techniques

In most instances histopathology identifies the nature of the lesion or tumour. Neoplastic – malignant - tumours are most frequently epithelial. A smaller number is neoplastic but non-epithelial, and includes lymphoproliferative disorders and soft tissue tumors. Histopathology is an adequate tool for solving differential diagnostic problems and typing of tumours. The differential diagnosis between anaplastic carcinomas, large-cell lymphoma, epithelioid stromal tumours and neuroendocrine tumours can be difficult but immunohistochemical stainings with antibodies against cytokeratins (CK), a marker for epithelial cells, CD117 a marker for gastrointestinal stromal tumors, chromogranin, a marker for endocrine cells and a common leucocyte marker can solve the problem. Antibodies to intermediate filaments such as the CKs can be potentially useful in other situations. CKs comprise a subfamily of more than 20 members. The relatively limited distribution of some CKs such as CK7 and CK20 and examination of coordinate expression of these two CKs can help in the differential diagnosis of carcinomas of unknown primary site.(Fig. 4)

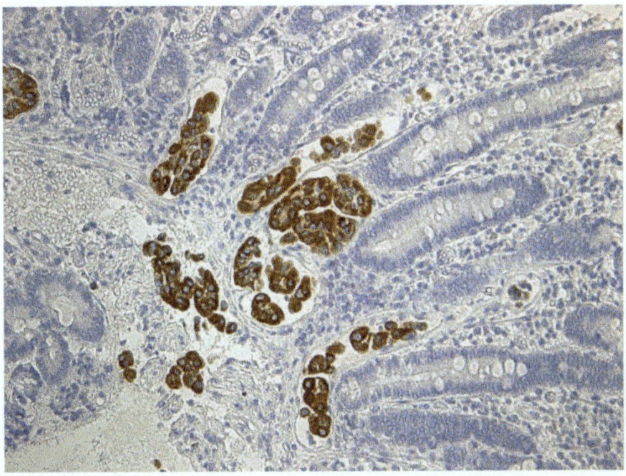

Figure 4. Microphotograph showing a rectal biopsy with Cytokeratin 7 positive immunohistochemistry demonstrating the presence of a breast cancer metastasis.

Immune histochemistry and cytogenetic analysis is essential for the management of lymphomas. Primary intestinal lymphomas should be sub-typed in B cell and T cell malignancies and classified according internationally validated classifications such as the recently published WHO.

Evaluating the proliferation fraction of the tumour cells using a marker such as Ki67 or MIB1 may provide some additional information on the biological behaviour of lymphomas. This is also true for endocrine tumours and gastrointestinal stromal tumours. Further ancillary techniques may include staining with antibodies against p53 for Barret's oesophagus or colitis-associated dysplasia. Currently a number of markers are under investigation for a more accurate identification of early neoplasia.

Histochemistry (histological special stains) searching for mucins or other substances, and occasionally electron microscopy and genetic markers can also be applied on biopsy samples. Many stainings can be performed on routinely formalin fixed material. Increasingly there is some overlap, between immune histochemistry and molecular techniques since genetic markers can be demonstrated also by immune histochemistry. This is for instance true for large-bowel cancers with microsatellite instability (MS), where the products of the DNA repair genes hMLH1, hMSH2 and MSH6, or the lack of them, can be demonstrated immune histochemically. These products do not however cover the whole range of MS. DNA or RNA extraction and genetic analysis remains important and there may even be a growing need.

5. The oesophagus

5.1. Inflammatory conditions

At present, there is no ideal scenario for a biopsy series for the diagnosis of gastro-oesophageal reflux disease (GORD). In general, it is accepted that changes in the squamous mucosa are usually found in the distal oesophagus close to the squamo-columnar junction. Biopsies from the squamous mucosa should be completed with biopsies from the cardia. Histological changes indicative of gastro-oesophageal reflux are indeed found at both sides of the squamo-columnar junction.[18-21] The diagnosis of this condition, called carditis, which occurs in the absence of signs of gastritis in the antrum and corpus due to Helicobacter pylori or other causes of gastritis implies also biopsies of antrum and corpus in order to exclude the presence of these causes. A biopsy run for GORD should therefore ideally include samples from the distal oesophagus, particularly from the Z-line and at 2 cm above, from the cardia distal to the Z-line and from the stomach.[22, 23] However, in most cases, peptic oesophagitis due to GORD - the most common inflammatory condition of the oesophagus - does not require biopsy diagnosis for those patients presenting with typical symptoms and macroscopic endoscopic alterations.[24]

Biopsies are mainly useful in patients presenting with normal endoscopy and abnormal acid exposure (non-erosive reflux disease – NERD), in patients with typical symptoms and normal endoscopy and pH-metry or in patients with atypical symptoms. The presence of "dilated intercellular spaces (DIS)" or of a combination of DIS with other microscopic features such as basal zone hyperplasia observed in GORD may confirm the suspected diagnosis of reflux.[21] There are however several other types of oesophagitis. The presence of an intense eosinophil infiltration must orient towards a diagnosis of eosinophilic oesophagitis. Eosinophilic oesophagitis can present a typical endoscopic pattern known as "ringed oesophagus" but the oesophagus can appear normal in up to 20% of the patients. It is important to recognise that the eosinophilic infiltration may have a heterogeneous distribution within the oesophagus. Therefore, when considering eosinophilic oesophagitis, it is critical to have biopsies from multiple areas, including the distal, mid, and proximal oesophagus.[25] Biopsies of the oesophagus are further indicated in the presence of oesophageal ulcers, erosions or an atypical aspect or topography and whenever an infectious aetiology is suspected. They can help to identify infections such as moniliasis, herpes and cytomegalovirus disease. (Fig. 5)

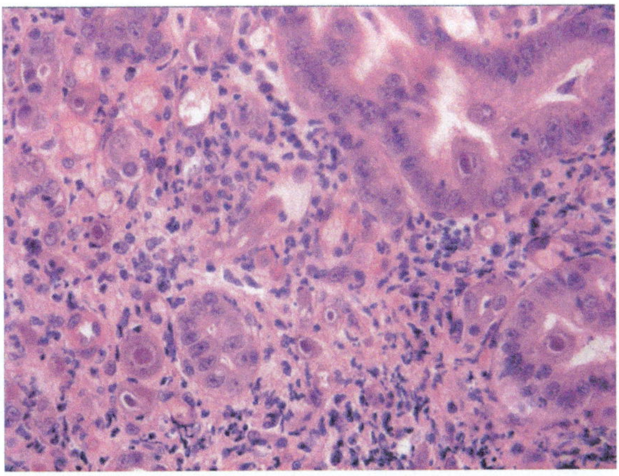

Figure 5. Gastric biopsy showing several Cytomegalovirus nuclear inclusions

Barrett's oesophagus presents a special problem. One definition of Barrett's oesophagus implies "endoscopic abnormalities suggestive of Barrett's oesophagus (endoscopically suspected oesophageal metaplasia) and the presence of columnar epithelium in biopsies. Barrett's oesophagus is a preneoplastic condition.[26] Effective management of the risk for oesophageal adenocarcinoma in Barrett's oesophagus requires precise detection of intestinal-type metaplasia and dysplasia. The detection of intestinal metaplasia is subject to significant sampling error.[27] (Fig. 6) Intestinal metaplasia increases with segment length of the Barrett's mucosa and detection improves with the number of biopsies taken.[28] Intestinal metaplasia can be missed easily when only one or two biopsies are obtained. Therefore it has been proposed to take multiple, closely spaced biopsies. One protocol proposes four-quadrant biopsies every 1 cm for circumferential metaplastic segments (in short segment Barrett's oesophagus) or 2 cm (in long segment Barrett's oesophagus).[3] In another study it was proposed that 8 random biopsies should be obtained. With 1 – 4 biopsies the yield of intestinal metaplasia was 35%.[6, 28] At the histological level, the detection of intestinal metaplasia can be increased by using mucin stains. or immunohistochemistry. It has been suggested that the presence of acidic mucins (blue on alcian blue stain) is a characteristic feature even in the absence of goblet cells. However, this theory has not been confirmed. Comparable disputed results have been obtained with immunohistochemical stains for CKs and MUC antigens.

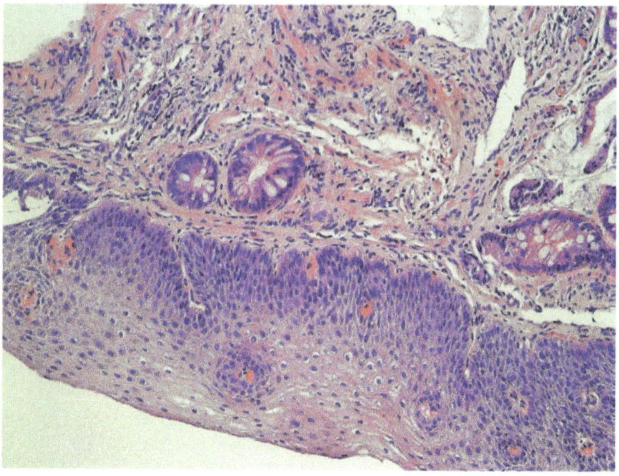

Figure 6. Oesophageal biopsy showing intestinal metaplasia in glands buried underneath the squamous epithelium

5.2. Neoplastic conditions

As the major risk of patients with Barrett's oesophagus is to develop an adenocarcinoma, there has been considerable interest in defining a subgroup of patients at risk. At the present time, the identification of dysplasia in endoscopic mucosal biopsies is the standard method to detect these patients. Systematic four-quadrant biopsy is considerably more effective for the detection of dysplasia in Barrett than non-systematic biopsy sampling.[29] Non-adherence to a protocol during surveillance leads to under-diagnosis or missed diagnosis because of sampling error.[30] However, problems with inter-observer agreement, particularly for low–grade dysplasia, on biopsy specimens have raised concern about the ability of pathologists to provide a consistent and accurate diagnosis upon which management decisions can be based.[31, 32] In order to reduce sampling errors, guidelines for the surveillance have been established by national and international societies. In the future, the diagnostic yield for dysplasia will however essentially be improved and sampling errors will be reduced by targeted biopsies. These can be obtained with the help of endoscopic procedures such as chromo-endoscopy and light- or laser-induced fluoroscopy.[33, 34]

High-grade dysplasia and early cancer can be treated by mucosal destructive or ablative techniques. Some techniques such as photodynamic therapy and laser therapy do not allow any histological study as their goal is complete destruction of the neoplastic tissue. Follow up biopsies can however show remnants of metaplastic and even neoplastic tissue buried underneath squamous epithelium. The frequency of buried metaplastic glands may be as high as 51% of cases. These glands may be difficult to identify on small endoscopic biopsies.

Endoscopic mucosal resection (EMR) is an ablative technique originally developed as a diagnostic procedure (strip-off biopsy) in the early 1980s but has now gained considerable attention as a potential curative form of therapy for patients with high grade dysplasia and superficial cancers. It is also a good tool for histological staging because the procedure allows to remove intact mucosa and submucosa enabling complete evaluation of mucosal and submucosal invasion. EMR as a diagnostic tool has been shown to be superior to mucosal biopsy and inter-observer agreement of Barrett's oesophagus related dysplasia is significantly better compared with biopsy specimens.[35] The presence of a double layer of muscularis mucosae, which is a hallmark of Barrett's oesophagus, is an important landmark. Only when invasion extends beyond the deeper layer (the genuine muscularis mucosae), a diagnosis of submucosal invasion is justified.[36]

Endoscopic biopsies are also commonly used for the diagnosis of cancer of the oesophagus and the distinction between squamous cell carcinoma and adenocarcinoma. Two samples can provide a positive diagnosis in 95.8% of cases. The addition of four samples increases the positive yield to 100%. There is no statistically significant difference in the yield according to the site and type of growth.[37] However, in strictures the diagnosis can be difficult. In this situation, the additional use of brush cytology may increase the diagnostic yield. Soft tissue tumours and lymphomas are less common in the oesophagus. The so-called Abrikosoff tumour or granular cell tumour, a relatively rare lesion, may present a problem as the overlying squamous epithelium can show hyperplasia which might be confused with neoplastic changes. The tumour itself is composed of aggregates of round cells with a characteristic granular cytoplasm showing S100 positivity with immunohistochemical stains. If the biopsy samples are too superficial, the diagnosis can however be difficult. Fine needle aspiration biopsy could be used for the former, although most soft tissue tumours of the oesophagus are not malignant. Brush cytology can be helpful for the diagnosis of infections.

6. The stomach

6.1. Inflammatory conditions

Throughout the GI tract, mucosal features such as redness, oedema, swelling, bleeding, erosions and ulcers can be observed. They reflect inflammation and tissue damage but may also be due to mucosal atrophy and epithelial metaplasia. Metaplasia is most readily detected endoscopically in the distal oesophagus but it is also common in the stomach. In the latter it may appear as small red depressions simulating erosions or aphthoid ulcers, as an irregular nodular area or as larger geographic red areas. The red colour and a depressed or nodular appearance can be explained by thinning of the mucosa due to atrophy and increased visibility of the vessels. Pathology is useful to confirm the endoscopic abnormality and probable diagnosis, or to exclude such abnormalities or give another explanation. A depressed red spot can indeed be a genuine erosion but it may also represent a vascular ectasia or a small area of mucosal atrophy. Inflammatory conditions in the stomach include gastritis and reactive gastropathy (chemical gastropathy, bile reflux). The latter is characterized by epithelial damage and a minimal inflammatory cell reaction. Several types of gastritis can be distinguished and histopathology plays a major role in this distinction. An aetiology-based classification was proposed in the Sydney system at the World Congress of Gastroenterology in 1990 and updated in 1994.[38, 39] The Sydney system also established the need for taking different biopsies of the gastric mucosa.[38] The guidelines include a) two biopsies of the corpus and two of the antrum for an overall assessment of the distribution of the gastritis and the distinction between antral gastritis, corpus gastritis and pan gastritis; b) one biopsy of the angulus because atrophic gastritis and intestinal metaplasia are related with the development of gastric cancer and occur most commonly at the angulus; c) the same area is the most appropriate area to look for the presence of dysplasia. In small children, this approach may however not be appropriate. Two samples from the stomach may be sufficient. Biopsy diagnosis should include the morphological site or sites, the morphological lesions present, and any potential cause. The sensitivity and specificity for the diagnosis of Helicobacter pylori gastritis are high, varying between 88 and 99% for the former and 90 and 100% for the specificity. The negative predictive value is near 100% for antral biopsies. Active gastritis, or gastritis with neutrophils is often Helicobacter pylori positive and will imply treatment, whether activity is mild, moderate or severe. Grading atrophy and intestinal metaplasia is less reproducible.[40] Staging of gastritis has been proposed among others by the so-called OLGA system but may be difficult to apply in routine practice.[41] Grading and staging could however be useful for the identification of patients at risk for cancer. In addition to the gastric biopsies ii seems reasonable to obtain, during the first diagnostic examination, also duodenal biopsies to look for the presence of mucous surface (gastric) metaplasia, a requirement for Helicobacter pylori colonisation of the duodenum which can induce duodenal ulcers, or for epithelial lymphocytosis. If the stomach biopsies are normal and duodenitis is found on histopathology, a Helicobacter pylori-induced duodenitis is highly unlikely. If the patient has lymphocytic gastritis of the antrum and epithelial lymphocytosis in the duodenum, a diagnosis of celiac disease should be suspected. Follow-up biopsies for gastritis can be considered when a treatment for HP has been given in order to assess eradication or when intestinal metaplasia and atrophy are very extensive.

Whenever special forms of gastritis are suspected multiple biopsies are needed. Histopathology can identify a variety of pathogens in infectious gastritis. Many of the special types lack endoscopic abnormalities. Lymphocytic gastritis can present as a hypertrophic variant with erosions and thickening of the gastric wall suggestive of Menetrier's disease. It can be diffuse or corporeal and correspond in these forms to varioliform gastritis. It can also be limited to the antrum and in this case includes various conditions (reflux gastritis, HP gastritis or coeliac disease) must be considered. [42] The histopathology of gastroduodenal Crohn's disease includes a wide spectrum of changes, including the presence of granulomas as well as focally enhanced (active) gastritis.[43] A correct diagnosis of Crohn's disease of the stomach can be reached more accurately when multiple samples of the suspected sites (n=5) and of normal sites are available. Granulomas can be detected in biopsies from macroscopically abnormal mucosa as well as in biopsies from normal mucosa. The frequency of detecting granulomas varies between 4.6% and 26% depending upon the presence of endoscopic lesions, the number of biopsies and the number of sections examined. Multiple biopsies will increase the diagnostic yield. Focally enhanced or focally active gastritis is typified by small collections of lymphocytes and histiocytes surrounding a small group of foveolae or gastric glands, often with infiltrates of neutrophils. Several studies have found that focally enhanced gastritis is common in adult

Crohn's disease patients. However, studies that used control groups have reported a prevalence of focally enhanced gastritis in non-IBD patients in up to 19.4%. Therefore, this type of gastritis may not be a good marker for the diagnosis of IBD or IBD-related gastritis in adults. [44, 45] It may still be a good marker in children although it may not reliably distinguish between Crohn's disease and ulcerative colitis. Some studies have found that focally enhanced gastritis is present in up to 20% of paediatric ulcerative colitis patients, suggesting that this type of gastritis is a marker of IBD in general in children.

Biopsies are less indicated for the diagnosis of vascular abnormalities. They can however be useful for the diagnosis of "gastric antral vascular ectasia" (GAVE). GAVE is a rare condition (prevalence approximately 3/10000 upper endoscopies), characterised by red spots in linear array in the antrum of the stomach. Based on the striped features from the antrum at endoscopy, the disorder has been called the "watermelon" stomach. The histological lesion consists of numerous dilated vessels in the mucosa, often with microthrombi, with fibromuscular hyperplasia and fibrohyalinosis of the perivascular lamina propria. The mucosa shows no or mild chronic inflammation or atrophy with intestinal metaplasia.[46] GAVE must be distinguished from "portal hypertensive gastropathy" and from "gastric vascular ectasia".[47]

6.2. Neoplastic conditions

In patients with marked atrophic gastritis or pernicious anaemia, the possibility of endocrine cell hyperplasia and dysplasia needs to be considered, and immunostains can readily answer this question. In patients with endocrine tumours (carcinoïds), the issue is whether these are sporadic, associated with atrophic gastritis, or even multiple endocrine neoplasia (MEN) and Zollinger-Ellison syndrome. Biopsies of adjacent gastric body mucosa will show whether there is hyperplasia of parietal cells without atrophy as in Zollinger Ellison and MEN, atrophy as seen in pernicious anemia, or normal mucosa as seen in sporadic endocrine tumours.

The macroscopic differential diagnosis between benign and malignant ulcers of the stomach is correct, on average, in only 75% of cases (52% to 94% of cases depending on the series reported in the literature).[3] Hence, the differential diagnosis can depend upon histology. Chromo-endoscopy with targeted biopsies will change the guidelines in the future.

In the series reported in the literature, the proportion of cancer-positive biopsies varies between 49% and 56% and about 25% of the biopsies are considered inadequate. A method of biopsy by quadrants with a technique that avoids the lesion to be covered by the bleeding from earlier biopsies reduces the number of unusable biopsies to 5.7% and increases the proportion of cancer-positive biopsies to 67%. An average of 7 - 10 biopsies is required to reach enough sensitivity and in order to avoid false negative results.[48, 49] When gastric lymphoma is suspected multiple biopsies are also required. If the lesion presents as an ulcer, biopsies from the edge (as for carcinoma) and the ulcer base should be obtained. Proper fixation (in order to allow additional tests such as immuno-histochemistry and Polymerase Chain Reaction) is absolutely indicated.

Histopathology is also very useful for the identification of metastases or secondary malignant involvement of the GI tract a problem which is becoming more common. Breast and melanoma are the most frequently found. Approximately 1 metastasis is observed per 3847 upper GI endoscopies and 1 lower metastasis per 1871 colonoscopies. The stomach and duodenum are the most common locations. Immune histochemistry for cytokeratin patterns and other markers can help to identify the primary origin if needed.

Overall a microscopic diagnosis of polyps (elevated lesions) depends on the type of the lesion and the size and number of biopsies. Polyps of epithelial origin can be diagnosed with classical pinch biopsies. They include benign lesions such as fundic gland polyps and neoplastic lesions such as adenomas or neuro-endocrine dysplasia. A complete evaluation may need larger snare biopsies and implies orientation. This is also needed for EMR specimens from early – superficial gastric cancer and adenomas. As in Barrett's oesophagus, a good orientation is essential for the assessment of the risk factors for residual tumour and the need for additional surgery. In contrast with the oesophagus, soft tissue tumours are more common in the stomach. These are usually gastrointestinal stromal tumours (GIST). These tumours show a positive staining with antibodies directed against CD117, DOG1 and often also for CD34 (87% positive cases in the stomach). They produce polypoid lesions with a smooth or ulcerated surface as a result of a submucosal process. Such a process can be inflammatory or tumoral and will often not be diagnosed adequately when the surface is intact and only mucosal biopsies are available (because of the superficial nature of these biopsies).

7. The duodenum

7.1. Inflammatory conditions

In the duodenum, inflammatory lesions include Helicobacter-associated disease, and other infections, malabsorption, drug-associated disease and the pathology of the papilla of Vater. Many GI diseases or systemic diseases (Helicobacter pylori, Crohn's disease, vasculitis, eosinophilic infiltrates) affect both the stomach and duodenum. Therefore, if duodenal biopsies are taken for any reason it is good to include biopsies of the antrum, in addition. Any duodenitis, inevitably raises the question of whether the condition may be associated with Helicobacter or drugs and biopsies of the antrum can solve this issue readily. Histopathology of the duodenum alone is indeed less useful for the diagnosis of Helicobacter pylori. Cytology is superior with a sensitivity which varies between 56% and 100% and a specificity between 58% and 93% depending on the coloration (modified Giemsa seems superior).[50]

Histopathology is certainly adequate for the diagnosis of other infections such as Giardia lamblia and strongyloides stercoralis.

A subtle increase of eosinophils in the duodenum may be associated with allergy and functional dyspepsia.[51]

Biopsy of the small intestine remains superior for the diagnosis of Whipple's disease and it is the gold standard for the diagnosis of celiac disease. Biopsies of the descending duodenum, rather than the more distal intestine seem sufficient for the diagnosis of celiac disease. Jumbo forceps have no marked advantage over standard size biopsies.[52] Due to the patchy nature of villous changes, multiple biopsies are necessary. It has been suggested that at least four endoscopic biopsies must be taken.[53, 54] Ideally, the specimens are oriented properly in order to allow adequate assessment of villous height and crypt depth. The specimens can therefore be immersed in the fixative after being placed on a Millipore filter paper, luminal side upwards.

The recognition of the spectrum of histological changes in celiac disease as classified by Marsh or modifications of this classification has provided a major advantage in the diagnosis. The earliest lesions have still a normal villous architecture but show intraepithelial lymphocytosis (>30-40 per 100 epithelial cells).[55] An intraepithelial lymphocytosis is not, however specific for celiac disease and may be seen in infective enteropathies, Crohn's disease, non steroidal anti-inflammatory drug usage, giardiasis and other conditions. Furthermore, celiac disease is not the only possible cause of subtotal or total villous atrophy. Other possibilities such as autoimmune enteropathy must be considered, especially in neonates, but also in adults. Serology remains therefore and important diagnostic tool. Histopathology is also essential for the diagnosis of rare congenital disorders such as microvillous inclusion disease and "tufting enteropathy" (also called intestinal epithelial dysplasia, with the term dysplasia used in its ethymological meaning of "malformation" ; the pathology is due to defects in cell adhesion due to defects in the EpCam gene).

7.2. Neoplastic conditions

Refractory sprue is a condition that appears to consist of several diseases, including collagenous sprue and enteropathy-type T-cell lymphoma (ETL). Histology can help identify these.[56]

Duodenal biopsies are also indicated in patients presenting with duodenal polyps. Many of these, especially in the first duodenum, are benign lesions and represent inflammatory polyps or ectopic gastric tissue.

Malignant small bowel tumours constitute less than 5% of GI malignancies. Four major different histological types of malignant small bowel tumours can be distinguished : adenocarcinomas, endocrine tumours, lymphomas and soft tissue tumours. Adenocarcinoma is the most common type. As in the large bowel, most adenocarcinomas arise from pre-existing adenomas that occur sporadically or in the context of familial adenomatous polyposis (FAP), hereditary nonpolyposis colorectal cancer (HNPCC) or variant syndromes. In patients with FAP "adenomas" are most commonly found in the duodenum. In a prospective study of 100 patients upper GI endoscopy revealed adenomatous polyps in the duodenum in 33. They occur mainly in the second part of the duodenum but may involve also the first and third part. A special staging system for duodenal polyposis has been designed whereby the lesions were subdivided in different stages according to the polyp number, size and histological type. The histological part of this system distinguishes the various types of polyps and grades of dysplasia. The types are : tubular/ hyperplastic/ inflammatory polyp = 1 point; tubulo-villous = 2 points; villous = 3 points; dysplasia is graded into mild = 1 point, moderate = 2, severe = 3. [57] Other polyps that may occur in the duodenum or sporadic hamartomas or Peutz-Jeghers polyps and polyps observed in other non-adenomatous polyposis syndromes.

Endocrine tumours of the small intestine include well differentiated neuro-endocrine tumours and malignant large cell neuro-endocrine carcinomas. In the GI tract, most endocrine tumours occur in the small bowel (29% of total) with the highest frequency in the ileum. Endoscopic biopsies are often negative because of the superficial nature of the samples.

Lymphomatous infiltrates in the GI tract are frequently found as part of a disseminated disease. Primary GI lymphoma defined as an extra-nodal lymphoma arising in the GI tract with bulk of the lesion in this site, is a rare disorder. These lymphomas represent 5 to 10% of all Non Hodgkin lymphomas. Despite the fact that the small intestine is the preferential part of the gut where the mucosa associated lymphoid tissue (MALT) is localized, less than 25% of the GI lymphomas affect the small intestine.

The duodenum is also the site of the papilla of Vater where the extra-hepatic bile and pancreatic ducts end. Tissue histopathology may be obtained during endoscopic retrograde cholangiopancreatography (ERCP) by brushing, biopsy, bile aspiration or a combination of these. Biopsies of the bile ducts have a specificity between 90% and 100% with a sensitivity between 43% and 81% for the diagnosis of cholangiocarcinoma. Brush cytology has a similar high specificity of nearly 100% but sensitivity is lower ranging from 18% - 60%. The low sensitivity is linked to low cellularity of many of these tumours. Repeated brushing may increase the yield. During ERCP, miniature cholangioscopes can be used and with these endoscopes, directed tissue biopsies can be obtained. The biopsies are usually smaller than standard forceps biopsies of the GI tract and may be inadequate in up to 28% of the samples. [58] However, with more modern equipment adequate tissue for examination can be obtained.[59]

8. The terminal ileum and colon

8.1. Inflammatory conditions

Ileocolonoscopy is an important tool for the diagnosis of diarrhoea and colitis. Several studies show that colonoscopy and biopsy is useful in the investigation of patients with chronic diarrhoea yielding a histological diagnosis in 22 –31% of patients who had a macroscopically normal colon at colonoscopy.[60-63] Histological diagnosis includes a variety of conditions such as spirochetosis, pseudomelanosis coli, collagenous colitis and lymphocytic colitis and variant forms.(Fig 7) The correct diagnosis of collagenous colitis implies multiple biopsies from different segments because thickening of the collagen layer can be discontinuous.[64] Histopathology can also help to identify amyloidosis and rare metabolic lysosomal or storage disorders such as Tangier disease and systemic diseases such as mastocytosis.[65]

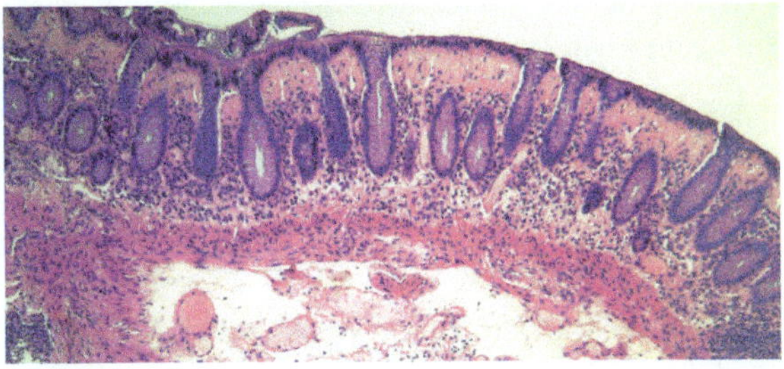

Figure 7. Biopsy from the colon showing thickening of the subepithelial collagen table in collagenous colitis

In inflammatory diarrhoea, a precise diagnosis and differential diagnosis between infections and IBD and between ulcerative colitis and Crohn's disease is important for therapy and follow up. Histopathology can identify a variety of pathogens such as amoeba, schistosoma and Cytomegalovirus. In transplant patients a diagnosis of Graft versus host disease or Cord Colitis can be confirmed and graded.[66] A correct diagnosis of ulcerative colitis can be made by the pathologist without clinical information in 64% of the cases with rectal biopsies only and in 74% of the cases when multiple biopsies from different segments of the colon, including the ileum are available.[10, 67] With clinical information a correct diagnosis is reached in more than 90% of the cases. A diagnosis of Crohn's disease on endoscopic samples of the colon relies particularly on the analysis of multiple biopsies from different segments of the colon including the ileum.[68] Analysis of multiple biopsies yields a positive diagnosis of Crohn's disease in 64% of the cases compared to 24% for one single rectal biopsy.[64, 69] Biopsies of the terminal ileum are mainly useful in patients with inflammatory diarrhoea.[70, 71] The differential diagnosis between infections and IBD relies on the distribution of the inflammatory infiltrate in the lamina propria and the presence of architectural changes. Focal or diffuse basal plasmacytosis is a strong predictor for the diagnosis of IBD, especially ulcerative colitis (occurring in over 70% of the patients). It is only rarely observed in infectious colitis (+/- 3% of the patients). Structural epithelial changes include the presence of an irregular surface, sometimes called pseudovillous or villiform surface and a disturbed crypt architecture.[72-74]

Atypical presentations such as ulcerative colitis with left-sided colitis and peri-appendicular inflammation or caecal patch are occasionally observed. However, the major clinical conditions where endoscopic and histological lesions may not be characteristic include initial onset of the disease, inflammatory diarrhoea in children, patients with liver disease and IBD, patients under treatment and patients presenting with severe, fulminant disease. Colonic biopsies from children between 1 and 10 years of age, presenting with new-onset ulcerative colitis show significantly less crypt branching, plasma cells in the lamina propria, cryptitis, crypt abscesses, and epithelial injury when compared with samples from adults. In 4 to 8% of cases the initial biopsy samples are completely normal. Rectal sparing has been well documented.[75, 76] Rectal sparing and patchy and focal inflammation are also more common in patients with primary sclerosing cholangitis (PSC) without clinically overt colitis, when compared to patients with ulcerative colitis without PSC.[77, 78]

When the differential diagnosis between ulcerative colitis and Crohn's disease can not be solved with endoscopic biopsies the patient should be categorized as "IBD unclassified".[79] Clinical and histo-pathological follow up will eventually solve the diagnosis in most cases.

During follow up of IBD, histopathology can identify persistent active inflammation in ulcerative colitis more reliably than endoscopy.[80] Persistent microscopic inflammation may be important in the pathogenesis of dysplasia in IBD.

A complication of Kock pouch and ileal pouch anal anastomosis (IPAA) is the development of a primary inflammation within the pouch which is associated with a clinical syndrome termed "pouchitis". This condition is common after surgery for ulcerative colitis, but can occur also after surgery for other indications. Pouch biopsy specimens from well functioning pouches can show mild villous shortening and chronic inflammation. The most consistent finding in pouchitis is ulceration. Grading of pouchitis depends on clinical features, endoscopic findings and histology. The degree of polymorphonuclear infiltration and the proportion of ulcerated area are items of the score. There are no guidelines for the number and location of biopsies from a pouch but there is some evidence that a biopsy, taken 5 cm above the ileoanal anastomosis from the posterior and anterior wall may be the most sensitive for a diagnosis of pouchitis. Pouchitis must be distinguished from "cuffitis" or "short-strip pouchitis", which is inflammation in the columnar cuff mucosa distal to the pouch. The top end of the anal canal is lined by columnar mucosa like that of the rectum. In a hand sewn pouch-anal anastomosis, this mucosa is stripped, albeit often incompletely since the junction between columnar epithelium and squamous or transitional epithelium is difficult to distinguish. Islands of columnar mucosa may be left behind.

Histology is also important for the differential diagnosis of eosinophilic disorders of the gastrointestinal tract. Eosinophils are constitutively present in the gastrointestinal mucosa outside the oesophagus and the precise normal numbers have not been defined. In the colon geographical and seasonal differences in numbers have been observed. In humans, appendix, caecum and ascending colon contain the highest numbers Therefore a diagnosis of eosinophilic (gastro-)enteritis is difficult. An intraepithelial position of eosinophils may be the most reliable marker of disease. Eosinophilic disorders can be separated into primary (idiopathic) and secondary diseases, primary having no known cause, and secondary due to other illnesses associated with eosinophilia such a infections, celiac disease, IBD and drug related pathology. A third situation is observed in the hypereosinophilic syndrome, a heterogeneous group of rare diseases defined by persistent blood eosinophilia for more than 6 months with evidence of organ involvement (blood eosinophilia > $1500/mm^3$).

Primary eosinophilic enteritis has been called allergic gastro-enteropathy, because a subset of patients have an associated allergic component. Although considered idiopathic, an allergic mechanism may be involved as most patients exhibit increased food-specific IgE levels.

8.2. Neoplastic conditions

Crohn's disease and ulcerative colitis carry an increased cancer risk. A pathway of "colitis – dysplasia – cancer" has been identified and this allows surveillance of patients with an increased risk (longstanding disease; extensive colitis; ulcerative colitis with primary sclerosing cholangitis…).(Fig. 8) It has been estimated that 33 to 64 biopsies are required to detect dysplasia with 90% and 95% probabilities respectively. Yet, with 20-40 biopsies less than 0.1% of the colorectal mucosa is covered.[81, 82] Current practice guidelines recommend that 4 biopsy specimens be taken from every 10 cm (0.05 % of the entire area of the colon) of diseased bowel in addition to macroscopically atypical lesions.[83] However, the detection rate of IBD-related dysplasia can substantially be improved with targeted biopsies obtained with the newly developed endoscopic techniques and this procedure should replace the random biopsy guidelines in the future.[84] Dysplasia in IBD can appear as polypoid lesions or as flat lesions. Polypoïd lesions can occur in a mucosa with signs of colitis, or in a mucosa with flat dysplasia. Therefore, biopsies should be obtained from the elevated lesion and from the surrounding tissue. The microscopic diagnosis of "dysplasia" is based on the presence of cytological and architectural abnormalities showing "unequivocal, non-invasive (confined within the basement membrane), neoplastic transformation of the epithelium excluding all reactive changes".[85] Biopsies positive for dysplasia can be subdivided into low-grade and high-grade. The grade of dysplasia is determined by the features of the most dysplastic portion. The two grade classification appears to be reproducible, although in general the agreement is better for high-grade dysplasia. Because of the diagnostic problems related to dysplasia ancillary techniques such as staining for p53 and AMACR can be applied on the tissue samples in order to improve the diagnosis. P53/AMACR coexpression seems to be of potential value for predicting neoplastic progression in ulcerative colitis patients with flat low grade dysplasia or indefinite lesions.[86]

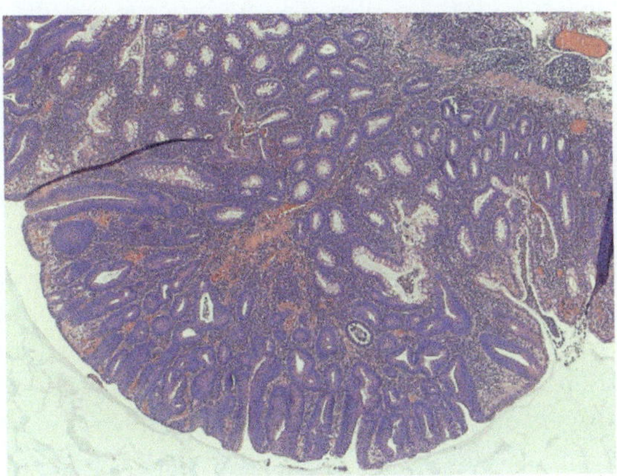

Figure 8. Raised polypoid lesion in a biopsy from a patient with ulcerative colitis showing microscopic features of dysplasia : DALM

Sporadic adenomas and polypoid "dysplasia" in IBD can be managed with endoscopic techniques and complete local excision appears to be adequate. Endoscopic resection specimens of IBD-related neoplasia should be handled properly, like all polypectomy specimens. They should be removed entirely if possible. Sporadic small polyps can be handled with a cold or hot biopsy forceps. While the latter can induce coagulation artefacts, the damage usually does not prevent adequate histological interpretation. Larger polyps should be oriented. The pathologist will identify the origin of the lesion, epithelial or not and the nature : neoplastic or not.

In recent years it has become clear that hyperplastic polyps are a heterogeneous group of lesions, now reported as "serrated lesions". They include benign polyps, so called (traditional) hyperplastic polyps which can be subdivided in several types (microvesicular type, goblet-cell-rich type and mucin-poor type) and lesions with a neoplastic potential. The distinction between the hyperplastic subtypes has a high inter-observer variation and therefore routine distinction of these subtypes is not necessary.[87] Among the lesions with a neoplastic potential, traditional serrated adenomas, with cytological dysplasia and sessile serrated adenomas or polyps have been identified. Both these lesions have a neoplastic potential through the serrated neoplastic pathway. In sessile serrated polyps, the epithelial cells show however some atypia or features of dysplasia.[88] Therefore a distinction is made between sessile serrated adenomas with and without dysplasia. A proper diagnosis of sessile serrated adenomas implies orientation of the endoscopic biopsy samples. The lesion is indeed characterized by dilatation of the crypts from top to bottom. Epithelial serration and dilatation are usually more prominent in the basal part of the crypts and this can not be evaluated properly on tangentially sectioned samples.

Histopathology allows grading of dysplasia in polyps and determination of the tubular or villous nature of the lesion. Tubular adenomas are by definition dysplastic and hence at least low-grade dysplastic lesions. Identification of high-grade dysplasia and intramucosal carcinoma is important. Endoscopic surveillance of patients with so-called "advanced adenoma" may need to be different from that performed in patients without advanced adenomas. In polyps, the occurrence of invasive cancer, must be differentiated from high-grade dysplasia, intramucosal cancer and entrapped (pseudo-invasive) mucosa. Only when cancer invades the submucosa, it is considered to have the potential to metastasize, although lymphangiogenesis can occur in the mucosa as shown in ulcerative colitis.[89] The established histopathological criteria that determine the treatment options of polypectomy versus subsequent surgical resection because of the risk of residual tumour are the status of the resection margin, the histological grade, lympho-vascular invasion, budding of cells and invasion into the submucosa below the stalk of the polyps but above the muscularis propria. Various staging systems have been proposed for this purpose.[7, 90]

As in the stomach and the small intestine, lymphomas and mesenchymal tumours can also occur in the colon and biopsies are suitable for a correct diagnosis.

9. Conclusions

Histopathology plays a critical role in GI practice. Endoscopic biopsies are important in order to establish, confirm or exclude a diagnosis suspected clinically or endoscopically, both in the absence and presence of endoscopic abnormalities. Biopsy diagnosis is greatly facilitated when the endoscopist provides adequate samples and understands the criteria used for histological diagnosis. Histopathology plays also a major role in the design of therapeutic strategy. A close collaboration between the endoscopist and the pathologist is therefore highly useful.

Author details

Karel Geboes[1*], Karen Geboes[2] and Anne Jouret-Mourin[3]

*Address all correspondence to: Karel.geboes@skynet.be

1 Department of Pathology, University of Leuven KUL, Leuven, Belgium

2 Department of Gastroenterology, Digestive Oncology, University of Gent, Gent, Belgium

3 Department of Pathology, Saint Luc Hospital, UCL, Brussels, Belgium

References

[1] Amado, R. G, Wolf, M, Peeters, M, et al. (2008). Wild-type KRAS is required for pnitumumab efficacy in patients with metastatic colorectal cancer. J Clin Oncol. , 26, 1626-1634.

[2] Rüschoff, J, Dietel, M, Baretton, G, Arbogast, S, et al. (2010). HER2 diagnostics in gastric cancer guideline validation and development of standardized immunohistochemical testing. Virchows Arch. , 457, 299-307.

[3] Mainguet, P, & Jouret, A. The collaboration between the endoscopist and the pathologist. ((1996). Acta Endoscop. , 26, 67-77.

[4] Geboes, K. La collaboration entre l'endoscopiste et le pathologiste. ((2005). Acta Endoscop. , 36, 245-56.

[5] Lauwers, G, Forcione, D. G, Nishioka, N. S, et al. (2009). Novel endoscopic therapeutic modalities for superficial neoplasms arising in Barrett's esophagus : a primer for surgical pathologists. Mod Pathol. , 22, 488-498.

[6] Flejou, J. F. Histological assessment of oesophageal columnar mucosa. ((2008). Best Pract Res Clin Gastroenterol. , 22, 671-686.

[7] Cooper, H. S. Pathology of the endoscopically removed malignant colorectal polyp. ((2007). Curr Diagn Pathol. , 13, 423-427.

[8] Weynand, B, Borbath, I, Galant, C, Piessevaux, H, & Deprez, P. H. (2011). Optimizing specimen collection and laboratory procedures reduces the non-diagnostic rate for endoscopic ultrasound-guided fine-needle aspiration of solid lesions of the pancreas. Cytopathology.

[9] Dejaco, C, Osterreicher, C, Angelberger, S, et al. (2003). Diagnosing colitis : a prospective study on essential parameters for reaching a diagnosis. Endoscopy. , 35, 1004-1008.

[10] Stange, E. F. Travis SPL, Vermeire S, et al. ((2006). European evidence-based consensus on the diagnosis and management of Crohn's disease : definitions and diagnosis. Gut. 55 Suppl I: ii15., 1.

[11] Faller, G, Berndt, R, Borchard, F, et al. (2003). Histopathological diagnosis of Barrett's mucosa and associated neoplasias. Results of a consensus conference of the Working Group for "Gastrointestinal Pathology of the German Society for pathology" on 22 September 2001. Pathology , 24, 9-14.

[12] Stein, H. J. (1996). Esophageal cancer: screening and surveillance. Results of a consensus conference held at the VIth world congress of the International Society for Diseases of the Esophagus. Dis Esophagus. 9: SS19., 3.

[13] Kiesslich, R, Fritsch, J, Holtmann, M, et al. (2003). Methylene blue-aided chromoendoscopy for the detection of intraepithelial neoplasia and colon cancer in ulcerative colitis. Gastroenterology , 124, 880-888.

[14] Kiesslich, R, & Neurath, M. F. (2004). Review : Potential of new endoscopic techniques : intravital staining and in vivo confocal endomicroscopy for the detection of premalignant lesions and early cancer in patients with ulcerative colitis. Acta Endoscopica , 34, 189-197.

[15] Kiesslich, R, Burg, J, Vieth, M, et al. (2004). Confocal laser endoscopy for diagnosing intraepithelial neoplasias and colorectal cancer in vivo. Gastroenterology , 127, 706-713.

[16] Inoue, H, Kudo, S, & Shiokawa, A. (2005). Technology Insight : laser-scanning confocal microscopy and endocytoscopy for cellular observation of the gastrointestinal tract. Nature clinical practice gasthep. , 2, 31-37.

[17] Jouret-mourin, A, Hoorens, A, Kockx, M, et al. (2011). Belgian guidelines for HER2 testing in gastric cancer. Belg J Med Oncol. , 5, 14-22.

[18] Riddell, R. H. (1996). The biopsy diagnosis of gastroesophageal reflux disease, "carditis," and Barrett's esophagus, and sequelae of therapy. Am J Surg Pathol. 20 Suppl 1: S, 31-50.

[19] Glickman, J. N, Fox, V, Antonioli, D. A, Wang, H. H, & Odze, R. D. (2002). Morphology of the cardia and significance of carditis in pediatric patients. Am J Surg Pathol. , 26, 1032-1039.

[20] Dent, J. (2007). Microscopic esophageal mucosal injury in nonerosive reflux disease. Clin Gastroenterol Hepatol. , 5, 4-16.

[21] Tytgat, G. (2008). The value of esophageal histology in the diagnosis of gastroesophageal reflux disease in patients with heartburn and normal endoscopy. Cur Gastroenterol Rep. , 10, 231-234.

[22] Vieth, M. (2008). Contribution of histology to the diagnosis of reflux disease. Best Pract Res Clin Gastroenterol., 22, 625-638.

[23] Takubo, K, Honma, N, Aryal, G, et al. (2005). Is there a set of histologic changes that are invariably reflux associated? Arch Pathol Lab Med. , 129, 159-163.

[24] Dent, J, Brun, J, Fendrick, A. M, et al. (1999). An evidence-based appraisal of reflux disease management- the Genval workshop report. Gut 44: SS16., 1.

[25] Chang, F, & Anderson, S. (2008). Clinical and pathological features of eosinophilic oesophagitis : a review. Pathology , 40, 3-8.

[26] Vakil, N, Van Zanten, S. V, Kahrilas, P, Dent, J, & Jones, R. (2006). The Montreal definition and classification of Gastroesophageal Reflux Disease : a global evidence-based consensus. Am J Gastroenterol. , 101, 1900-1920.

[27] Weinstein, W. M, & Ippoliti, A. F. (1996). The diagnosis of Barrett's esophagus: goblets, goblets, goblets. Gastrointest Endosc. , 44, 91-95.

[28] Gatenby, P. A, Ramus, J. R, Caygill, C. P, Shepherd, N. A, & Watson, A. (2008). Relevance of the detection of intestinal metaplasia in non-dysplastic columnar-lined esophagus. Scand J Gastroenterol. , 43, 524-530.

[29] Abela, J, Going, J. J, Mackenzie, J. F, Mckernan, M, Mahoney, O, & Stuart, S. RC. ((2008). Systematic four-quadrant biopsy detects Barrett's dysplasia in more patients than non-systematic biopsy. Am J Gastroenterol. , 103, 850-855.

[30] Peters, F. P, Curvers, W. L, Rosmolen, W. D, et al. (2008). Surveillance history of endoscopically treated patients with early Barrett's neoplasia : nonadherence to the Seattle biopsy protocol leads to sampling error. Dis Esophagus , 21, 475-479.

[31] Reid, B. J, Haggitt, R. C, Rubin, C. E, et al. (1985). Criteria for dysplasia in Barrett's esophagus: a cooperative consensus study. Gastroenterology 88: 1552 (abstract).

[32] Sagan, C, Fléjou, J. F, Diebold, M. D, & Potet, F. Le Bodic MF. ((1994). Reproductibilité des critères histologiques de dysplasie sur muqueuse de Barrett. Gastroenterol Clin Biol. , 18, 31-34.

[33] Gossner, L, Pech, O, May, A, Vieth, M, Stolte, M, & Ell, C. (2006). Comparison of methylene blue-directed biopsies and four-quadrant biopsies in the detection of

high-grade intraepithelial neoplasia and early cancer in Barrett's esophagus. Dig Liver Dis. , 38, 724-729.

[34] Curvers, W. L, & Kiesslich, R. Bergman JJGHM. ((2008). Novel imaging techniques in the detection of oesophageal neoplasia. Best Pract Res Clin Gastroenterol. , 22, 687-720.

[35] Mino-kenudson, M, Hull, M. J, Brown, I, et al. (2007). EMR for Barrett's esophagus-related superficial neoplasms offers better diagnostic reproducibility than mucosal biopsy. Gastrointest Endosc. , 66, 667-669.

[36] Geboes, K, Ectors, N, Geboes, K. P, & Lambert, R. (2005). Intraepithelial neoplasia, dysplasia and early cancer of the digestive tract : Modifications in terminology. Current Cancer Therapy Reviews , 1, 145-155.

[37] Lal, N, Bhasin, D. K, Malik, A. K, Gupta, N. M, Singh, K, & Mehta, S. K. (1992). Optimal number of biopsy specimens in the diagnosis of carcinoma of the oesophagus. Gut , 33, 724-726.

[38] Price, A. B. (1991). The Sydney System : Histological division. J Gastroenterol and Hepatol. , 6, 209-222.

[39] Dixon, M. F, Genta, R. M, Yardley, J. H, & Correa, P. (1996). Classification and grading of gastritis : the updated Sydney System. Am J Surg Pathol. , 20, 1161-1181.

[40] Nichols, L, Sughayer, M, De Girolami, P. C, et al. (1991). Evaluation of diagnostic methods for Helicobacter pylori gastritis. Am J Clin Pathol. , 95, 769-773.

[41] Rugge, M, & Correa, P. DiMario F, et al. ((2008). The Olga staging of gastritis: a tutorial. Dig & Liver disease , 40, 650-658.

[42] Haot, J, Jouret, A, Willette, M, Gossuin, A, & Mainguet, P. B. (1990). Lymphocytic gastritis : prospective study of its relationship with varioliform gastitis. Gut, 31; , 282-285.

[43] Oberhuber, G, Puspok, A, Oesterreicher, C, et al. (1997). Focally enhanced gastritis : a frequent type of gastritis in patients with Crohn's disease. Gastroenterology , 112, 698-706.

[44] Xin, W, & Greenson, J. K. (2004). The clinical significance of focally enhanced gastritis. Am J Surg Pathol, , 28, 1347-1351.

[45] Yao, K, Yao, T, Iwashita, A, et al. (2000). Microaggregate of immunostained macrophages in noninflamed gastroduodenal mucosa: a new useful histological marker for differentiating Crohn's colitis from ulcerative colitis. Am J Gastroenterol. , 95, 1967-1973.

[46] Gilliam, J. H, Geisinger, K. R, Wu, W. C, et al. (1989). Endoscopic biopsy is diagnostic in gastric antral vascular ectasia. The "Watermelon stomach". Dig Dis Sci. , 34, 885-888.

[47] Misra, V, Misra, S. P, Dwivedi, M, et al. (1997). Histomorphometric study of portal hypertensive enteropathy. Am J Clin Pathol. , 108, 652-657.

[48] Vyberg, M, Hougen, H. P, & Tonnesen, K. (1983). Diagnostic accuracy of endoscopic gastrobiopsy in carcinoma of the stomach. Acta Path Microbiol Immunol Scand (A). , 91, 483-487.

[49] Misiewicz, J. J. Tytgat GNJ, Goodwin CS, Price AB, Sipponen P, Strickland RG ((1990). The Sydney system : a new classification of gastritis. Proceedings of the 9th World Congress of Gastroenterology. Sydney, Australia, , 1-10.

[50] Debongnie, J. C, Delmee, M, Mainguet, P, Beyaert, C, Haot, J, & Legros, G. (1992). Cytology : a simple, rapid, sensitive method in the diagnosis of Helicobacter pylori. Am J Gastroenterol. , 87, 20-23.

[51] Walker, M. M, Salehian, S. S, Murray, C. E, Rajendran, A, Hoare, J. M, Negus, R, Powell, N, & Talley, N. J. (2010). Implications of eosinophilia in the normal duodenal biopsy- an association with allergy and functional dyspepsia. Aliment Pharmacol Ther. 31; , 1129-1136.

[52] Mee, A. S, Burke, M, Vallon, A. G, Newman, J, & Cotton, P. B. (1985). Small bowel biopsy for malabsorption : comparison of diagnostic adequacy of endoscopic forceps and capsule biopsy specimens. Br Med J. , 291, 769-772.

[53] Green PHRRostami K, Marsh MN. ((2005). Diagnosis of coeliac disease. Best Pract Res Clin Gastroenterol. , 19, 389-400.

[54] Dickson, B. C, Streutker, C. J, & Chetty, R. (2006). Coeliac disease : an update for pathologists. J Clin Pathol. , 59, 1008-1016.

[55] Ensari, A. (2010). Gluten sensitive enteropathy (celiac disease) : controversies in diagnosis and classification. Arch Pathol Lab Med. , 134, 826-836.

[56] Brousse, N. Meijer JWR. ((2005). Malignant complications of coeliac disease. Best Pract Res Clin Gastroenterol. , 19, 401-412.

[57] Spigelman, A. D, Williams, C. B, Talbot, I. C, & Domizio, P. Phillips RKS. ((1989). Upper gastrointestinal cancer in patients with familial adenomatous polyposis. Lancet ii: , 783-785.

[58] Van Caillie, M. A, Geboes, K, Van Eyken, P, & Van Steenbergen, W. (2006). The diagnostic value of intraductal biopsy of the extrahepatic bile ducts. Tijdschr Geneesk. , 62, 1035-1043.

[59] Nguyen, K. Sing Jr JT. ((2008). Review of endocopic techniques in the diagnosis and management of cholangiocarcinoma. World J Gastroenterol. , 14, 2995-2999.

[60] Prior, A, Lessels, A. M, & Whorwell, P. J. (1987). Is biopsy necessary if colonoscopy is normal? Dig Dis Sci. , 32, 673-676.

[61] Whitehead, R. (1990). Colitis : Problems in definition and diagnosis. Virchows Archiv Pathol Anat. , 417, 187-190.

[62] Marshall, J. B, Singh, R, & Diaz-arias, A. A. (1995). Chronic, unexplained diarrhea : are biopsies necessary if colonoscopy is normal? Am J Gastroenterol. , 90, 372-376.

[63] Shah, R. J, Fenoglio-preiser, C, Bleau, B. L, & Giannella, R. A. (2001). Usefulness of colonoscopy with biopsy in the evaluation of patients with chronic diarrhea. Am J Gastroenterol. , 96, 1091-1095.

[64] Geboes, K. (2008). Lymphocytic, collagenous and other microscopic colitides : pathology and the relationship with idiopathic inflammatory bowel diseases. Gastroenterol Clin Biol. , 32, 689-694.

[65] Kirsch, R, Geboes, K, Shepherd, N. A, et al. (2008). Systemic mastocytosis involving the gastrointestinal tract : Clinicopathologic and molecular study of five cases. Mod Pathol. , 21, 1508-1516.

[66] Herrera, A. F, Soriano, G, Bellizzi, A. M, Hornick, J. L, Ho, V. T, Ballen, K. K, Baden, L. R, Cutler, C. S, Antin, J. H, Soiffer, R. J, & Marty, F. M. (2011). Cord colitis syndrome in cord-blood stem-cell transplantation. N Engl J Med. , 365, 815-854.

[67] Bentley, E, Jenkins, D, Campbell, F, & Warren, B. F. (2002). How could pathologists improve the initial diagnosis of colitis? Evidence from an international workshop. J Clin Pathol. , 55, 955-960.

[68] Dejaco, C, Osterreicher, C, Angelberger, S, et al. (2003). Diagnosing colitis : a prospective study on essential parameters for reaching a diagnosis. Endoscopy , 35, 1004-1008.

[69] Stange, E. F. Travis SPL, Vermeire S, et al. ((2008). European evidence-based consensus on the diagnosis and management of ulcerative colitis : Definitions and diagnosis. J Crohn's & Colitis , 2, 1-23.

[70] Mchugh, J. B, Appelman, H. D, & Mckenna, B. J. (2007). The diagnostic value of endoscopic terminal ileum biopsies. Am J Gastroenterol. , 102, 1084-1089.

[71] Geboes, K. (2007). The strategy for biopsies of the terminal ileum should be evidence based. Am J Gastroenterol. , 102, 1090-1092.

[72] Schumacher, G, Kollberg, B, & Sandstedt, B. (1994). A prospective study of first attacks of inflammatory bowel disease and infectious colitis. Histologic course during the 1st year after presentation. Scand J Gastroenterol. , 29, 318-332.

[73] Jenkins, D, Balsitis, M, Gallivan, S, et al. (1997). Guidelines for the initial biopsy diagnosis of suspected chronic idiopathic inflammatory bowel disease. The British Society of Gastroenterology Initiative. J Clin Pathol. , 50, 93-105.

[74] Seldenrijk, C. A, Morson, B. C, et al. (1991). Histopathological evaluation of colonic mucosal biopsy specimens in chronic inflammatory bowel disease : diagnostic implications. Gut , 32, 1514-15.

[75] Markowitz, J, Kahn, E, Grancher, K, et al. (1993). Atypical rectosigmoid histology in children with newly diagnosed ulcerative colitis. Am J Gastroenterol. , 88, 2034-2037.

[76] Robert, M. E, Tang, L, Hao, M, et al. (2004). Patterns of inflammation in mucosal biopsies of ulcerative colitis. Perceived differences in pediatric populations are limited to children younger than 10 years. Am J Surg Pathol. , 28, 183-189.

[77] Loftus EV JrHarewood GC, Loftus CG, et al. ((2005). PSC-IBD : a unique form of inflammatory bowel disease associated with primary sclerosing cholangitis. Gut , 54, 91-96.

[78] Perdigoto, R, & Wiesner, R. H. LaRusso NF, et al. ((1991). Inflammatory bowel disease associated with primary sclerosing cholangitis: Incidence, severity and relationship to liver disease. Gastroenterology 100:A238.

[79] Geboes, K, Colombel, J. F, Greenstein, A, et al. (2008). Indeterminate colitis : A review of the concept- What's in a name? Inflamm Bowel Dis. , 14, 860-867.

[80] Geboes, K, Riddell, R, Öst, Ä, Jensfelt, B, Persson, T, & Löfberg, R. (2000). A reproducible grading scale for histological assessment of inflammation in ulcerative colitis. Gut , 47, 404-409.

[81] Rosenstock, E, Farmer, R. G, Petras, R, et al. (1985). Surveillance for colonic carcinoma in ulcerative colitis. Gastroenterology. , 89, 1342-1346.

[82] Rubin, C. E, Haggitt, R. C, et al. (1992). DNA-aneuploidy in colonic biopsies predicts future development of dysplasia in ulcerative colitis. Gastroenterology. , 103, 1611-1620.

[83] Kornbluth, A, & Sachar, D. B. (1997). Ulcerative colitis practice guidelines in adults. American College of Gastroenterology, Practice Parameters Committee. Am J Gastroenterol. , 92, 204-211.

[84] Kiesslich, R, Fritsch, J, Holtmann, M, et al. (2003). Methylene blue-aided chromoendoscopy for the detection of intraepithelial neoplasia and colon cancer in ulcerative colitis. Gastroenterology. , 124, 880-888.

[85] Riddell, R. H, Goldman, H, Ransohoff, D. F, et al. (1983). Dysplasia in inflammatory bowel disease : Standardized classification with provisional clinical applications. Hum Pathol, , 14, 931-968.

[86] Van Schaik FDMOldenburg B, Offerhaus JA, Schipper MEI, Vleggaar FP, Siersema PD et al. ((2012). Role of immunohistochemical markers in predicting progression of dysplasia to advanced neoplasia in patients with ulcerative colitis. Inflamm Bowel Dis. , 18, 480-488.

[87] Yantiss, R. K. (2007). Serrated colorectal polyps and the serrated neoplastic pathway : emerging concepts in colorectal carcinogenesis. Curr Diagn Pathol. , 13, 456-466.

[88] Jouret-mourin, A, & Geboes, K. Serrated lesions of the colorectum : a new entity : What should an endoscopist know about it? ((2012). Acta Gastroenterol Belg. , 76, 197-202.

[89] Kaiserling, E, Kröber, S, & Geleff, S. (2003). Lymphatic vessels in the colonic mucosa in ulcerative colitis. Lymphology. , 36, 52-61.

[90] Ueno, H, Mochizuki, H, Hashiguchi, Y, et al. (2004). Risk factors for an adverse outcome in early invasive colorectal carcinoma. Gastroenterology , 127, 385-394.

Chapter 2

Adhesion Prevention Strategies in Laparoscopic Surgery

George Pados, Anastasios Makedos and Basil Tarlatzis

Additional information is available at the end of the chapter

1. Introduction

Adhesions are defined as abnormal attachments between tissues and organs [1]. Intra-abdominal adhesions may be classified as congenital or acquired [2]. Congenital adhesions are a consequence of embryological anomaly in the development of the peritoneal cavity. Acquired adhesions result from the inflammatory response of the peritoneum that arises after intra-abdominal inflammatory processes (e.g. acute appendicitis, pelvic inflammatory disease, exposure to intestinal contents and previous use of intrauterine contraceptive devices), radiation and surgical trauma [3]. It has been reported that the majority of acquired adhesions (about 90%) are post-surgical [2].

Factors associated with the formation of post-surgical adhesions include tissue trauma, infection, ischaemia,reaction to foreign bodies (sutures, powder from gloves, gauze particles etc.), haemorrhage, tissue overheating or desiccation and exposure to irrigation fluids [4]. The incidence of intra-abdominal adhesions ranges from 67% to 93% after general surgical abdominal operations and from 60% to 90% after gynecological procedures. Not unexpectedly, adhesion formation is considered one of the most common post-operative complications [2,5]. Post-surgically, many adhesions may be asymptomatic or can lead to a broad spectrum of clinical problems, including intestinal obstruction, chronic pelvic or abdominal pain and female infertility, requiring re-admission and often additional surgery, while at the same time they can complicate future surgical procedures [6]. Adhesion-related re-operations are a common consequence of gynecological procedures and adhesiolysis is followed by a high incidence of adhesion reformation and *de-novo* adhesion formation [7].

The major strategies for adhesion prevention in gynecological surgery aim at the optimization of surgical technique and use of adhesion-prevention agents. Laparoscopic surgery in gynecology represents the most innovative surgical approach, compared with laparotomy since it has been shown from a large number of clinical, but also experimental studies, that is associated with less development of *de novo* adhesions. Without any doubt, the most important factor is the operating surgeon, whose attention to proper surgical technique will serve as a mainstay for adhesion formation.

2. Mechanism of adhesion development

The mechanism of adhesion formation represents a variation of the physiological healing process [8]. The process of peritoneal healing differs from that of other tissues. Peritoneal defects heal by a process of metaplasia from the underlying mesenchyme, partly from migration of epithelial cells from the free peritoneal fluid and minimally through proliferation of epithelial cells from the defect's edges. Consequently, peritoneal wounds need the same time to heal regardless of their size, in contrast with other tissues, such as the skin, where large injuries take longer to heal than do small injuries [9]. There is no difference between peritoneal healing and adhesion formation for the first 3 days after peritoneal injury. Injuries to the peritoneum cause a disruption of stromal mast cells, resulting in the release of histamine and vasoactive cinins. Also as a response to trauma, various cytokines, such as interleukin (IL)-1, IL-6 and tumor necrosis factor-a (TNF-a) are locally released. The cytokines attract and activate macrophages to secrete vasodilating substances, which in turn, cause an increase in capillary permeability, leading to the formation of fibrous exudate [10]. Platelets are an important component of the inflammatory exudate and have the ability to adhere it to the traumatized surfaces. The platelet degranulation releases adrenaline, transforming growth factor b and serotonin and contribute to the production of prostaglandins and leukotrienes. The chemokines direct the migration of cells to the injury site, while platelets contribute to the initial fibrin clot and to the initiation of the coagulation process [11]. The activation of the coagulation cascade leads to the transformation of the inactive prothrombin into thrombin that triggers the conversion of fibrinogen into monomers of fibrin, which interact and polymerize. The initially soluble polymer becomes insoluble by coagulation factors such as factor XIIIa [12]. The exudate coagulates within 3 h and forms a fibrinous material that plugs the defective area and generates attachments between adjacent tissue surfaces. The presence of blood and post-operative bleeding increases the fibrin deposition. Most of the fibrin depositions will disperse by fibrinolysis. The fibrinous mass that will remain, results in the organization and formation of adhesions [8]. Polymorphonuclear cells, macrophages, fibroblasts and mesothelial cells migrate and proliferate into the fibrinous exudate. Macrophages increase in number, change function and secrete a variety of substances that recruit mesothelial cells onto the injured surfaces. Mesothelial cells form islands, proliferate and cover the injured area. All these cells release a variety of substances such as plasminogen activator, plasminogen activator inhibitor, arachidonic acid metabolites,reactive oxygen species, cytokines, IL-1, IL-6, tumor necrosis factor-a, prostaglandin E2, collagenase, elastase and the transforming growth factors leukotriene B4 a and b(TGFa and TGFb). These factors modulate the process of peritoneal healing and adhesion formation [12-14].

The deposition is the key step for the healing process and the balance between deposition and degradation will determine normal peritoneal healing or adhesion formation. The fibrin absorption is controlled by fibrinolysis. The inactive plasminogen is converted to plasmin through tissue plasminogen activator (tPA) and urokinase type plasminogen activator (uPA). The tPA is present in both mesothelium and submesothelial blood vessels of serosal and peritoneal membranes[12,15]. The fibrinolytic activity normally begins three days after peritoneal injury and increases to a maximum by day 8. Therefore, those adhesions that will be formed are in place by day 8, when mesothelial regeneration has been completed [8]. Normal peritoneum has a high fibrolytic activity in order to prevent adhesion formation between different tissue surfaces. During the inflammatory process, IL-1 and IL-6 stimulate epithelial and inflammatory cells to release plasminogen activator inhibitor 1 and 2 (PAI-1 and PAI-2), which inhibit fibrinolytic activity [16]. Patients with extensive adhesions have been found to have an overexpression of PAI-1 in the peritoneum [17]. Also, the deficient blood supply, the reduced tissue oxygenation and the release of reactive oxygen species that frequently co-exist with surgical trauma, decrease the peritoneal fibrinolytic activity [9,18].

3. Adhesion prevention

In order to prevent the development and reformation of post-operative intra-abdominal adhesions a variety of surgical techniques and adjuvants have been proposed. Agents, that in theory can modify the mechanism of adhesion formation, have been evaluated in experimental trials and many of them have been advocated for use during surgery in humans. Surgical techniques are focused on the limitation of surgical trauma, prevention of ischaemia and exposure of peritoneal cavity to foreign materials (Table 1). Improvement of surgical techniques can potentially reduce adhesion formation but cannot eliminate it. Anti-adhesive agents can be classified as pharmacological agents, systemic or intra-peritoneal, and intra-peritoneal barriers (solid or liquid). Pharmacological agents (Table 2) target the modification of inflammatory reaction (limitation of fibrin deposition), amplification of fibrin absorption and suppression of fibroblast activity. Barriers (Table 3) are used in order to prevent traumatized peritoneal surface apposition during the healing process so as to prevent tissue adherence [17,19].

Achieving excellent haemostasis and avoiding local ischaemia
Avoiding foreign bodies (talc, starch)
Avoiding peritoneum suturing or use of fine non-reactive suture
Minimizing surgical trauma
Minimizing tissue handling
Reducing drying or overheating of tissues
Reducing infection risk
Removing intra-peritoneal blood deposits

Table 1. Surgical techniques for prevention of adhesion formation

Fibrinolytic agents	Fibrinolysin
Anticoagulants	Papain
Anti-inflammatory	Streptokinase, streptodornase
agents	Urokinase
Antibiotics	Hyaluronidase
Other agents	Chymotrypsin, trypsin, pepsin
	Elastase
	Recombinant tissue plasminogen activator
	Citrates
	Oxalates
	Heparin
	Corticosteroids
	Antihistamines
	Non-steroidal anti-inflammatory drugs
	Tetracycline
	Cephalosporin
	Progesterone
	Oestrogens
	Gonadotrophin-releasing hormone agonists
	Antiproliferative agents
	Aromate inhibitors
	Statins
	Melatonin

Table 2. Pharmacological anti-adhesive agents

4. Laparoscopy and adhesions

The development of operative laparoscopy in gynaecology was associated with the expectation of reduced adhesion formation. Therefore, a large number of experimental and human clinical trials has been performed, which have shown that, compared with laparotomy, laparoscopic surgery is associated with less development of adhesions [17,20,21]. Reduction of adhesion formation is facilitated by minimal tissue handling and trauma, avoidance of exposure to foreign bodies (powder from gloves, gauze particles, e.t.c.) and prevention of air pollution in the peritoneal cavity that leads to the reduction of tissue drying. Pneumoperitoneum via increased intra-abdominal pressure has a tamponade effect that facilitates haemostasis, limits the use of diathermy and formation of ischaemic areas. In addition, laparoscopy is associated with a lower incidence of post-operative infection [21,22]. On the other hand, it has been advocated that the beneficial effect of laparoscopy in adhesion formation might be reduced by the use of pneumoperitoneum with CO2 [12]. CO2 pneumoperitoneum is associated with increased intra-abdominal pressure that compresses the splanchnic veins, reducing the blood flow by elevating vascular resistance. This stasis leads to a reduction in tissue oxygenation, anaerobic cell metabolism, acidosis and production of reactive oxygen species. The clinical impact of reactive oxygen species remains unclear but there is evidence that they are associated with increased adhesion formation [23]. Moreover it has been recently proposed that a low intra-peritoneal pressure (IPP) (8 mmHg) may be better than the standard IPP (12 mmHg) to minimize the adverse impact on the surgical peritoneal environment during a CO2 pneumoperitoneum [24].

Solid barriers	Omental grafts
(membranes, gel)	Peritoneal grafts
Endogenous tissue	Bladder strips
Fluid barriers	Fetal membranes
Exogenous material	Various oils
	Liquid paraffin
	Amniotic fluid
	Dextran
	Crystalloid solutions
	Icodextrin 4%
	Polyglycan esters
	Silicone
	Vaseline
	Gelatin
	Metal foils
	Elastic and silk foils
	Expanded
	polytetrafluoroethylene
	Oxidized regenerated
	cellulose
	Hyaluronic acid
	Carboxymethylcellulose
	Polyethylene glycol
	Polylactide
	Fibrin, **N,O**carboxymethylchitosan

Table 3. Anti-adhesive barier methods.

5. Pharmacological agents

A wide variety of pharmacological agents (Table 2) have been used in attempts to prevent or attenuate the formation of post-surgical adhesions, but none of them has been found to be effective. The use of drugs for adhesion prevention has some obstacles that affect their efficacy. Ischaemia and inadequate blood supply are important factors in adhesion formation and these also decrease systemic drug delivery inhibiting their effectiveness. Peritoneum has an extremely rapid absorption mechanism, that limits the half life and efficacy of many intra-peritoneally administered agents. Anti-adhesion agents must not affect normal wound healing, which has steps in common with adhesion formation (fibrinous exudate, fibrin deposition, fibroblast activity and proliferation) [19,25]. The clinical effectiveness of these agents has been evaluated in a systematic review and meta-analysis that analysed data from relevant randomized controlled trials (RCT) published up to 2005 [26].

6. Non-steroidal anti-inflammatory drugs

Non-steroidal anti-inflammatory drugs (NSAID) affect adhesion formation by several mechanisms. They act by modifying arachidonic acid metabolism and altering cyclooxygenase activities. This results in decreased vascular permeability, platelet aggregation, and coagulation and enhanced macrophage function. A number of locally and systemically administered NSAID have been used in experimental trials.

No relevant clinical trials assessing the effectiveness of NSAID in adhesion prevention have been published to date in patients undergoing gynaecological surgery. Their clinical efficacy is questionable probably because of inadequate concentrations at the sites of surgical trauma or by rapid absorption from the peritoneal membrane [3,19,27].

7. Corticosteroids and antihistamines

Corticosteroids alter the inflammatory response by reducing vascular permeability and decreasing cytokine and chemotactic factor secretion. Antihistamines inhibit fibroblast proliferation and stabilize lysosomal membranes and histamine secretion. Corticosteroids have been used alone or plus antihistamines by intra-peritoneal or systemic administration or by flushing through Fallopian tubes post-operatively and were effective in many, but not all, experimental models. In the limited data from RCT [28,29,30], no significant beneficial effect was detected with the use of corticosteroids (systemic, intra-peritoneal or Fallopian tube flushing) in the deterioration of adhesion score at second-look laparoscopy or on the probability of clinical pregnancy. However, limited data suggest that the addition of post-operative steroids to systemic intra-operative steroids might be associated with a favourable outcome both in terms of adhesion score deterioration (increase) or improvement (reduction) [31]. On the other hand, adverse events such as suppression of the pituitary–adrenal axis, immunosuppression and delayed wound healing have been reported with the use of corticosteroids [19,32,33]. Regarding antihistamines, only one RCT has evaluated the role of oral promethazine in the prevention of adhesion formation after pelvic surgery. In that study, no significant difference was detected either in deterioration or improvement of adhesion score in patients who received promethazine as compared with those who did not [31].

8. Progesterone and oestrogens

Progesterone has been used for the prevention of post-operative adhesions. Administration of progesterone resulted in less adhesion formation in animal models, but does not appear to be effective in humans. Oestrogens have been associated with increased adhesion formation in animal models. It was demonstrated that a hypo-oestrogenic state, produced by gonadotrophin-releasing hormone agonists or aromatase inhibitors such as tamoxifen and anastrazole, decrease development of post-operative adhesions in experimental models [3,34,35]. This hypothesis, however, has never been tested in humans.

9. Anticoagulants – Fibrinolytics

Anticoagulants such as heparin can reduce adhesion formation by inhibition of the coagulation cascade and promotion of fibrinolysis [36]. The use of heparin for intra-peritoneal irrigation in a dose that can reduce adhesion formation was associated with haemorrhage and delayed wound healing, but low-dose heparin irrigation showed no benefit in adhesion reduction [3,19,37]. In the only available RCT, heparin delivery with oxidized regenerated cellulose failed to demonstrate a superior effect compared with oxidized regenerated cellulose alone [38]. Furthermore, in experimental trials, the combination of carboxymethylcellulose or 32% dextran 70 plus heparin failed to reduce adhesion formation [38,39,40].

Fibrinolytic agents as streptokinase, elastase and tissue plasminogen activator produced by recombinant DNA techniques (rtPA) can contribute in adhesion prevention directly by reducing the fibrinous mass and indirectly by stimulating plasminogen activator activity. Systemic administration of anticoagulants is impeded by lack of safety. The concentrations of fibrinolytic agents required to prevent adhesion formation are too close to the anticoagulatory concentrations and increase the risk for post-operative haemorrhage and delayed wound healing. Intra-peritoneal administration is ineffective due to rapid absorption by the peritoneal membrane [3,25,41]. The use of carboxymethylcellulose gel and oxidized regenerated cellulose as a carrier to deliver rtPA intra-peritonealy was not associated with a reduction of adhesion formation in animal models [42,43].

A recent study has investigated the impact of gonadotropin-releasing hormone analogue (GnRH-a) on coagulation and fibrinolytic activities and its effectiveness in the prevention of pelvic adhesion after myomectomy in thirty-two infertile women. Patients treated with GnRH-a showed significant decrease in plasminogen activator inhibitorPAI, thrombin activatable fibrinolysis inhibitor (TAFI), factors V, and VIII and increased protein C (PC), but no significant change in plasminogen and α2-antiplasmin levels compared with control group, suggesting a possible critical role of the GnRH-a therapy in preventing postoperative adhesion development [44].

10. Antibiotics

Antibiotics are commonly used for prophylaxis against post-operative infections and hence the inflammatory response that leads to adhesion formation. Peritoneal irrigation with antibiotic solutions does not reduce adhesion formation, while it has been shown that in some cases it may promote them [45].

11. Other pharmacological regimens

Many other agents, such as apoprotin, noxytioline, growth factor inhibitors and modulators, phosphatidylcholine, thiazolidinediones, colchicine and calcium channel blockers, have been utilized in experimental trials. The intra-peritoneal administration of noxytioline is the only one of these interventions that has been tested in the context of a RCT and no significant difference was identified in terms of reduction of adhesions and clinical pregnancy rates in patients who were administered intra-peritoneal noxytioline and the control group [29]. There is no data from RCT to support the conclusion that any of the other agents is efficacious in preventing the development of post-operative adhesions [19,46,47].

12. Anti-adhesive barriers

The failure of pharmacological regimens to prevent adhesion formation has led to the revival of the barrier technique. With the barrier technique, traumatized peritoneal surfaces are kept separated, during mesothelial regeneration, thus precluding adherence of adjacent organs and tissues and reducing the development of adhesions. The separation can be achieved by the use of solid (films or gels) or fluid barriers [19,25]. Anti-adhesive barriers are currently the most useful adjuvant for prevention of post-operative adhesion formation. Numerous substances (Table 3) have been used as mechanical barriers to separate tissue surfaces. Most of these materials are of historical interest only and had no effect or even aggravated adhesion formation [48,49]. An anti-adhesive agent should be effective, safe, economical and easy to use in both open and laparoscopic surgery [50]. The clinical effectiveness of several of these agents has been evaluated in two recent Cochrane reviews [26,51].

13. Solid barriers

Solid barriers are placed over one or between two traumatized surfaces providing a separation that averts tissue apposition during the critical period of fibrin formation and mesothelial regeneration following surgical trauma. It should be noted though, that solid barriers have some significant drawbacks. They are often ineffective in the presence of blood, have a complex preparation and application, do not conform easily to the shape of pelvic organs, need suturing and are difficult to use via laparoscopic surgery. Their benefits are also limited to the site of application and do not prevent the development of adhesions at sites of indirect trauma. So the surgeon has to surmise where adhesions will be formed in order to choose the placement sites and optimize barrier efficacy [52]. Not infrequently, this proves to be a challenging task, since, for example, midline laparotomy initiates a generalized peritoneal response that can lead to adhesion formation distant from surgical trauma [53].

14. Expanded polytetrafluoroethylene

Expanded polytetrafluoroethylene (Preclude, Gore-Tex Surgical Membrane; Johnson and Johnson, Arlington, TX) is a non-absorbable, non-reactive, synthetic material that

inhibits cellular migration and tissue adherence. In the only available RCT, it has been shown to be associated with fewer post-operative de-novo adhesions after myomectomy when compared with no treatment [54]. Moreover, when compared with oxidized regenerated cellulose, Preclude was found to be more effective in terms of adhesion reformation after adhesiolysis [55]. However, in another RCT, no evidence of a beneficial effect of Preclude was demonstrated in the de-novo formation of adhesions after laparoscopic myomectomy when compared to oxidized regenerated cellulose [56]. Expanded polytetrafluoroethylene has the disadvantages that it must be sutured in place, is difficult to use in laparoscopic surgery and, ideally, requires a subsequent surgical procedure for removal after the injury has healed [57]. The use of Preclude in Europe is limited and it has been withdrawn from the market in USA after the development of the absorbable barriers [25].

15. Oxidized regenerated cellulose

Oxidized regenerated cellulose (Interceed (TC7); Johnson and Johnson) is the first degradable barrier that was used in clinical practice and represents a modification of its precursor Surgicel, which has been used as a haemostatic agent for a long time. It is a mesh designed to be placed over or between traumatized surfaces. About 8 h after the application in the peritoneal cavity, it becomes a viscous gel and finally it is degraded to monosaccharides and completely absorbed in about 2 weeks [3,22]. Oxidized regenerated cellulose use in laparoscopic surgery is feasible [8]. In order to evaluate the efficacy of oxidized regenerated cellulose in the prevention of the development of post-surgical adhesions, many studies have been carried out. A meta-analysis of 11 relevant RCT [51] has shown that the barrier is safe and reduces significantly the incidence of de-novo adhesions, as well as the reformation of adhesions as compared with no treatment in laparoscopy [58-62]. In laparotomy, the available RCT [63-68], when meta-analysed [51], demonstrated that a significant reduction in the reformation (or mixture) of adhesions can be expected with the use of oxidized regenerated cellulose as compared with the no treatment group. The product is site specific, thus the efficacy is limited to surgical situations where raw surfaces can be completely covered with the mesh and its benefit is limited to the site of barrier placement. The fundamental disadvantage is that it becomes ineffective when the entire area is not completely haemostatic. The presence of small amounts of blood in the peritoneal cavity or post-operative bleeding results in blood permeating the mesh, fibrin deposition and, finally, adhesion formation [8,69,70]. In addition, as reported previously, the combination of oxidized regenerated cellulose plus heparin resulted in a significant reduction of adhesion formation and reformation in experimental models. This improvement in efficacy was not confirmed in clinical trials [36,38,40]. Oxidized regenerated cellulose has been approved by the US Food and Drink Administration (FDA) for use in open surgery in the USA [69].

16. Hyaluronic acid

Hyaluronic acid (HA) is a linear polysaccharide with repeating disaccharide units that are composed of sodium D-glucuronate and N-acetyl-D-glucosamine. It is a naturally occurring component of many body tissues and fluids, where it provides mechanically protective and physically supportive roles [69]. Various combinations of HA have been used for the prevention of adhesion formation. HA and carboxymethylcellulose (Seprafilm; Genzyme, Cambridge, Massachusetts, USA) is an absorbable membrane that dissolves and forms a hydrophilic gel approximately 24 h after placement. It is a site-specific barrier and acts by separating mechanically opposite tissue surfaces and lasts for 7 days. The HA is completely cleared from the body within 4 weeks, but the absorption of carboxymethylcellulose is not well known. It does not conform to the shape of pelvic organs as well as oxidized regenerated cellulose and is usually used to prevent adhesions between the incision of anterior abdominal wall and bowel or omentum [71,72]. Its use in laparoscopic procedures is difficult. In a blind prospective, randomized, multicentre study, the treatment of patients after myomectomy with Seprafilm significantly reduced the extent and area of post-operative uterine adhesions [72]. Potential side effects include induced foreign body reaction, higher incidence of pulmonary emboli and intra-peritoneal abscess formation, but these findings were not statistically significant in the relevant trials [3,73]. High cost is another limitation because, for an effective protection from intestinal obstruction, a mean of 4.5 sheets per patient is required [25]. Seprafilm has been approved by the FDA for use in open surgery in the USA [22]. Ferric hyaluronate 0.5% gel (Intergel; Gynecare, Sommerville, New Jersey, USA) is a viscous gel that provides a broader coverage than previous site-specific agents. It was shown to be easy to use in open and laparoscopic surgery. In relevant prospective randomized trials, ferric hyaluronate was associated with a significant reduction of severity and extent of post-operative adhesions and statistically significant improvement of the American Fertility Society (AFS) and modified AFS scores at second-look laparoscopy [69,74,75]. It was withdrawn from the market in 2003 because of problems with late onset post-operative pain and rare reports of sclerosing peritonitis [25,76]. Low-viscosity 0.04% HA combined with phosphate-buffered saline (Sepracoat; Genzyme) is a bioabsorbable macromolecular dilute solution of HA that is cleared from the body in less than 5 days. The solution is applied in the peritoneal cavity before any tissue manipulation in order to protect peritoneal surfaces from indirect trauma and finally before the end of the procedures [3,77,78]. In a blind, prospective, randomized, placebo-controlled multicentre study, where patients had undergone open gynecological procedures, low-viscosity 0.04% HA resulted in a statistically significant reduction of adhesions, as well as of the mean adhesion score, at second-look laparoscopy. However, it was not effective in reducing post-operative adhesion formation at sites of direct surgical trauma [78]. It has been approved by the FDA for use in open surgery in the USA [22]. HA cross-linked to HA (Hyalobarrier Gel; Baxter, Bracknell, UK) is a site-specific highly viscous gel is considered as easy to use in laparoscopic and open surgery. In a prospective, randomized, controlled study where the rate of post-surgical adhesions after laparoscopic myomectomy was examined, cross-linked HA resulted in significantly more adhesion-free patients [79]. Pregnancy rates at 6 and 12 months after laparoscopic myomectomy were significantly higher in patients treated with cross-linked HA [80]. In another randomized trial, adhesion-free patients after laparoscopic myomectomy were greater in the treatment group but the difference was not statistically significant. The incidence and severity of adhesions was similar in both groups, but a significant reduction of uterine adhesions was found in the treatment group [81]. When the data from the two aforementioned studies were combined, a statistically significant reduction of adhesions during second-look laparoscopy was detected in the group of patients treated with HA-cross-linked HA as compared with the control group. Auto-cross-linked internal ester form of HA (ACP gel; Fidia Advanced Biopolymers, AbanoTerme, Italy) has the biocompatibility of the original polymer but higher viscosity and extended residence. It is a gel that has been shown to be efficacious in reducing abdominal adhesions in experimental models [82,83]. Two prospective randomized controlled trials have been published so far by the same group regarding the use of ACP gel for the prevention of intrauterine adhesions after hysteroscopic surgery. In these studies, ACP gel has been associated with a significant reduction in the incidence and the severity of subsequent intrauterine adhesions [84,85]. A stratified analysis of these two studies confirmed this finding by demonstrating a significant reduction in the proportion of patients with adhesions at second-look hysteroscopy. Cross-linked thiol-modified HA with 4% polyethyleneglycoldiacrylate (Carbylan-S and Carbylan-SX; CarbylanBioSurgery, Palo Alto, CA, USA) is a bioabsorbable solution of HA. Carbylan-S is a hydrogel and Carbylan-SX has two formats, a sprayable gel and a hydrogel film. In animal models, Carbylan- S containing mitomycin C and Carbylan-SX were effective in prevention of post-operative intra-abdominal adhesions [52,86].

17. Polylactide

Polylactide (copolymer of 70:30 poly(L-lactide-CO-D, L-lactide; SurgiWrap, MacroporeBiosurgeryinc., San Diego, USA) is a bioabsorbable film with a long absorption period (up to 6 months). It is metabolized to lactic acid and finally to CO2 and exhaled through the respiratory system. It requires suturing in order to avoid its loss from the site. In preclinical studies, polylactide appears to be effective in the reduction of adhesion formation, but there are no data currently for safety and efficacy in humans [87,88].

18. Polyethylene glycol

Polyethylene glycol (SprayGel; Confluent Surgical, Waltham, Massachusetts, USA). It is a synthetic hydrogel formed when two polyethylene glycol-based liquids are sprayed together with an air assisted sprayer at the target tissue, where they cross-link and form a hydrogel barrier. One liquid is clear and one is coloured with methylene blue in order that facilitate its application. The gel remains intact for approximately 5–7 days and then gradually breaks down by hydrolysis and is cleared through the kidneys [89]. Drawbacks of the product are the intricacy of preparation and application, the time required to cover the target tissue and the high cost. In a prospective randomized controlled phase-III trial, in 40 patients undergoing myomectomy, polylactide resulted in a significant decrease in the mean tenacity score. The extent of adhesions was increased in the control group but the difference was not significant. Also, the proportion of adhesion-free patients at second-look laparoscopy was increased in the treatment group but the difference was not statistically significant [89]. It has been approved for use in laparoscopic and open surgery in Europe, but by the FDA only for use in open surgery in USA [22,25].

19. Carboxymethylcellulose

Carboxymethylcellulose is a high-molecular-weight polysaccharide, derivative of cellulose. The mechanism of its absorption is not well known. It has been used in combination with rtPA and with HA. A composite gel of carboxymethylcellulose and polyethylene oxide (Oxiplex; FzioMed, San Luis Obispo, CA, USA) is a viscoelastic gel, which acts as a barrier between tissues that inhibits protein deposition and thrombus formation [74]. The gel is absorbed by 6 weeks, but in cases where large amounts of gel were applied in multiple layers to the surgically treated sites or in cases of stage-IV endometriosis, small collections of gelatinous material were noted in areas of gel application or in areas deep in the cul-de-sac [90]. In two blind randomized controlled trials, where patients underwent adnexal surgery, carboxymethylcellulose and polyethylene oxide showed a significant improvement of AFS score in the treated group, but not in all clinical situations. It did not appear to provide this benefit to patients with grade-IV endometriosis [74,91]. Another double-blind prospective randomized controlled trial has shown that the mean AFS score for patients in the treatment group was unchanged, while in control patients an increased AFS score was noted [91]. No statistical pooling was feasible for these three studies, since the data were not analysed and presented per randomization unit (they were analysed per adnexa and not per patient). It is easy to use in laparoscopic surgery and it has been approved in Europe for use in abdominal and pelvic surgery [25].

20. Fibrin glue

Fibrin glue (Tissucol; Baxter International, Deerfield, IL, USA) is a biological product. Fibrin glue is made by mixing human fibrinogen with bovine thrombin, calcium and factor XIII

[92]. Obviously, the use of human blood products raises a theoretical risk for transmission of infectious diseases. According to the pathogenesis of adhesions, application of fibrin glue at the traumatized peritoneal surfaces should increase adhesion formation. Possibly, fibrin glue application confines fibrin deposition and averts the development of attachments between opposing tissue surfaces. In animal studies, the use of fibrin glue has been shown to decrease adhesion formation and reformation but clinical data are limited. Fibrin glue has not been approved by the FDA for use in USA [22,47]. So far, no relevant data from trials in humans have been published.

21. Carboxymethylchitosan

N,O-carboxymethylchitosan (Adhes-X, Chitogenics, New Jersey, USA) is a purified derivative of chitin obtained from the exoskeleton of shrimp and has similar structure to hyaluronic acid and carboxymethylcellulose [93]. The product comprises both a clear gel and a solution. The gel is placed initially at the sites of surgical trauma where it is tamped with a laparoscopic instrument and subsequently the solution is placed at the same places. Its efficacy and safety have been confirmed in some animal models. A prospective randomized controlled study, performed on 34 patients undergoing laparoscopy for various gynaecological indications, demonstrated a decrease in the recurrence, extent and severity of adhesions and a decrease of de-novo adhesion formation at second-look laparoscopy, but none of these findings were statistically significant [94].

22. Fluid barriers

Fluids constitute an ideal barrier agent because their action is not limited to the site of application. Their function is provided by hydrofloration of intra-peritoneal structures in the liquid that is infused into the peritoneal cavity at the end of the surgical procedure. Hydrofloration provides a temporary separation between raw peritoneal surfaces allowing independent healing without the formation of adhesions. Possibly, fluid circulation in the peritoneal cavity contributes to the prevention of adhesion formation by diluting fibrinous exudates released from traumatized surfaces. Fluid barriers may prevent adhesion formation both at the traumatized area and elsewhere in the pelvis. The instillation of fluids in the peritoneal cavity may be associated with some undesirable side effects, such as leakage from the incision, labial oedema, feeling of fluid moving around, abdominal discomfort, abdominal distension and complications such as pulmonary and peripheral oedema. Large volumes of intra-peritoneal fluids may decrease the peritoneum ability to confront bacterial infections [3,17,76].

23. Crystalloid solutions

Crystalloid solutions (Ringer's lactate, NaCl 0.9%) are rapidly absorbed by the peritoneal cavity, at a rate of 30–50 ml/h. Consequently, 24 h after the surgery, minimal or no crystalloid solution would be left in the peritoneal cavity. The instillation of crystalloids does not seem to result in decreased adhesion formation. They are commonly used but they are not approved for use as anti-adhesive agents [25,69,95]. Crystalloids have also been used in various combinations with heparin, steroids, antihistamines and other pharmacological agents in randomized controlled trials, but none of them has been found effective in decreasing post-operative adhesion formation or improving pregnancy rates [96].

24. Dextran

Dextran (32% dextran 70; Hyskon; Pharmacia, Piscataway, New Jersey, USA) is a 1–6-linked dextrose polymer. A summary [26] of the available data from relevant RCT [37,97-99] demonstrated a decreased proportion of patients with adhesions at second-look laparoscopy in the group that received 32% dextran 70, as compared with the group that did not. However, despite the fact that the patients with improvement and deterioration in the adhesion score at second-look laparoscopy were increased and decreased, respectively, in the treatment group, when compared with the control group, this difference was not statistically significant. In addition, its use was associated with significant side effects as pulmonary and peripheral oedema caused by its osmotic properties, liver function abnormalities, pleural effusion and, rarely, allergic reactions or anaphylactic shock and disseminated intra-vascular coagulation. It has not been approved for use as an anti-adhesive agent [3,17,100,101].

25. Polyglycan esters

Polyglycanesters (Adcon-P; Gliatech, Cleveland, Ohio) is a viscous bioabsorbable solution. Its prototypes Adcon-L and Adcon-T/N were found effective for adhesion prevention in spinal and neurosurgical procedures. Experimental studies have shown that application of Adcon-P effectively reduces development of post-operative intra-abdominal adhesions. There are no data for the safety and the efficacy of this product in humans [102].

26. Icodextrin

Icodextrin 4% (Adept; Shire Pharmaceuticals, Basingstoke, Hampshire, UK) is a 1–4-linked glucose polymer. Icodextrin 4% is a clear isomolar solution and does not predispose to infection. It is absorbed gradually via the lymphatic system into the systemic circulation, where it is digested to oligosaccharides by amylase. Amylase is absent from the human peritoneal cavity. Preclinical studies had shown significant reduction of post-operative adhesions and confirmed the safety of icodextrin 4%. It was indicated that the agent was more effective in adhesion reduction when used as both an irrigant and post-operative instillate [103]. In a small double-blind prospective randomized multicentre study, icodextrin 4% resulted in the reduction of incidence, severity and extent of adhesions but these results were not statistically significant [104]. However, recently, in the largest prospective randomized double-blind multicentre study for an anti-adhesive agent, icodextrin 4% has been shown to result in a significant reduction of incidence, severity and extent of adhesions and a significant improvement of AFS score. Also the study showed that icodextrin 4% prevents the deterioration of pre-existing adhesions, considering that patients with the higher number of adhesion lysed at initial surgery had the greater reduction in adhesion incidence [95]. A stratified analysis of these two studies revealed a statistically significant effect oficodextrin 4% use on the de-novo formation of adhesions, as well as on the proportion of patients with an improvement of the adhesion score at second-look laparoscopy [105]. Simultaneously with clinical trials, a European patients registry (ARIEL) was created allowing surgeons to record and report the experiences of the use of icodextrin 4% in open and laparoscopic gynaecological and general surgery. The registry provides feedback on routine use in 4620 patients (2882 that underwent gynaecological and 1738 general surgery). The general consensus is that it is easy to use in both open and laparoscopic surgery, it is well tolerated by patients and the incidence of adverse events is considered similar to the control group [76,106]. Low cost is another advantage of icodextrin 4%. Adept (1.5 litre bags) are about half the price of each sheet of Interceed or Seprafilm and it is about four times cheaper than one SprayGel package [50]. Icodextrin 4% has been approved for use in open and laparoscopic surgery in Europe and it was the first anti-adhesive agent that has been approved by the FDA for use in laparoscopic surgery in the USA [25,76,91,95].

27. Conclusions

Development of post-operative adhesion is a widespread consequence of surgical trauma and healing following open or laparoscopic gynecological surgery and is associated with significant complications. At present, the main strategy to avoid formation and reformation of adhesions is focused on the use of careful surgical techniques and anti-adhesive agents. Reduction of adhesion formation after laparoscopic surgery in comparison to the more conventional approach by laparotomy can be attributed to less tissue manipulation, less tissue drying, avoidance of insertion of foreign bodies such as talc from the surgical gloves, fibers from the gauzes e.t.c. On the other hand pneumoperitoneum during laparoscopy exerts a tamponade effect that facilitates hemostasis, so minimizing the use of electrocautery, which is known that leads to the formation of ischaemic areas and therefore predisposing to adhesion formation. The use of CO2 for pnemoperitoneum may lead to adhesion formation, since its use is associated with reduction in tissue oxygenation, acidosis and release ofreactive oxygen species, which are considered adhesiogenic. Therefore, the addition of oxygen, the heating of the insufflatedCO2 or the alternative use of other gases (i.e. helium) may be beneficial in terms of reduction of *de novo* adhesion formation. At the end of each operation an «underwater» examination should be used in order to document complete intra-peritoneal hemostasis, since it has been clearly demonstrated that incomplete hemostasis is associated with adhesion formation.

Finally, several anti-adhesive agents are used during laparoscopic intrventions, in order to minimizepostoperative adhesions. These fall into two main categories, which include pharmacological agents and barrier methods. Limited data support the use of the former, either locally or systemically. Barriers, which mechanically separate the opposed serosal surfaces and exert their beneficial action, at least partly, because they remain in place beyond the critical 3-day point, at which competition of fibrinolytic activityandfibrosis will lead to adhesion formation. The tissue separation can be achieved either by the use of solid (films or gel) or fluid barriers. The clinical effectiveness of several of these agents has been thoroughly evaluated in two recent Cochrane reviews by Metwally et al [26] and Ahmad et al [51].

Author details

George Pados, Anastasios Makedos and Basil Tarlatzis

1st Dept. of OB-GYN, School of Medicine, Aristotle University of Thessaloniki, «Papageorgiou» General Hospital, N. Efkarpia, Greece

References

[1] Holmdahl, L., Risberg, B., Beck, D.E., et al. Adhesions: pathogenesis and prevention-panel discussion and summary. Eur. J. Surg. Suppl. 1997; 56: 62.

[2] Menzies, D., Ellis, H. Intestinal obstruction from adhesions – how big is the problem? Ann. R. Coll. Surg. Engl. 1992; 72: 60–63.

[3] Liakakos, T., Thomakos, N., Fine, P.M., Dervenis, C., Young, R.L. Peritoneal adhesions: etiology, pathophysiology, and clinical significance. Recent advances in prevention and management.Dig. Surg. 2001; 18: 260–273.

[4] Menzies, D. Peritoneal adhesions. Incidence, cause, and prevention. Surg. Annu. 1992; 24: 27–45.

[5] Operative Laparoscopy Study Group. Postoperative adhesion development after operative laparoscopy: evaluation at early second-look procedures. Fertil. Steril. 1991; 55: 700–704.

[6] Lower, A.M., Hawthorn, R.J., Clark, D., et al. Adhesion- related readmissions following gynaecological laparoscopy or laparotomy in Scotland: an epidemiological study of 24 046 patients. Hum. Reprod. 2004;19: 1877–1885.

[7] Diamond, M.P., Freeman, M.L. Clinical implications of postsurgical adhesions. Hum. Reprod. Update. 2001; 7: 567–576.

[8] Pados, G.A., Devroey, P. Adhesions. Curr. Opin. Obstet. Gynecol. 1992; 4: 412–418.

[9] DiZerega, G.S. Biochemical events in peritoneal tissue repair. Eur. J. Surg. Suppl. 1997; 10: 16.

[10] Badia, J.M., Whawell, S.A., Scott-Coombes, D.M., Abel, P.D., Williamson, R.C., Thompson, J.N. Peritoneal and systemic cytokine response to laparotomy. Br. J. Surg. 1996;83: 347–348.

[11] Boland, G.M., Weigel, R.J. Formation and prevention of postoperative abdominal adhesions. J. Surg. Res. 2006; 132: 3–12.

[12] Binda, M.M., Molinas, C.R., Koninckx, P.R. Reactive oxygen species and adhesion formation: clinical implications in adhesion prevention. Hum. Reprod. 2003; 18: 2503–2507.

[13] Drollette, C.M., Badawy, S.Z. Pathophysiology of pelvic adhesions. Modern trends in preventing infertility. J. Reprod. Med. 1992; 37: 107–121.

[14] Rodgers, K.E., diZerega, G.S. Function of peritoneal exudate cells after abdominal surgery. J. Invest. Surg. 1993; 6: 9–23.

[15] Dano, K., Andreasen, P.A., Grondahl-Hansen, J., Kristensen, P., Nielsen, L.S., Skriver, L. Plasminogen activators, tissue degradation, and cancer. Adv. Cancer Res. 1985; 44: 139–266.

[16] Buckman, R.F., Woods, M., Sargent, L., Gervin, A.S. A unifying pathogenetic mechanism in the etiology of intraperitoneal adhesions. J. Surg. Res. 1976; 20: 1–5.

[17] Sutton, C. Adhesions and their prevention. Obstet. Gynaecol. 2005; 7: 168–176.

[18] Raftery, A.T. Effect of peritoneal trauma on peritoneal fibrinolytic activity and intraperitoneal adhesion formation. An experimental study in the rat. Eur. Surg. Res. 1981;13:397–401.

[19] Risberg, B. Adhesions: preventive strategies. Eur. J. Surg. Suppl. 1997;32: 39.

[20] Lundorff, P., Hahlin, M., Kallfelt, B., Thorburn, J., Lindblom, B. Adhesion formation after laparoscopic surgery in tubal pregnancy: a randomized trial versus laparotomy. Fertil. Steril. 1991;55: 911–915.

[21] Schafer, M., Krahenb hl, L., Buchler, M.W. Comparison of adhesion formation in open and laparoscopic surgery. Dig. Surg. 1998; 15: 148–152.

[22] The Practice Committee of the ASRM. Control and prevention of peritoneal adhesions in gynecologic surgery. Fertil. Steril. 2006;86: S1–S5.

[23] de Souza, A.M., Wang, C.C., Chu, C.Y., Lam, P.M., Rogers, M.S. The effect of intra-abdominal pressure on the generation of 8-iso prostaglandin F2alpha during laparoscopy in rabbits. Hum. Reprod. 2003;18: 2181–2188.

[24] Matsuzaki S, Jardon K, Maleysson E, D'Arpiani F, Canis M, Botchorishvili R. Impact of intraperitoneal pressure of a CO2 pneumoperitoneum on the surgical peritoneal environment. Hum Reprod. 2012;27(6): 1613-23.

[25] Trew, G: Postoperative adhesions and their prevention. Rev. Gynaecol. Perinat. Pract. 2006;6: 47–56.

[26] Metwally, M., Watson, A., Lilford, R., Vandekerckhove, P. Fluid and pharmacological agents for adhesion prevention after gynaecological surgery. Cochrane Database Syst Rev, CD001298, 2006.

[27] Luciano, A.A., Hauser, K.S., Benda, J. Evaluation of commonly used adjuvants in the prevention of postoperative adhesions. Am. J. Obstet. Gynecol. 1983;146: 88–92.

[28] Jansen, R.P. Failure of intraperitoneal adjuncts to improve the outcome of pelvic operations in young women. Am. J. Obstet. Gynecol. 1985;153: 363–371.

[29] Querleu, D., Vankeerberghen-Deffense, F., Boutteville, C. The effect of noxytioline and systemic corticosteroids in infertility surgery. A prospective randomized study. (Traitement adjuvant des plastiestubaires. Etude prospective randomisee des corticoides par voiegeneraleet de la noxytioline). J. Gynecol. Obstet. Biol. Reprod. 1989;18: 935–940.

[30] Rock, J.A., Siegler, A.M., Meisel, M.B. The efficacy of postoperative hydrotubation: a randomized prospective multicenter clinical trial. Fertil. Steril. 1984;42(2): 373–376.

[31] Jansen, R.P. Controlled clinical approaches to investigating the prevention of peritoneal adhesions. Prog. Clin. Biol. Res. 1990;358: 177–192.

[32] Granat, M., Schenker, J.G., Mor-Yosef, S., Rosenkovitch, E., Castellanos, R.C., Galili, U. Effects of dexamethasone on proliferation of autologous fibroblasts and on the immune profile in women undergoing pelvic surgery for infertility. Fertil. Steril. 1983;39: 180–186.

[33] Harris, W.J., Daniell, J.F: Use of corticosteroids as an adjuvant in terminal salpingostomy. Fertil. Steril. 1983;40: 785–789.

[34] Kaya, U., Oktem, M., Zeyneloglu, H.B., Ozen, O., Kuscu, E. Impact of aromatase inhibitors on adhesion formation in a rat model. Fertil. Steril. 2007;87: 934–939.

[35] Montanino-Oliva, M., Metzger, D.A., Luciano, A.A. Use of medroxyprogesterone acetate in the prevention of postoperative adhesions. Fertil. Steril. 1996;65: 650–654.

[36] Diamond, M.P., Linsky, C.B., Cunningham, T. Adhesion reformation: reduction by the use of Interceed (TC7) plus heparin. J. Gynecol. Surg. 1991;7(a): 1–6.

[37] Jansen, R.P.Failure of peritoneal irrigation with heparin during pelvic operations upon young women to reduce adhesions. Surg. Gynecol. Obstet. 1988;166: 154–160.

[38] Reid, R.L., Hahn, P.M., Spence, J.E., Tulandi, T., Yuzpe, A.A., Wiseman, D.M. A randomized clinical trial of oxidized regenerated cellulose adhesion barrier (Interceed, TC7) alone or in combination with heparin. Fertil. Steril.1997; 67: 23–29.

[39] Diamond, M.P., Linsky, C.B., Cunningham, T., et al. Synergistic effects of INTERCEED(TC7) and heparin in reducing adhesion formation in the rabbit uterine horn model. Fertil. Steril. 1991;55(b): 389–394.

[40] Reid, R.L., Lie, K., Spence, J.E., Tulandi, T., Yuzpe, A. Clinical evaluation of the efficacy of heparin-saturated Interceed for prevention of adhesion reformation in the pelvic sidewall of the human. Prog. Clin. Biol. Res. 1993;381: 261–264.

[41] Doody, K.J., Dunn, R.C., Buttram Jr., V.C. Recombinant tissue plasminogen activator reduces adhesion formation in a rabbit uterine horn model. Fertil. Steril. 1989;51: 509–512.

[42] Bothin, C. Counteracting postsurgical adhesions – the effect of combining oxidized regenerated cellulose and tissue plasminogen activator. Int. J. Fertil. Menopausal Stud. 1995;40: 102–105.

[43] Gehlbach, D.L., O'Hair, K.C., Parks, A.L., Rosa, C. Combined effects of tissue plasminogen activator and carboxymethylcellulose on adhesion reformation in rabbits. Int. J. Fertil. Menopausal Stud. 1994;39: 172–176.

[44] Di Nardo MA, Annunziata ML, Ammirabile M, Di Minno MN, Ruocco AL, De Falco M, Di Lieto A.Pelvic adhesion and gonadotropin-releasing hormone analogue: effects of triptorelin acetate depot on coagulation and fibrinolytic activities. Reprod Sci. 2012;19(6):615-22.

[45] Rappaport, W.D., Holcomb, M., Valente, J., Chvapil, M. Antibiotic irrigation and the formation of intraabdominal adhesions. Am. J. Surg. 1989;158: 435–437.

[46] Demirturk, F., Aytan, H., Caliskan, A., et al. The effect of rosiglitazone in the prevention of intra-abdominal adhesion formation in a rat uterine horn model. Hum. Reprod. 2006;21: 3008–3013,.

[47] Hellebrekers, B.W., Trimbos-Kemper, G.C., van Blitterswijk, C.A., Bakkum, E.A., Trimbos, J.B. Effects of five different barrier materials on postsurgical adhesion formation in the rat. Hum. Reprod. 2000;15: 1358–1363.

[48] Arora, M., Jaroudi, K.A., Hamilton, C.J., Dayel, F. Controlled comparison of intercede and amniotic membrane graft in the prevention of postoperative adhesions in the rabbit uterine horn model. Eur. J. Obstet. Gynecol. Reprod. Biol. 1994;55: 179–182.

[49] Seifer, D.B., Diamond, M.P., DeCherney, A.H. An appraisal of barrier agents in the reduction of adhesion formation following surgery. J. Gynecol. Surg. 1990; 6: 3–10.

[50] Trew, G., Lower, A. Consensus in adhesion reduction management. Obstetr. Gynaecol. 2004; 6: 1–2.

[51] Ahmad, G., Duffy, J.M., Farquhar, C., et al. Barrier agentsfor adhesion prevention after gynaecological surgery. Cochrane Database Syst Rev, CD000475, 2008.

[52] Liu, Y., Li, H., Shu, X.Z., Gray, S.D., Prestwich, G.D. Crosslinkedhyaluronan hydrogels containing mitomycin C reduce postoperative abdominal adhesions. Fertil. Steril. (Suppl. 1). 2005; 83:1275–1283.

[53] Becker, J.M., Stucchi, A.F.Intra-abdominal adhesion prevention: are we getting any closer? Ann. Surg. 2004;240: 202–204.

[54] Myomectomy ASG. An expanded polytetrafluoroethylene barrier (Gore-Tex Surgical Membrane) reduces post-myomectomy adhesion formation. The Myomectomy Adhesion Multicenter Study Group. Fertil. Steril. 1995;63: 491–493.

[55] Haney, A.F., Hesla, J., Hurst, B.S., et al. Expanded polytetrafluoroethylene (Gore-Tex Surgical Membrane) is superior to oxidized regenerated cellulose (Interceed TC7+) in preventing adhesions. Fertil. Steril. 1995;63: 1021–1026.

[56] Korell, M. Reduction of adhesion by INTERCEED Barrier and Gortex Surgical Membrane after laparoscopic myomectomy, Moglichkeiten der Adhasionprophylaxe, Munich, 1994.

[57] Farquhar, C., Vandekerckhove, P., Watson, A., Vail, A., Wiseman, D: Barrier agents for preventing adhesions after surgery for subfertility. Cochrane Database Syst Rev, CD000475, 2000.

[58] Keckstein, J., Ulrich, U., Sasse, V., Roth, A., Tuttlies, F., Karageorgieva, E. Reduction of postoperative adhesion formation after laparoscopic ovarian cystectomy. Hum. Reprod. 1996;11: 579–582.

[59] Mais, V., Ajossa, S., Marongiu, D., Peiretti, R.F., Guerriero, S., Melis, G.B. Reduction of adhesion reformation after laparoscopic endometriosis surgery: a randomized trial with an oxidized regenerated cellulose absorbable barrier. Obstet. Gynecol. 1995;86(a): 512–515.

[60] Mais, V., Ajossa, S., Piras, B., Guerriero, S., Marongiu, D., Melis, G.B. Prevention of de-novo adhesion formation after laparoscopic myomectomy: a randomized trial to evaluate the effectiveness of an oxidized regenerated cellulose absorbable barrier. Hum. Reprod. 1995;10(b): 3133–3135.

[61] Saravelos, H., Li, T.C. Post-operative adhesions after laparoscopic electrosurgical treatment for polycystic ovarian syndrome with the application of Interceed to one ovary: a prospective randomized controlled study. Hum. Reprod. 1996;11: 992–997.

[62] Wallwiener, D., Meyer, A., Bastert, G. Adhesion formation of the parietal and visceral peritoneum: an explanation for the controversy on the use of autologous and alloplastic barriers? Fertil. Steril. 1998;69: 132–137.

[63] Azziz, R. Microsurgery alone or with INTERCEED Absorbable Adhesion Barrier for pelvic sidewall adhesion re-formation. The INTERCEED (TC7) Adhesion Barrier Study Group II. Surg. Gynecol. Obstet. 1993;177: 135–139.

[64] Franklin, R.R. Reduction of ovarian adhesions by the use of Interceed. Ovarian Adhesion Study Group. Obstet. Gynecol. 1995;86: 335–340.

[65] Li, T.C., Cooke, I.D. The value of an absorbable adhesion barrier, Interceed, in the prevention of adhesion reformation following microsurgical adhesiolysis. Br. J. Obstet. Gynaecol. 1994;101: 335–339.

[66] Nordic APSG. The efficacy of Interceed(TC7)* for prevention of reformation of postoperative adhesions on ovaries, fallopian tubes, and fimbriae in microsurgical operations for fertility: a multicenter study. Nordic Adhesion Prevention Study Group. Fertil. Steril. 1995;63: 709–714.

[67] Sekiba, K. Use of Interceed(TC7) absorbable adhesion barrier to reduce postoperative adhesion reformation in infertility and endometriosis surgery. The Obstetrics and Gynecology Adhesion Prevention Committee. Obstet. Gynecol. 1992;79: 518–522.

[68] Van Geldorp, H. Interceed absorbable adhesion barrier reduces the formation of postsurgical adhesions after ovarian surgery. Fertil. Steril. 1994;273: 213–214.

[69] Johns, D.B., Keyport, G.M., Hoehler, F., diZerega, G.S. Reduction of postsurgical adhesions with Intergel adhesion prevention solution: a multicenter study of safety and efficacy after conservative gynecologic surgery. Fertil. Steril. 2001;76: 595–604.

[70] Larsson, B. Efficacy of Interceed in adhesion prevention in gynecologic surgery: a review of 13 clinical studies. J. Reprod. Med. 1996;41: 27–34.

[71] Beck, D.E. The role of Seprafilmbioresorbable membrane in adhesion prevention. Eur. J. Surg. Suppl. 1997;49: 55.

[72] Diamond, M.P.Reduction of adhesions after uterine myomectomy by Seprafilm membrane (HAL-F): a blinded, prospective, randomized, multicenter clinical study. Seprafilm Adhesion Study Group. Fertil. Steril. 1996;66: 904–910.

[73] Klingler, P.J., Floch, N.R., Seelig, M.H., Branton, S.A., Wolfe, J.T., Metzger, P.P. Seprafilm-induced peritoneal inflammation: a previously unknown complication. Report of a case. Dis. Colon Rectum 1999;42: 1639–1643.

[74] Lundorff, P., Donnez, J., Korell, M., Audebert, A.J., Block, K., diZerega, G.S. Clinical evaluation of a viscoelastic gel for reduction of adhesions following gynaecological surgery by laparoscopy in Europe. Hum. Reprod. 2005;20: 514–520.

[75] Thornton, M.H., Johns, D.B., Campeau, J.D., Hoehler, F., DiZerega, G.S. Clinical evaluation of 0.5% ferric hyaluronate adhesion prevention gel for the reduction of adhesions following peritoneal cavity surgery: open-label pilot study. Hum. Reprod. 1998;13: 1480–1485.

[76] Sutton, C., Minelli, L., Garcıa, E., et al.Use of icodextrin 4% solution in the reduction of adhesion formation after gynaecological surgery. Gynecol. Surg. 2005;2: 287–296.

[77] Burns, J.W., Skinner, K., Colt, J., et al. Prevention of tissue injury and postsurgical adhesions by precoating tissues with hyaluronic acid solutions. J. Surg. Res. 1995;59: 644–652.

[78] Diamond, M.P. Reduction of de novo postsurgical adhesions by intraoperative precoating with Sepracoat (HAL-C) solution: a prospective, randomized, blinded, placebo-controlled multicenter study. The Sepracoat Adhesion Study Group. Fertil. Steril. 1998;69: 1067–1074.

[79] Pellicano, M., Bramante, S., Cirillo, D., et al. Effectiveness of autocrosslinked hyaluronic acid gel after laparoscopic myomectomy in infertile patients: a prospective, randomized, controlled study. Fertil. Steril. 2003;80: 441–444.

[80] Pellicano, M., Guida, M., Bramante, S., et al: Reproductive outcome after autocrosslinked hyaluronic acid gel application in infertile patients who underwent laparoscopic myomectomy. Fertil. Steril. 2005;83: 498–500.

[81] Mais, V., Bracco, G.L., Litta, P., Gargiulo, T., Melis, G.B. Reduction of postoperative adhesions with an auto-crosslinkedhyaluronan gel in gynaecological laparoscopic surgery: a blinded, controlled, randomized, multicentre study. Hum. Reprod. 2006;21: 1248–1254.

[82] Belluco, C., Meggiolaro, F., Pressato, D., et al. Prevention of postsurgical adhesions with an autocrosslinkedhyaluronan derivative gel. J. Surg. Res. 2001;100: 217- 221.

[83] De Iaco, P.A., Stefanetti, M., Pressato, D., et al. A novel hyaluronan-based gel in laparoscopic adhesion prevention: preclinical evaluation in an animal model. Fertil. Steril. 1998;69: 318– 323.

[84] Acunzo, G., Guida, M., Pellicano, M., et al. Effectiveness of auto-cross-linked hyaluronic acid gel in the prevention of intrauterine adhesions after hysteroscopicadhesiolysis: a prospective, randomized, controlled study. Hum. Reprod. 2003;18: 1918–1921.

[85] Guida, M., Acunzo, G., Di SpiezioSardo, A., et al. Effectiveness of auto-crosslinked hyaluronic acid gel in the prevention of intrauterine adhesions after hysteroscopic surgery: a prospective, randomized, controlled study. Hum. Reprod. 2004;19:1461–1464.

[86] Liu, Y., Shu, X.Z., Prestwich, G.D. Reduced postoperative intra-abdominal adhesions using Carbylan-SX, a semisynthetic glycosaminoglycan hydrogel. Fertil. Steril. 2007;87: 940–948.

[87] Zong, X., Li, S., Chen, E., et al. Prevention of postsurgery- induced abdominal adhesions by electrospunbioabsorbablenanofibrouspoly(lactide-co-glycolide)-based membranes. Ann. Surg. 2004;240: 910–915.

[88] Avital, S., Bollinger, T.J., Wilkinson, J.D., Marchetti, F., Hellinger, M.D., Sands, L.R. Preventing intra-abdominal adhesions with polylactic acid film: an animal study. Dis. Colon Rectum 2005;48: 153–157.

[89] Mettler, L., Audebert, A., Lehmann-Willenbrock, E., Schive-Peterhansl, K., Jacobs, V.R. A randomized, prospective, controlled, multicenter clinical trial of a sprayable, site-specific adhesion barrier system in patients undergoing myomectomy. Fertil. Steril. 2004;82: 398–404.

[90] Young, P., Johns, A., Templeman, C., et al. Reduction of postoperative adhesions after laparoscopic gynecological surgery with Oxiplex/AP Gel: a pilot study. Fertil. Steril. 2005; 84: 1450–1456.

[91] diZerega, G.S., Verco, S.J., Young, P., et al. A randomized, controlled pilot study of the safety and efficacy of 4% icodextrin solution in the reduction of adhesions following laparoscopic gynaecological surgery. Hum. Reprod. 2002;17: 1031–1038.

[92] Evrard, V.A., De Bellis, A., Boeckx, W., Brosens, I.A. Peritoneal healing after fibrin glue application: a comparative study in a rat model. Hum. Reprod. 1996;11: 1877–1880.

[93] Krause, T.J., Zazanis, G.A., McKinnon, R.D. Prevention of postoperative adhesions with the chitin derivative N–O–carboxymethylchitosan. Wound Repair Regen. 1996;4: 53–57.

[94] Diamond, M.P., Luciano, A., Johns, D.A., Dunn, R., Young, P., Bieber, E. Reduction of postoperative adhesions by N, O-carboxymethylchitosan: a pilot study. Fertil. Steril. 2003;80: 631–636.

[95] Brown, C.B., Luciano, A.A., Martin, D., Peers, E., Scrimgeour, A., diZerega, G.S. Adept (icodextrin 4% solution) reduces adhesions after laparoscopic surgery for adhesiolysis: a double- blind, randomized, controlled study. Fertil. Steril. 2007;88: 1413–1426.

[96] Wiseman, D.M., Trout, J.R., Franklin, R.R., Diamond, M.P. Meta-analysis of the safety and efficacy of an adhesion barrier (Interceed TC7) in laparotomy. J. Reprod. Med. 1999;44: 325–331.

[97] Adhesion Study Group. Reduction of postoperative pelvic adhesions with intraperitoneal 32% dextran 70: a prospective, randomized clinical trial. Fertil. Steril. 1983;40: 612–619.

[98] Larsson, B., Lalos, O., Marsk, L., et al.Effect of intraperitoneal instillation of 32% dextran 70 on postoperative adhesion formation after tubal surgery. Acta Obstet. Gynecol. Scand. 1985;64: 437–441.

[99] Rosenberg, S.M., Board, J.A. High-molecular weight dextran in human infertility surgery. Am. J. Obstet. Gynecol. 1984;148: 380–385.

[100] Ricaurte, E., Hilgers, T.W. Safety of intraperitoneal 32% dextran 70 as an antiadhesion adjuvant. J. Reprod. Med. 1989;34: 535–539.

[101] Watson, A., Vandekerckhove, P., Lilford, R. Pharmacological adjuvants during infertility surgery: a systematic review of evidence derived from randomized controlled trials. Hum. Fertil. 1999; 2: 149–157.

[102] Oncel, M., Remzi, F.H., Senagore, A.J., Connor, J.T., Fazio, V.W. Application of Adcon-P or Seprafilm in consecutive laparotomies using a murine model. Am. J. Surg. 2004;187: 304–308.

[103] Verco, S.J., Peers, E.M., Brown, C.B., Rodgers, K.E., Roda, N., diZerega, G. Development of a novel glucose polymer solution (icodextrin) for adhesion prevention: preclinical studies. Hum. Reprod. 2000;15: 1764–1772.

[104] diZerega, G.S., Coad, J., Donnez, J. Clinical evaluation of endometriosis and differential response to surgical therapy with and without application of Oxiplex/AP* adhesion barrier gel. Fertil. Steril. 2007;87: 485–489.

[105] Pados G, Venetis CA, Almaloglou K, Tarlatzis BC. Prevention of intra-peritoneal adhesions in gynaecological surgery: theory and evidence. Reproductive BioMedicine Online. 2010;21: 290– 303.

[106] Menzies, D., Pascual, M.H., Walz, M.K., et al. Use of icodextrin 4% solution in the prevention of adhesion formation following general surgery: from the multicentre ARIEL Registry. Ann. R. Coll. Surg. Engl. 2006;88: 375–382.

Chapter 3

Anesthetic Management for Laparoscopic Cholecystectomy

Somchai Amornyotin

Additional information is available at the end of the chapter

1. Introduction

Laparoscopic surgery aims to minimize trauma of the interventional process but still achieve a satisfactory therapeutic result. It is commonly performed because of various advantages such as reduced postoperative pain, faster recovery and more rapid return to normal activities, shorter hospital stay, and reduced postoperative pulmonary complications. The operative technique requires inflating gas into the abdominal cavity to provide a surgical procedure. An intra-abdominal pressure (IAP) of 10-15 mmHg is used. Carbon dioxide (CO_2) is commonly used because it does not support combustion, is cleared more rapidly than other gases, and is highly soluble in blood. However, the disadvantage of CO_2 is that the absorption of CO_2 can cause hypercapnia and respiratory acidosis [1].

Laparoscopic cholecystectomy (LC) procedure offers several advantages such as a reduction in stress response, postoperative pain, postoperative wound infection rate, intraoperative bleeding, impairment of respiratory function and pulmonary complications, short recovery time, and cosmetic appearance [1,2]. LC reduces hospital stay but has no overall effect on postoperative mortality [3]. The risk factors for perioperative complications in patients undergoing LC can be estimated based on patient characteristics, clinical findings and the surgeon's experience [4]. The advantages should to be balanced with potential adverse effects caused by CO_2 pneumoperitoneum.

The physiological effects of intra-abdominal CO_2 insufflation combined with the variations in patient positioning can have a major impact on cardiorespiratory function. In addition, the sequential effects of anesthesia combine to produce a characteristic hemodynamic response. A thorough understanding of these physiological changes is fundamental for optimal anesthetic care. Several anesthetic techniques can be performed for LC. General anesthesia using balanced anesthetic technique including intravenous drugs, inhalation agents and muscle relaxants is usually used. Short acting drugs such as propofol, atracurirm, vecuronium, sevoflurane or desflurane represent the maintenance drugs of choice. Preprocedure assessment and preparation, appropriate monitoring and a high index of suspicion can result in early diagnosis and treatment of complications.

2. Pathophysiological effects during laparoscopic cholecystectomy

2.1. Physiological effects of pneumoperitoneum

Carbon dioxide was shown to be affected by raising the intra-abdominal pressure (IAP) above the venous pressure which prevents CO_2 resorption leading to hypercapnia. Hypercapnia activates the sympathetic nervous system leading to an increase in blood pressure, heart rate, arrhythmias and myocardial contractility as well as it also sensitizes myocardium to catecholamines [5]. Increased IAP may compress venous vessels causing an initial increase in preload, followed by a sustained decrease in preload.

2.2. Respiratory effects

The changes in pulmonary function during LC include reduction in lung volumes, decrease in pulmonary compliance, and increase in peak airway pressure [6]. Increased IAP shifts the diaphragm cephalad and reduces diaphragmatic excursion, resulting in early closure of smaller airways leading to intraoperative atelectasis with a decrease in functional residual capacity. Additionally, the upward displacement of diaphragm leads to preferential ventilation of nondependent parts of lung, which results in ventilation-perfusion (V/Q) mismatch with a higher degree of intrapulmonary shunting. Oxygenation is minimally affected with no significant change in alveolar arterial oxygen gradient [7]. Higher IAP reduces the thoracic compliance and may cause pneumothorax and pneumomediastinum due to the increased in alveolar pressures [6].

2.3. Cardiovascular effects

Hemodynamic changes include the alterations in arterial blood pressure, arrhythmias and cardiac arrest. These cardiovascular changes depend on the interaction of several factors including patient positioning, neurohumoral response and the patient factors such as cardiorespiratory status and intravascular volume. The principal responses are an increase in systemic vascular resistance, mean arterial blood pressure and myocardial filling pressures, with little change in heart rate [2]. CO_2 pneumoperitoneum is associated with increased preload and afterload in patients undergoing LC. It also decreased heart performance (fractional shortening), but does not affect cardiac output [8]. The patients with normal cardiovascular function are able to well tolerate these hemodynamic changes. At IAP levels greater than 15 mmHg, venous return decreases leading to decreased cardiac output and hypotension [9]. However, these changes are short lived and have no statistical significance at 10 minutes from the time that the patient undergoes pneumoperitoneum [10].

Bradyarrhythmias are attributed to vagal stimulation caused by insertion of the needle or the trocar, peritoneal stretch, stimulation of the fallopian tube during bipolar electrocauterization, or carbon dioxide embolization [11]. These may induce cardiovascular collapse during laparoscopy even in the healthy patients. Increased concentrations of CO_2 and catecholamines can create tachyarrhythmias. Paroxysmal tachycardia and hypertension, followed by ventricular fibrillation, have been reported [12].

2.4. Effects of other systems

Increases in IAP, cardiovascular responses to peritoneal insufflations, changes in patient position and alterations in CO_2 concentration can alter intracranial pressure (ICP) and cerebral perfusion. ICP shows a significant further increase. Cerebral blood flow has been shown to increase significantly during CO_2 insufflation.

Pneumoperitoneum reduces renal cortical and medullary blood flow with an associated reduction in glomerular filtration rate (GFR), urinary output and creatinine clearance [2]. The reduction of renal blood flow may be due to a direct pressure effect on renal cortical blood flow and renal vascular compression as well as an increase in antidiuretic hormone (ADH), aldosterone and renin. Pretreatment with an ADH antagonist improves urine output and urea excretion despite an unaltered GFR.

Increased in IAP reduces femoral venous blood flow. This is due to increased pressure on the inferior vena cava and iliac veins, which reduces venous blood flow in the lower extremetries. It also has been shown to reduce the portal blood flow, which may lead to transient elevation of liver enzymes.

The C-reactive protein and interleukin-6 levels are less elevated after laparoscopy compared to the open surgery, suggesting an attenuation of the surgical inflammatory response [13].

Patient positions can further compromise cardiac and respiratory functions, can increase the risk of regurgitation and can result in peripheral nerve injuries. Head-up position reduces venous return, cardiac output, cardiac index and mean arterial blood pressure as well as an increase in peripheral and pulmonary vascular resistance [5,14]. Head-down position increases volume and cardiac output back towards normal. Respiratory function is impaired because of the cephalad shifting of diaphragm is exaggerated. Intracranial pressure is increased.

3. Anesthetic management

3.1. Preoperative assessment

The general health status of each patient must be evaluated. History and physical examinations are generally sufficient techniques. The patients with cardiorespiratory diseases require additional investigation. To aid in assessment risk, the American Society of Anesthesiologists (ASA) has developed a classification system for patients, which categorizes individuals on a general health basis. In this preoperative assessment, there are no differences in a routine practice between the laparoscopy and the open surgery.

3.2. Patient monitoring

Appropriate patient selection with proper monitoring to detect and reduce complications must be used to ensure optimal anesthesia care during LC. Standard intraoperative monitoring including noninvasive blood pressure, electrocardiogram, pulse oximeter, airway pressure, end tidal carbon dioxide ($ETCO_2$), body temperature and peripheral nerve stimulation is routinely used. Invasive hemodynamic monitoring may be appropriate in the patients with hemodynamic unstable or those with compromised cardiopulmonary function [1].

$ETCO_2$ is most commonly used as a noninvasive indicator of $PaCO_2$ in evaluating the adequacy of ventilation. Careful consideration should be taken for the gradient between $PaCO_2$ and the tension of CO_2 in expired gas ($PECO_2$) because of V/Q mismatch. However, in the patients with compromised cardiopulmonary function, the gradient between $PaCO_2$ and $PECO_2$ increases to become unpredictable. Direct arterial blood gas analysis may be considered to detect hypercarbia. Generally, the airway pressure monitor is routinely used during intermittent positive pressure ventilation. The high airway pressure can help detection of excessive elevation in IAP.

3.3. Anesthetic techniques

Various anesthetic techniques can be performed for LC. However, general anesthesia with endotracheal intubation for controlled ventilation is the most common anesthetic technique. In short procedures and in certain patients, ventilation using supraglottic airway device can be used as an alternative. General anesthesia without endotracheal intubation can be used safely and effectively with a ProSeal laryngeal mask airway in non-obese patients [15]. The use of laryngeal mask airway results in less sore throat and provide smoother emergence with less post-extubation coughing compared with endotracheal intubation [16].

3.3.1. General anesthesia

General anesthesia using balanced anesthesia technique including inhalation agents, intravenous drugs and muscle relaxant drugs is usually used. The uses of rapid and short acting volatile anesthetics such as sevoflurane and desflurane as well as rapid and short acting intravenous drugs such as propofol, etomidate, remifentanil, fentanyl, atracurium, vecuronium and rocuronium are commonly used and have allowed anesthesiologists to more consistently achieve a recovery profile. Propofol is effective and safe even in children and elderly patients [17-21].

Ventilation should be adjusted to keep $ETCO_2$ of around 35 mmHg by adjusting the minute ventilation [1]. In patients with chronic obstructive pulmonary disease and in patients with a history of spontaneous pneumothorax or bullous emphysema, an increase in respiratory rate rather than tidal volume is preferable to avoid increased alveolar inflation and reduce the risk of pneumothorax [22].

Furthermore, the use of an auditory evoked potential or Bispectral index monitor to titrate the volatile anesthetics leads to a significant reduction in the anesthetic requirement, resulting in a shorter postanesthesia care stay and an improved quality of recovery from the patient's perspective [23].

Combination of local anesthetic wound infiltration, intraperitoneum spray of local anesthetic, paracetamol and non-steroidal anti-inflammatory drugs or cyclooxygenase 2 inhibitors provides the most effective pain relief, which can be supplemented with small doses of opioids.

3.3.2. Regional anesthesia

Several advantages of regional anesthesia technique are quicker recovery, decreased postoperative nausea and vomiting, fewer hemodynamic changes, less postoperative pain, shorter hospital stay, early diagnosis of complications, improved patient satisfaction and cost effectiveness [24]. This anesthetic technique requires a cooperative patient, low IAP to reduce pain and ventilation disturbances, gentle surgical technique and a supportive operating room staff. However, regional anesthesia technique is not commonly used for LC. This technique should be performed in combination with other anesthetic techniques. Local anesthetic infiltration at the trocar site combined with general anesthesia significantly reduces postoperative pain and decreases medication usage costs [25]. Additionally, subcostal transversusabdominis block provides superior postoperative analgesia, improves theater efficiency by reducing time to discharge from the recovery unit and reduces opioid requirement following LC [26]. Bilateral paravertebral blockade at T5-6 level combined with general anesthesia can be used for LC [27].

Mehta and college had been conducted a prospective, randomized, controlled trial to compare spinal anesthesia with the gold standard general anesthesia for elective LC in the healthy patients. Their study demonstrated that spinal anesthesia was adequate and safe for LC in otherwise healthy patients and offered better postoperative pain control than general anesthesia without limiting the recovery [28]. The interim analysis of a controlled randomized trial is also confirmed [29]. Thoracic epidural anesthesia with 0.75% ropivacaine and fentanyl for elective LC is also efficacious and has preserved ventilation and hemodynamic changes within physiological limits during pneumoperitoneum with minimal treatable side effects [30]. In addition, epidural anesthesia might be applicable for LC. However, the incidence rate of intraoperative referred pain is high, and so careful patient recruitment and management of shoulder pain should be considered [31].

4. Intraoperative complications

Misplacement of the needle can lead to intravascular, subcutaneous tissue, preperitoneal space, bowel, and omentum. Inadvertent insufflation of gas into intravascular vessels, tear of abdominal wall or peritoneal vessels, can produce to gas embolism. Although, it is rare but it is a potentially lethal complication and can result in severe hypotension, cyanosis, arrhythmias and asystole. Subcutaneous emphysema may occur after direct subcutaneous gas insufflations. The majority of subcutaneous emphysema has no specific intervention. It can resolve soon after the abdomen is deflated and nitrous oxide is discontinued to ovoid expansion of closed space.

Pneumothorax can occur when the airway pressure is high. The gas traverses into the thorax through the tear of visceral peritoneum, parietal pleura during dissection, or spontaneous rupture of pre-existing emphysematous bulla [1]. Pneumothorax can be asymptomatic or can increase the peak airway pressure, decrease oxygen saturation, hypotension, and even cardiac arrest in severe cases. The treatment is according to the severity of cardiopulmonary compromise [32].

Extension of subcutaneous emphysema into thorax and mediastinum can lead to pneumomediastinum. Pneumopericardium can occur when the gas is forced through the inferior vena cava into the mediastinum and pericardium. Their managements depend on the severity of the cardiovascular dysfunction.

The other complications can be presented. Accidental insertion of the trocar or needle into the major or minor vessels, gastrointestinal tract injuries and urinary tract injuries can occur [32].

5. Postoperative period

The efficacy of post-anesthesia care units is therefore important to facilitate return to normal functions. In the early postoperative period, respiratory rate and $ETC0_2$ of laparoscopic patients breathing spontaneously are higher as compared with open surgery. So, the ventilation requirement is increased. The patients with respiratory dysfunction can have problems excreting excessive CO_2 load, which results in more hypercapnia. Additionally, the patients with cardiovascular diseases are more prone to hemodynamic changes and instabilities.

Although LC results in less discomfort compared with the open surgery, postoperative pain still can be considerable. Several medications used intraoperatively for prevention and treatment of postoperative pain are the uses of local anesthesia, opioids, nonsteroidal anti-inflammatory drugs, and multimodal analgesia techniques. Additionally, preprocedure administration of parecoxib is clinically effective [33].

Postoperative nausea and vomiting (PONV) is a common and distressing symptom following LC. The use of multimodal analgesia regimens and the reduction of opioid doses are likely to reduce the incidence of PONV. Propofol-based anesthesia has been associated with reduced PONV [34]. Ondansetron has been found to provide effective prophylaxis against PONV [35]. Administration of ondansetron at the end of surgery produces a significantly greater anti-emetic effect compared to pre-induction dosing. Reduced preoperative anxiety by providing more information should also relieve postoperative adverse effects in order to promote faster and better postoperative recovery period.

6. Summary

Laparoscopic cholecystectomy has proven to be a major advance in the treatment of patients with symptomatic gall bladder diseases. Several advantages from this procedure are minimal tissue trauma, reduction of postoperative pain, quicker recovery, shortening the hospital stay. Pneumoperitoneum induces intraoperative cardiorespiratory changes. Arterial CO_2 increases because of CO_2 absorption from the pneumoperitoneum. Improved knowledge of pathophysiological changes in the patients allows for successful anesthetic management. Proper patient selection and preparation as well as adequate monitoring should be performed. General anesthesia and controlled ventilation comprise the accepted anesthetic technique. Balanced anesthesia technique including inhalation agent, intravenous drug and muscle relaxant is commonly used. Intraoperative complications may arise due to physiologic changes associated with patient positioning and pneumoperitoneum. Multimodal analgesic regimen combining opioids, non-steroidal anti-inflammatory drugs, and local anesthetic infiltration is the most effective regimen for postoperative pain management.

Author details

Somchai Amornyotin

Department of Anesthesiology and Siriraj GI Endoscopy Center, Faculty of Medicine, Siriraj Hospital, Mahidol University, Bangkok, Thailand

References

[1] Gerges FJ, Kanazi GE, Jabbour-Khoury SI. (2006). Anesthesia for laparoscopy: a review. Journal of Clinical Anesthesia 2001; 18(1): 67-78.

[2] Leonard IE, Cunningham AJ. Anesthetic consideration for laparoscopic cholecystectomy. Best Practice & Research Clinical Anesthesiology 2002; 16(1): 1-20.

[3] McMahon AJ, Fischbacher CM, Frame SH, MacLeod MC. Impact of laparoscopic cholecystectomy: a population-based study. Lancet 2000; 356(11): 1632-1637.

[4] Giger UF, Michel JM, Opitz I, et al. Risk factors for perioperative complications in patients undergoing laparoscopic cholecystectomy: analysis of 22,953 consecutive cases from the Swiss Association of laparoscopic and thoracoscopic surgery database. Journal of American College of Surgeons 2006; 203(5): 723-728.

[5] Gutt CN, Oniu T, Mehrabi A, et al. Circulatory and respiratory complications of carbon dioxide insufflations. Digestive Surgery 2004; 21(2): 95-105.

[6] Rauh R, Hemmerling TM, Rist M, Jacobi KE. Influence of pneumoperitoneum and patient positioning on respiratory system compliance. Journal of Clinical Anesthesia 2001; 13(5): 361-365.

[7] Sharma KC, Brandstetter RD, Brensilver JM, Jung LD. Cardiopulmonary physiology and pathophysiology as a consequence of laparoscopic surgery. Chest 1996; 110(3): 810-815.

[8] Larsen JF, Svendsen FM, Pedersen V. Randomized clinical trial of the effect of pneumoperitoneum on cardiac function and hemodynamics during laparoscopic cholecystectomy. British Journal of Surgery 2004; 91(7): 848-854.

[9] Odeberg S, Ljungqvist O, Svenberg T, et al. Hemodynamic effects of pneumoperitoneum and the influence of posture during anesthesia for laparoscopic surgery. ActaAnaesthesiologicaScandinavica 1994; 38(3): 276-283.

[10] Zuckerman RS, Heneghan S. The duration of hemodynamic depression during laparoscopic cholecystectomy. Surgical Endoscopy 2002; 16(8): 1233-1236.

[11] Sprung J. Abdelmalak B, Schoenwald PK. Recurrent complete heart block in a healthy patient during laparoscopic electrocauterization of the fallopian tube. Anesthesiology 1998; 88(5): 1401-1403.

[12] Cheong MA, Kim YC, Park HK, et al. Paroxysmal tachycardia and hypertension with or without ventricular fibrillation during laparoscopic adrenalectomy: two case reports in patients with noncatecholamine-secreting adrenocortical adenomas. Journal of Laparoendoscopic& Advanced Surgical Techniques A 1999; 9(3): 277- 281.

[13] Grabowski JE, Talamini MA. Physiological effects of pneumoperitoneum. Journal of Gastrointestinal Surgery 2009; 13(5): 1009-1016.

[14] Hirvonen EA, Poikolainen EO, Paakkonen ME, Nuutinen LS. The adverse hemodynamic effects of anesthesia, head-up tilt, and carbon dioxide pneumoperitoneum during laparoscopic cholecystectomy. Surgical Endoscopy 2000; 14(3): 272-277.

[15] Maltby JR, Beriault MT, Watson NC, Liepert D, Fick GH. The LMA-ProSeal is an effective alternative to tracheal intubation for laparoscopic cholecystectomy. Canadian Journal of Anesthesia, 2002; 49(8): 857-862

[16] Cook TM, Lee G, Nolan JP. The ProSeal laryngeal mask airway: a review of the literature. Canadian Journal of Anesthesia 2005; 52(7): 739-760.

[17] Amornyotin S. Chalayonnavin W, Kongphlay S. Assisted sedation for percutaneous endoscopic gastrostomy in sick patients in a developing country. Gastroenterology Insights 2010; 2(e5): 17-20.

[18] Amornyotin S. Prakanrattana U, Chalayonnavin W, Kongphlay S, Kachintorn U. (2010). Propofol based sedation does not increase perforation rate during colonoscopic procedure. Gastroenterology Insights 2010; 2(e4): 13-16.

[19] Amornyotin S. Chalayonnawin W, Kongphlay S. Propofol-based sedation does not increase rate of complication during percutaneous endosopic gastrostomy procedure. Gastroenterology Research and Practice 2011 Article ID 134819; 6 pages, doi: 10.1155/2011/134819.

[20] Amornyotin S, Srikureja W, Pausawasdi N, Prakanrattana U, Kachintorn U. Intravenous sedation for gastrointestinal endoscopy in very elderly patients of Thailand. Asian Biomedicine 2011; 5(4): 485-491.

[21] Amornyotin S. Kachintorn U, Chalayonnawin W, Kongphlay S. Propofol-based deep sedation for endoscopic retrograde cholangiopancreatography procedure in sick elderly patients in a developing country. Therapeutics and Clinical Risk Management 2011; 7: 251-255.

[22] Salihoglu Z, Demiroluk S, Dikmen Y. Respiratory mechanics in morbid obese patients with chronic obstructive pulmonary disease and hypertension during pneumoperitoneum. European Journal of Anaesthesiology 2003; 20(8): 658-661.

[23] Recart A, Gasanova I, White PF, et al. (2003). The effect of cerebral monitoring on recovery after general anesthesia: a comparison of the auditory evoked potential and Bispectral index devices with standard clinical practice. Anesthesia Analgesia 2003; 97(6): 1667-1674.

[24] Collins LM, Vaghadia H. Regional anesthesia for laparoscopy. Anesthesiology Clinic of North America 2001; 19(1): 43-55.

[25] Hasaniya NW, Zayed FF, Faiz H, Severino R. Preinsertion local anesthesia at the trocar site improves perioperative pain and decreases costs of laparoscopic cholecystectomy. Surgical Endoscopy 2001; 15(9): 962-964.

[26] Tolchard S, Davies R, Martindale S. Efficacy of the subcostal transversusabdominis plane block in laparoscopic cholecystectomy: comparison with conventional port-site infiltration. Journal of Anaesthesiology Clinical Pharmacology 2012; 28(3): 339-343.

[27] Naja MZ, Ziade MF, Lonnqvist PA. General anesthesia combined with bilateral paravertebral blockade (T5-6) vs. general anesthesia for laparoscopic cholecystectomy: a prospective, randomized clinical trial. European Journal of Anaesthesiology 2004; 21(6): 489-495.

[28] Mehta PJ, Chavda HR, Wadhwana AP, Porecha MM. Comparative analysis of spinal versus general anesthesia for laparoscopic cholecystectomy: a controlled, prospective, randomized trial. Anesthesia: Essays and Researches 2010; 4(2): 91-95.

[29] Tzovaras G, Fafoulakis F, Pratsas K, et al. Spinal vs general anesthesia for laparoscopic cholecystectomy: an interim analysis of a controlled randomized trial. Archives of Surgery 2008; 143(5): 497-501.

[30] Gupta A, Gupta K, Gupta PK, Agarwal N, Rastogi B. Efficacy of thoracic epidural anesthesia for laparoscopic cholecystectomy. Anesthesia: Essays and Researches 2011; 5(2): 138-141.

[31] Lee JH, Huh J, Kim DK, et al. Laparoscopic cholecystectomy under epidural anesthesia: a clinical feasibility study. Korean Journal of Anesthesiology 2010; 59(6): 383-388.

[32] Joshi GP. Complications of laparoscopy. Anesthesiology Clinic of North America 2001; 19(1): 89-105.[33]

[33] Amornyotin S, Chalayonnawin W, Kongphlay S. A randomized controlled trial of preprocedure administration of parecoxib for therapeutic endoscopic retrograde cholangiopancreatography. Journal of Pain Research 2012; 5: 251-256.

[34] Fujii Y. Management of postoperative nausea and vomiting in patients undergoing laparoscopic cholecystectomy. Surgical Endoscopy 2011; 25(3): 691-695.

[35] Wu SJ, Xiong XZ, Cheng TY, Lin YX, Cheng NS. Efficacy of ondansetronvs metoclopramide in prophylaxis of postoperative nausea and vomiting after laparoscopic cholecystectomy: a systematic review and meta-analysis. Hepatogastroenterology 2012; 59(119), Doi: 10.5754/hge11811 [Epub ahead of print]

Chapter 4

Cleaning, Disinfection and Sterilization of Heat-Sensitive Endoscopes

Norman Miner

Additional information is available at the end of the chapter

1. Introduction

High level disinfection is a process that kills high numbers of all types of vegetative non-spore forming bacteria (Gram-positive and Gram-negative), fungi, all types of viruses (hydrophylic and lipophylic), and mycobacteria (TB), but not necessarily high numbers of bacterial spores in the relatively brief exposure time for disinfection. Sterilization is a process that kills all types of microbes including highly resistant bacterial spores. Sterilization usually requires a much longer exposure time than disinfection. Gastroscopes, colonoscopes, urethroscopes, and cystoscopes normally do not break the barrier between non-sterile areas of the body and sterile areas, and therefore high level disinfection is the commonly accepted practice for these endoscopes. Bronchoscopes are a possible exception as they may enter into the sterile bronchioles, although they make that entrance through the non-sterile nasal passages where they likely become contaminated with the flora of the oral-nasal body cavities. Endoscopists, and certainly patients, all agree that endoscopes and their accessories such as biopsy forceps should be thoroughly cleaned of all body fluids and any possible microbes between patients, even if not technically sterilized.

2. Methods

Unless endoscopes can be completely dried after disinfection, creating an environment where microbes cannot survive or multiply, or there is laboratory culturing evidence that endoscopes still contain very few or no microbes, they should be disinfected and rinsed again in the morning before first use. Any microbes that might remain in the endoscopes after disinfection, or be introduced into the endoscopes by means of non-sterile rinse water, could multiply overnight or over a weekend or holiday to unsafe numbers, or begin to form a biofilm within the channels of the endoscope. Certain microbes such as Staphylococcus aureus, Pseudomonas aeruginosa, or Escherichia coli can divide every 60 minutes or faster in dark, moist, and warm conditions. Just 10 or 20 microbes remaining in an endoscope at 4:00 PM can multiply to about one million colony forming units by the time of the 1st case at about 8:00 AM the next day, and many more if the starting number is higher than "just 10 or 20" if there is enough substrate to sustain a population that size. The hospital laboratory or a contract laboratory/microbiologist can be a valuable ally to know by testing how many microbes are in the channels of an endoscope after a cleaning/disinfecting procedure, or after a storage interval. It takes only a few minutes for a microbiologist to flush recovery solutions through an endoscope, and then assay those fluids to validate the numbers, if any, of microbes within the channels of an endoscope. At intervals of about three or four months, or after newly trained personnel begin to process and disinfect endoscopes, or the disinfecting procedure is modified, a sampling of the endoscopes should be cultured to validate that the endoscopes are indeed disinfected, and any numbers of bacteria in the endoscopes are very low. B.T. Petersen, et. al. is another publication regarding methods for reprocessing flexible endoscopes [1].

3. Cleaning endoscopes

The initial cleaning step happens in the Procedure Room when the insertion tube is removed from the patient and wiped with a gauze pad saturated with a disinfectant, and the internal air, suction, and water channels are flushed with water. This initial cleaning step removes much of the organic soil and probably removes and kills at least 99% of any microbes on the endoscope. The endoscope is then transported in a plastic bin to the reprocessing room and tested for possible leaks. The control valves are removed, and the endoscope and all parts (valves) are submerged in a deep stainless steel sink (or plastic basin) with about two or three gallons of warm tap water with a disinfectant-detergent solution. The endoscope should be cleaned within about 30.0 min of leaving the procedure room, and not allowed to dry. Organic soil and microbes are much more difficult to remove and to kill after they become dry than when they are wet. A disinfectant-detergent cleaning solution is a concentrate of a low-foaming surfactant (detergent) and disinfectant. These disinfectant-detergent cleaning solutions are concentrates intended and labeled to be diluted in the range of 1:16 to 1:32. The label will give the exact dilution to be used, and also identify that the solution will kill Gram-positive and Gram-negative bacteria, fungi, and hydrophylic and lipophylic viruses, (and possibly even mycobacteria and some spores or spore-forming bacteria, depending on the particular disinfectant-detergent chosen). Labels that use the scientific names of microbes can be difficult for non-microbiologists to understand. The hospital laboratory, or any microbiologist, can help to translate the label into common terms such as Gram positive or Gram negative bacteria, fungi, and viruses. The disassembled valves should be flexed and lightly brushed with the disinfectant-detergent cleaning solution (cleaning solution), the exterior of the endoscope should be wiped with a soft cloth saturated with the cleaning solution, and the biopsy or working channel of the endoscope should be filled with the cleaning solution and brushed the entire length several times with a tight-fitting brush. Insert the brush into the channel until the brush emerges from the channel. Brush the channel repeatedly about three or four times. Allow the brush to emerge from the channels submerged within the cleaning solution to avoid a splattering of microbes in the air. The air-water channel is too small to brush, and care should be taken to ensure that this small channel is not blocked and is filled with the cleaning solution. This wiping and brushing of all parts of the endoscope with the cleaning solution should continue for about 5.0 min which allows the disinfectant to kill many of any contaminating microbes. This cleaning procedure is completed by triple-rinsing all parts and sections of the endoscope with fresh warm tap water. Some cleaning solutions contain enzymes, and enzymes are not antimicrobial, and are not compatible with disinfectants. Enzymes require at least body temperature (35 °C) and many minutes to function. Enzymes are proteins, and it is proteins such as blood and tissues that are being removed from the endoscopes. For those reasons, especially the fact that enzyme-detergent combinations are not antimicrobial, and are not compatible with disinfectants, these enzyme-detergent combinations are not recommended by this author for cleaning endoscopes. Enzyme products are useful as a soak to dissolve clogged air/water channels that are too narrow to be brushed. The purpose of using a disinfectant-detergent cleaning solution during this cleaning stage is to remove organic soil (blood, mucous, fecal matter), and lower the number of microbes on the endoscope in advance of the final stage of disinfecting or sterilizing, and to protect the technician and the environment from a splattering of wash water containing potentially infectious microbes.

4. High level disinfection of the endoscope

After the endoscope and all of its parts have been cleaned as described above in a disinfectant-detergent cleaning solution, and thoroughly triple-rinsed with tap water to remove the disinfectant-detergent, the rinsed endoscope should then be soaked in a high level disinfectant at the labeled exposure time and temperature for any particular high level disinfectant. A high level disinfectant is a disinfectant that is labeled to kill all Gram-Positive and Gram-Negative vegetative bacteria, all fungi, all mycobacteria (TB), and all types of viruses, hydrophylic and lipophylic, within the labeled exposure time and temperature. High level disinfectants are also able to kill bacterial spores and spore-forming bacteria, although it takes a longer time to kill high numbers of bacterial spores than to kill vegetative microbes. After the initial disinfection and rinse in the procedure room, and the procedure of cleaning the endoscope with the disinfectant-detergent cleaning solution, the number of spore-forming bacteria on the endoscope should be very low, and thus this disinfecting procedure will also remove and kill many bacterial spores.

5. Sterilization of an endoscope

The procedure to sterilize an endoscope contains all the steps for cleaning and high level disinfection of an endoscope as described above, but the exposure time for sterilization is longer than for disinfection in order to kill spores and spore-forming bacteria [2]. The label of the high level disinfectant will identify the sterilization soak time, which can be many hours. Also, the final rinse should be with sterilized water rather than ordinary tap water. Air should be forced through the internal channels with a syringe to dry them, and the endoscope should be stored in some sterile manner such as covering the endoscope with a sterile wrap or cloth. Hang the endoscope so it can further drip dry.

6. Protective clothing

Although care is taken to not splash contaminated water from an endoscope during reprocessing, there will be some splash and splatter as brushes emerge from the internal channels, and otherwise. Personnel should wear a plastic face shield covering the eyes, nose, and mouth; hair covering; elbow-length rubber gloves; and long-sleeved, waterproof gowns or coats.

7. Examples of disinfectant-detergent cleaning solutions

A disinfectant-detergent cleaning solution will be a concentrate intended to be diluted with tap water, usually 16- or 32-fold. The detergent should be anionic or non-ionic, low foaming, and easily rinsed from the endoscope. Use the lowest concentration (highest dilution) recommended to facilitate rinsing and removal of the disinfectant-detergent solution. There are dozens of these disinfectant-detergents listed on the US Environmental Protection Agency (EPA) web site. Local Sales Representatives will also be able to provide written descriptions and access to disinfectant-detergent concentrates. They contain modified phenolic chemicals (phenylphenol, amylphenol, etc); quaternary ammonium chemicals (dimethyl benzyl ammonium chloride); sodium hypochlorite/bleach; iso- or ethyl alcohol; or other common disinfectants. These disinfectant-detergents are being used in the cleaning stage to clean organic material from the endoscopes by way of the detergent, to lower the bioburden of microbes on the endoscope by way of the disinfectant, and to provide some respite to the environment and to the operator from the microbes inevitably splashed with the cleaning water. Several endoscopes can be cleaned in a basin filled with the diluted disinfectant-detergent at one time. Discard/drain the disinfectant-detergent cleaning solution after each endoscope cleaning procedure. The basin could be repeatedly drained and filled with tap water to triple rinse the endoscopes, or additional basins could be used for rinse water.

8. Examples of high level disinfectants

High level disinfectants are able to kill high numbers of all vegetative bacteria, fungi, viruses, and mycobacteria within a relatively brief exposure time such as about 10.0 min to

20.0 min at temperatures of about 20 °C to about 25 °C. The label of the high level disinfectant will have an exposure time and temperature. However, if the cleaning procedure used a disinfectant-detergent which would have killed large numbers of microbes, the high level disinfectant exposure time can be shortened to 20.0 min. With a longer exposure time such as hours, a high level disinfectant can also kill highly resistant forms of bacterial spores. Alkaline glutaraldehyde solutions (Cidex Solution), solutions of glutaraldehyde enhanced with isopropanol (Aldahol High Level Disinfectant), and peracetic acid solutions are high level disinfectants. The sterilization time for Ortho-Phthalaldehyde (OPA) is 32 hours, which is not practical, and OPA is not labelled as a sterilant. Alkaline glutaraldehyde solutions with and without isopropanol, and peracetic acid solutions are highly soluble in water, and thus are easily rinsed from endoscopes. OPA has a low solubility in water, and is difficult to rinse away from endoscopes with any practical number of rinses [3]. Trade names of some high level disinfectants are Cidex Activated Dialdehyde Solution, Aldahol High Level Disinfectant [4], Rapicide High Level Disinfectant, Resert XL HLD, and Acecide High Level Disinfectant.

9. Automatic endoscope reprocessing machines

Automatic endoscope reprocessing (AER) machines are available. Some of these AER machines also claim to be able to clean the endoscopes as well as to disinfect them. The cleaning action of the cleaning solution for these AER machines is by force rather than by brush, and this author is skeptical that such forceful rinsing is able to clean the channels of endoscopes as well as a brush. If an AER machine is used, the endoscope should be manually brushed before it is placed into the machine. Duodenoscopes have an elevator wire channel that must be manually cleaned regardless of a final clean in a machine.

10. Protection from irritating disinfectant vapors

Glutaraldehyde solutions, glutaraldehyde-isopropanol solutions, and peracetic acid solutions all have irritating and sensitizing chemical vapors. These solutions should be contained and used in a manner to protect workers from the irritating and sensitizing chemical vapors. This can be done by soaking the cleaned endoscope in a covered container of the disinfectant, and/or working in a hood that ventilates the chemical vapors through a filter to remove the vapors, or ventilates the vapors to outside air. If a hood is not available, a small fan can be positioned to blow the chemical vapors away from the operator. Any spilled high level disinfectant should be immediately cleaned up. Serious and effective efforts must be made to ventilate and eliminate and protect personnel from the vapors of glutaraldehyde, OPA, and peracetic acid.

11. Biofilms

The interior channels of endoscopes can be convoluted, and the air-water channel is too narrow to brush. Therefore it is possible over time for the channels of an endoscope to develop a film of microbes, called a biofilm. Endoscope channels that contain a biofilm cannot be disinfected [5]. Detection of a biofilm is one reason why endoscopes should be periodically cultured. Biofilms can be removed by soaking the endoscope and all of its channels in an enzyme detergent for a prolonged period of time such as one or two hours, followed by vigorous brushing of the channels. After this prolonged soaking, brushing and rinsing procedure, the endoscope should again be cultured to determine that the biofilm has been removed. The hospital laboratory or a contract microbiologist can be the Endoscopists best friend, and the only way to know for certain that procedures lead to a disinfected endoscope is to culture the endoscope, at least periodically.

Author details

Norman Miner

MicroChem Laboratory, Inc.Euless, Texas, USA

References

[1] Petersen, B T, Chennat, J, Cohen, J, Cotton, P B, Greenwald, D A, et.al. Multisociety guideline on reprocessing flexible gastrointestinal endoscopes. Infect. Control and Hosp. Epidem. 2011, 33: pp 527 – 537.

[2] Miner N, Harris V, Ebron T, Cao T. Sporicidal activity of disinfectants as one possible cause for bacteria in patient-ready endoscopes. Gastroenterol Nurs.2009; 30: 285-90.

[3] Miner N, Harris V, Lukomski N, Ebron T. Rinsability of ortho-phthalaldehyde from endoscopes. Diagnost and TherapEndosc. 2012; 2012: Article 853781.

[4] Miner N, Harris V, Cao T D, Ebron T, and Lukomski N. Aldahol High Level Disinfectant. Amer J Infect Control. 2010; 38: No.3, 205 – 211.

[5] Pajkos A, Vickery K, Cossart Y. Is biofilm accumulation on endoscope tubing a contributor to the failure of cleaning and decontamination? J Hosp Infect. 2004; 58: 224 – 9.

Section 2

Head and Neck

Narrow Band Imaging (NBI) — Endoscopic Method for Detection of Head and Neck Cancer

Petr Lukes, Michal Zabrodsky, Jan Plzak,
Martin Chovanec, Jaroslav Betka, Eva Foltynova and
Jan Betka

Additional information is available at the end of the chapter

1. Introduction

The most common head and neck malignancy is squamous cell carcinoma (SCC). It is well recognized that these tumours may arise in multiple sites, either synchronously or metachronously [1]. The surgical and oncological treatment of large tumours leads to a significant mutilation of the affected individual. The results are not only cosmetic, but also functional defects, such as swallowing, chewing, breathing disorders and voice production deterioration. Early detection of these tumours is therefore one of the most important factors of treatment success [2].

Efforts to achieve the earliest detection of malignant disease have led to the development of new endoscopic examination methods. Lesions few millimetres in diameter are in most cases impossible to detect using conventional white light endoscopy. This led to the introduction of special endoscopic methods that allow detection of lesions of millimetre dimensions. New techniques such as autofluorescence [3], contact endoscopy and optical coherence tomography (OCT) [4] are increasingly used in ENT practice. In the last few years, NBI (Narrow Band Imaging) method has been introduced [5]. This diagnostic tool was already proved as a useful screening method in other endoscopic fields (e.g. gastroenterology) [6]. Superficial mucosal lesions that would be missed by regular white light endoscopy, can be identified, in view of their neoangiogenetic pattern of vasculature, using the narrow-band imaging in head and neck mucosa.

2. The principles of NBI endoscopy

The best case scenario for early detection of mucosal SCC would be at the stage of dysplasia or carcinoma in situ (CIS). These early lesions are difficult to detect in white light endoscopy, if they are less then 1 cm in diameter [7]. In the oesophagus, these lesions can be easily detected by Lugol chromoendoscopy, where squamous dysplasia and CIS appear as Lugol voiding lesions [8]. This is not suitable for ivestigation of upper aerodigestive tract due to severe mucosal irritation caused by Lugol solution [7]. Chromoendoscopy is able to show differences in epithelium quality. NBI shows differences in epithelium quality and changes of mucosal vascularization. NBI is an optical image enhancement technology that enhances vessels in the mucosal surface and patterns of the mucosa using the characteristics of light spectrum [6]. It is a non-invasive technique that can be carried out in the outpatient clinic without need of general anaesthesia. NBI system consists of the same components as conventional videoendoscopic systems - light source, camera unit and camera head or chip equipped videoendoscope. In addition, NBI system contains a special image processor and a lighting unit with special filters that narrow frequency range of emitted light to 400-430 nm (centered at 415 nm) and 525-555 nm (centered at 540 nm) bands. It relies on the principle of depth of light penetration. In contrast to red light, 415 nm wavelenght light has less penetration and less scattering thus enhancing image resolution. The blue filter is designed to correspond to the peak absorption spectrum of haemoglobin to enhance the image of capillary vessels (IPCL - Intraepithelial Papillary Capillary Loops) on mucosal surface. 540 nm wavelenght light penetrates deeper and highlights the submucosal vascular plexus. The reflection is captured by a charge coupled device chip (CCD), and an image processor creates a composite pseudo-colour image, which is displayed on a monitor, enabling NBI to enhance mucosal contrast without the use of dyes [9] (Figure 1). In the resulting image the mucosal microvascularization is displayed brown and submucosal vessels cyan (Figure 2). Vascular structures are displayed with greater contrast to the epithelium than in white light illumination [10]. In detection of surface mucosal changes characteristic for neoplastic lesions (e.g. dysplasia, ca in-situ, carcinoma) epithelial abnormalities (thickening, changes in the surface layer) and vascular changes can be better observed in NBI. In developing neoangiogenesis IPCL changes occur (expansion, extension and changes of course). These changed IPCL are noticeable in the NBI as brown dots irregularly distributed in the demarcated area of altered epithelium [6]. It is possible to detect lesions measuring a few millimetres in diameter.

3. The use of NBI endoscopy in ENT

Typical suspect finding in NBI image is defined as well demarcated brownish area, exhibiting scattered brown dots within this area on close view [11] (Figure 3). Brown dots are caused by expansion of IPCL, which is due to neoangiogenesis in tumour growth. The finding of brown dots, spread freely in the mucosa of e.g. post-irradiation oedema, without boundary line of altered epithelium, must be carefully distinguished. Such image can not be judged as suspect for neoplasia (Figure 4).

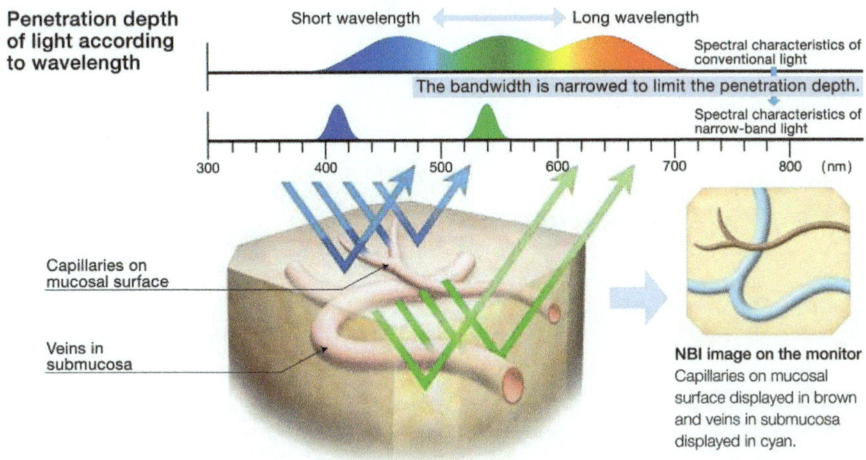

Figure 1. NBI principles (with permission of OLYMPUS CZECH GROUP).

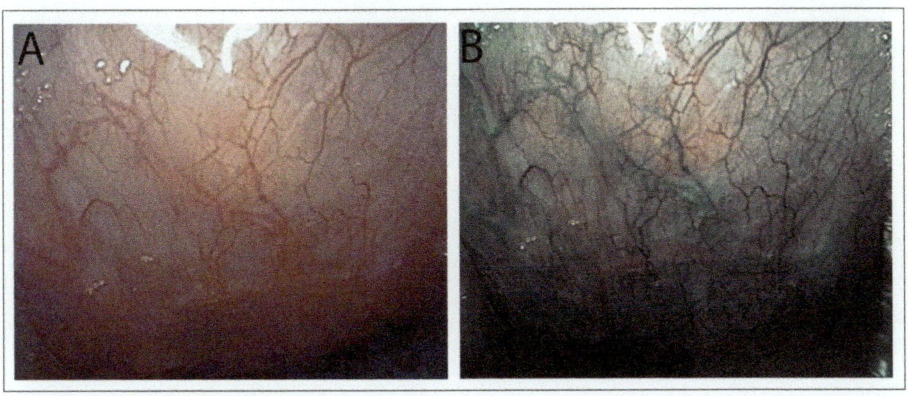

Figure 2. Healthy nasopharyngeal mucosa in white light (A) and NBI (B), mucosal blood vessels displayed in brown and submucosal vessels in cyan.

Recently, NBI was used for diagnosis of oral [12], oropharyngeal [13], hypopharyngeal [14], nasopharyngeal [15] and laryngeal [16] pathologies. NBI is used for screening and for follow-up after chemo- and/or radiotherapy treatment of head and neck SCC [17]. Some authors also used NBI intraoperatively to perform targeted biopsies of most suspect areas and also to determine the safe limits of resection margins [17] (Figure 5).

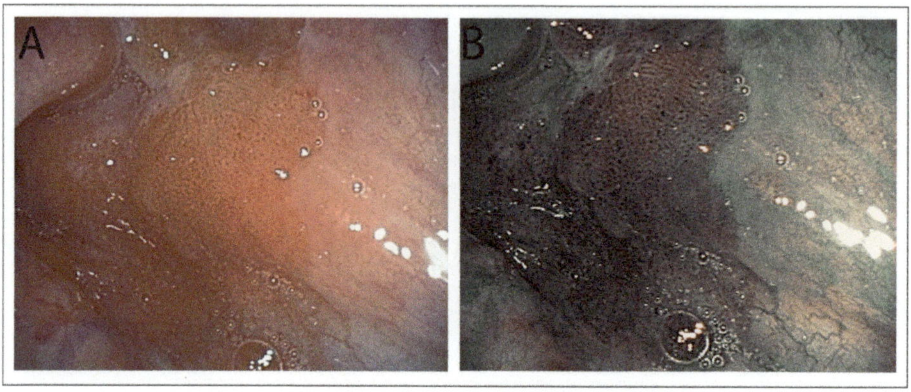

Figure 3. Mucosal spread of squamous cell carcinoma in vallecula in white light (A) and NBI (B). Clear boundary line between tumour and healthy mucosa and scattered brown dots are well visible in NBI.

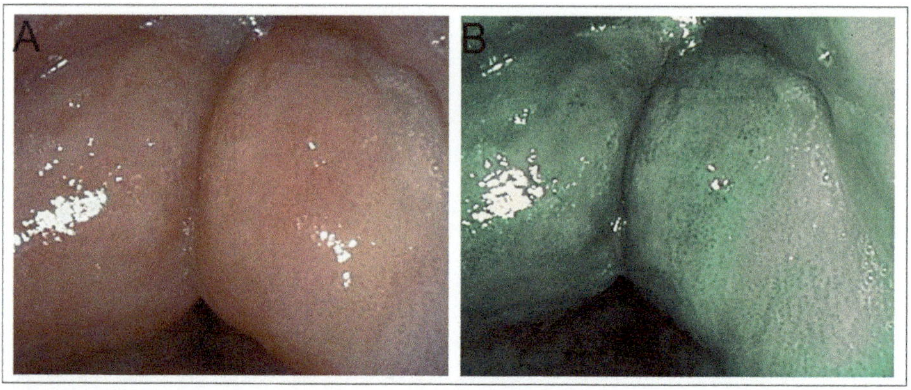

Figure 4. Post-radiotherapy mucosal oedema of the arythenoids in white light (A) and NBI (B). Non-suspect image of brown dots.

For NBI endoscopy both flexible and rigid videoendoscopic systems are used in ENT. For outpatient practice ultra-thin flexible videoendoscopes were developed with distal end diameter of 3-4 mm, and also ultra-thin bronchoscopes or gastroscopes with the diameter of the distal end of less than 5 mm are used. These scopes are suitable for transnasal insertion and therefore allow to examine the nasal sinuses, nasopharynx, oropharynx, hypopharynx, oesophagus, larynx, trachea and bronchi and provides better results than conventional transoral examination. Transnasal examination can be performed under local anaesthesia of the nasal mucosa and throat or without any anaesthesia [18]. Improved contrast between mucosal epithelium and blood vessels helps to visualize mucosal lesions few millimetres in

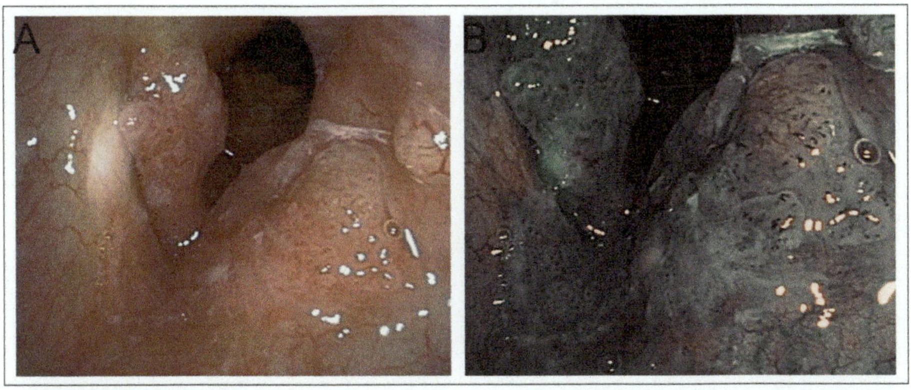

Figure 5. Bilateral carcinoma of the vocal folds in white-light (A) and NBI (B). Supraglottic spread of the cancer is clearly visible on NBI image.

diameter (Figure 6). The sensitivity and specificity of flexible NBI endoscopy in follow-up of head and neck SCC patients were reported 91,3 - 100% and 91,6 - 98% respectively [17,11].

Rigid telescopes are also used in the outpatient service during the examination of the nasal cavities, nasopharyngx, oropharynx and oral cavity. Rigid angled telescopes (0 º, 30 º and 70 º) yielded significant improvement in the diagnostic possibilities of direct laryngoscopy under general anaesthesia [19,20]. They allow a thorough examination of all areas of the larynx and even the front commissure and subglottic area. Sensitivity and specificity of NBI examination can be significantly increased in combination with high definition (HDTV) magnifying endoscopy [21].

4. Magnifying endoscopy and endoscopy with high-definition (HDTV)

Development of mucosal malignancies is accompanied by changes of IPCL in terms of their extension, expansion, irregularities of calibre, loss of regular arrangement and in the last stage of tumourigenesis complete loss of vascular microarchitecture [22]. Standard endoscopes, however, does not permit a more accurate display of these changes. They are displayed as irregularly dispersed brown dots in NBI endoscopy. Certain magnification and image resolution is needed to obtain better visibility of IPCL changes [9]. Recent development in endoscopic techniques has led to the introduction of so-called magnifying endoscopy, which, combined with high-definition television (HDTV) allows to display the vascular microarchitecture in vivo. Till now, malignant lesions were determined only on the basis of histological examination. Rigid magnifying telescopes, which allow observing the surface of the mucosa from a distance of few millimetres (e.g. combined with direct laryngoscopy) in combination with HDTV camera head, allow diagnosing the malignancy with high probability prior the conclusion of histology examination. Different classifications of IPCL changes were proposed

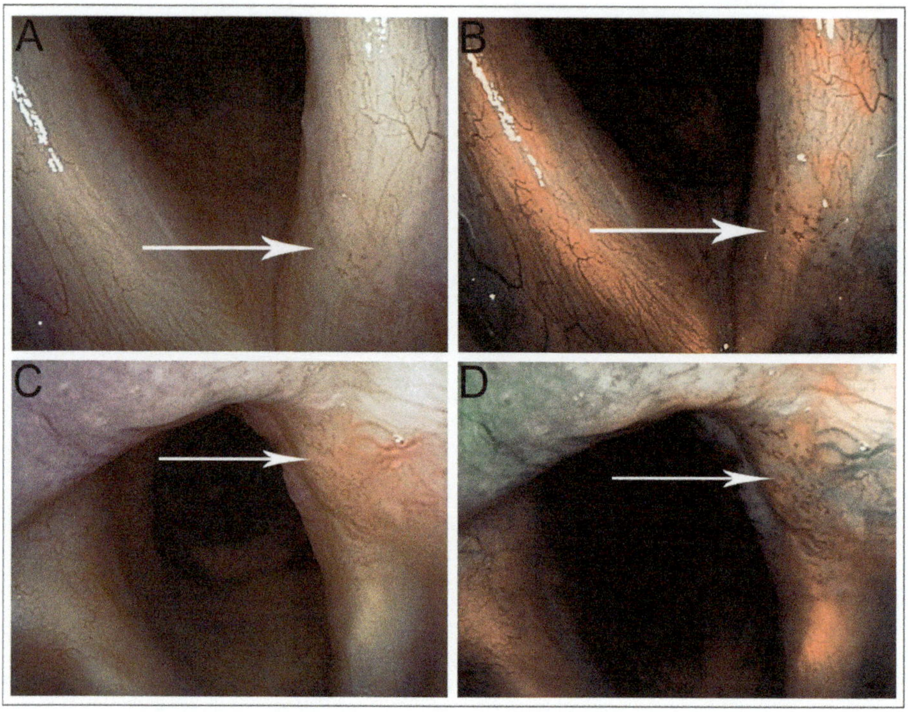

Figure 6. Larynx - the left vocal cord dysplasia in white light (A) and NBI (B), arrows point demarcated area of altered epithelium with the presence of brown dots. Another dysplastic lesion in the same patient in the posterior part of the vocal cord in white light (C) and NBI (D).

for oesophagus and pharynx [23], oral cavity [12] and larynx [16]. In oesophagus and pharynx the IPCL changes are graded as Type I (normal IPCL) to Type V (cancer IPCL). Type V is further subdivided into 4 sublevels. According to these levels, the depth of cancer invasion into the mucosa and submucosal tissue can be evaluated [23]. For oral cavity just Type I (normal IPCL) to Type IV (cancer IPCL) grades are proposed [12] (Figure 7, 8).

5. Limits of NBI endoscopy

In some cases even NBI endoscopy examination does not bring the expected results. Since NBI is an optical method based on observation of the mucosal surface, conditions that prevent a direct view of the clear mucous membrane may limit or completely baffle the examination. Most often this is due to stagnant saliva or sticky mucus, especially in patients with a history of oncology treatment. Also, lesions that are characterized by a high layer of hyperkeratosis prevent visualization of mucosal vascularization – eg. verrucous carcinomas [24].

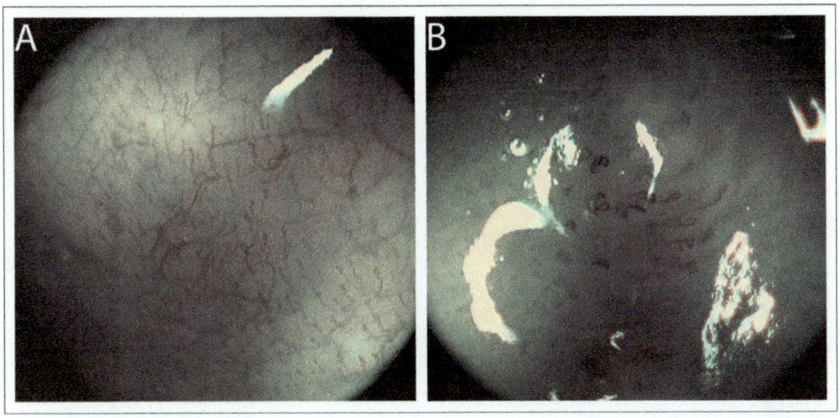

Figure 7. HDTV NBI magnifying endoscopy, the buccal mucosa. Normal (Type I) intraepithelial papillary capillary loops - IPCL (A), enlarged and irregular dysplastic IPCL (Type III) (B).

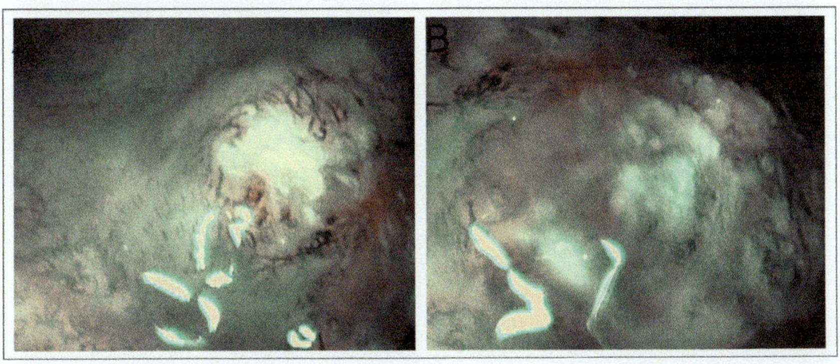

Figure 8. Advanced tumour of apex of tongue – HDTV NBI, complete collapse of IPCL microarchitecture (Type IV) is visible.

NBI endoscopy brings great results in case of clear observable mucosa. Benign findings such as vocal cord polyps, nodules or granulomas are clearly recognizable. Blood vessels run paralelly to the mucosal surface and do not form brown dots (Figure 9), in contrast to malignant changes that typically show presence of these dots.

Nevertheless, most false positive results of NBI endoscopy were reported in case of laryngeal papillomatosis [11]. In these cases, demarcated lesions with scattered brown dots are often found. The discrimination from cancerous lesions could be very difficult using non-magnifying NBI endoscopy (Figure 10).

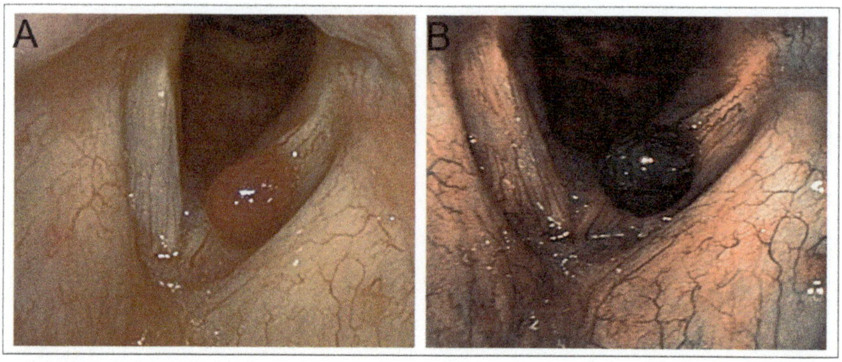

Figure 9. Benign polyp of vocal cord in white-light (A) and NBI (B). Blood vessels run paralelly to the mucosal surface. No brown dots are visible.

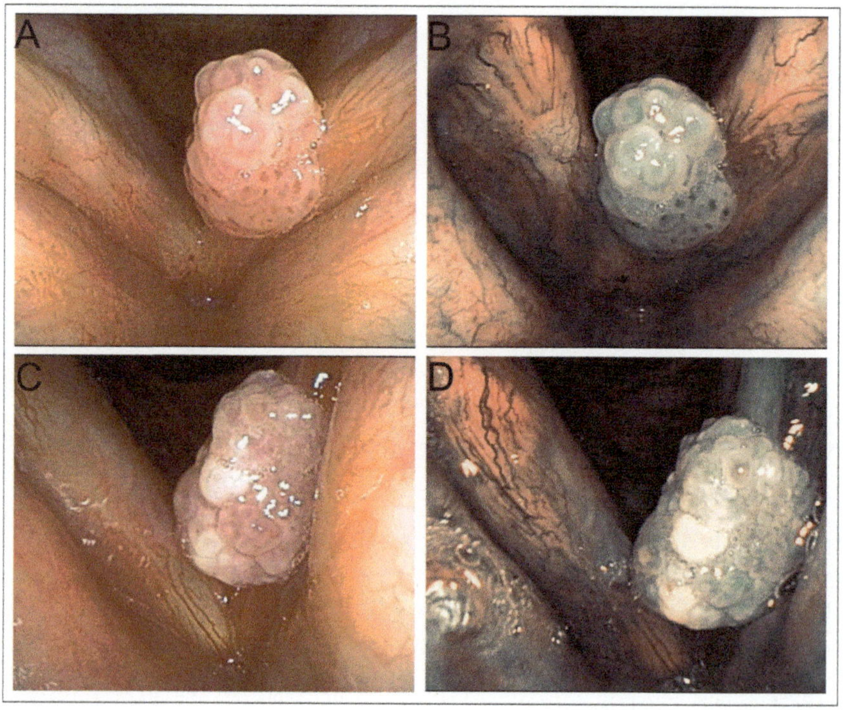

Figure 10. Laryngeal papilloma in white-light (A) and NBI (B). Verrucous cancer of the vocal fold in white-light (C) and NBI (D). Discrimination of these lesions can be very difficult

Utilization of HDTV NBI magnifying endoscopy can improve the diagnostic accuracy. The papillomas are characterised by forming multiple papillae covered by squamous epithelium with a central axis vessel in each papilla [25]. The microarchitecture of these lesions is often rather regular. On the other hand, the cancerous lesions are characterised by lost of regularity of IPCL shape and also by disruption of the microarchitecture regularity [26] (Figure 11, 12).

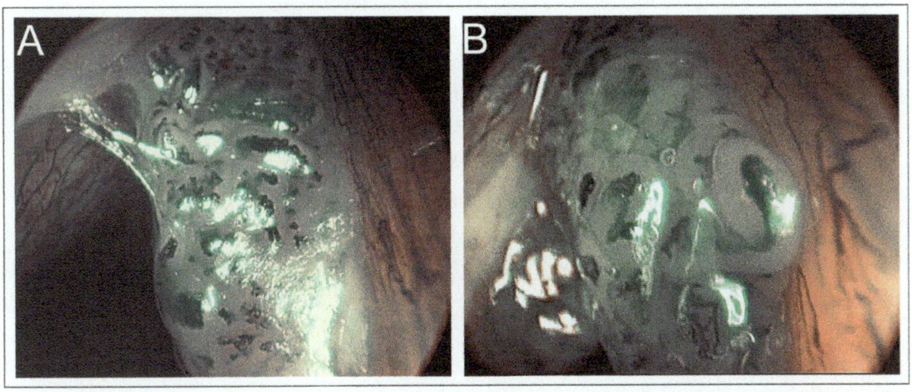

Figure 11. Laryngeal papilloma in HDTV NBI magnifying endoscopy(A, B). Multiple regular papillae covered by squamous epithelium with a central axis vessel are typical for papillomas.

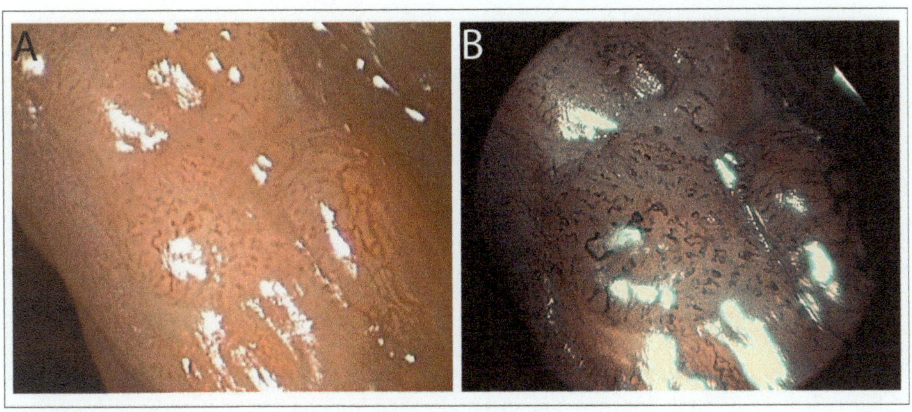

Figure 12. Spinocellular carcinoma of the vocal cord in HDTV magnifying endoscopy in white light (C) and NBI (D). Complete disruption of vascular microarchitecture and IPCL irregularities are clear signs of carcinoma.

6. Conclusions

NBI is an advanced endoscopic imaging technique that allows early detection of small superficial mucosal lesions that are undetectable using the conventional white-light endoscopy. NBI is increasingly used in otorhinolaryngology as a convenient screening method for detection of new diseases, but also for follow-up of patients after treatment for head and neck malignant tumours, when early detection of possible recurrence is crucial. Intraoperatively, it can be used as a helpful tool for targeting biopsies, determining the tumour spread and safe resection margins. Using magnifying HDTV endoscopy in combination with NBI dramatically improves the sensitivity and specificity of endoscopic examination. The main advantage is its use particularly in direct laryngoscopy under general anaesthesia in combination with rigid angled telescopes that allow determining the malignancy with high probability during the operation as well as the exact extent of disease.

NBI endoscopy investigation can be limited in cases of stagnant saliva, sticky mucus or high layer of hyperkeratosis. In these situations the clear mucosal surface can be impossible to observe, therefore the advantages of NBI method could be lost. NBI endoscopy achieves high sensitivity and specificity, yet can lead to false positive findings, most frequently in the case of laryngeal papillomatosis. Finding of brown dots there may be mistakenly interpreted as tumour neovasculature. Utilization of HDTV NBI magnifying endoscopy contributes to better differentiation of these lesions.

Acknowledgements

Supported by grant IGA MZ CR NT11544 and the project for conceptual development of research organization 00064203.

All photographs were captured by the author using OLYMPUS EXERA II system.

Author details

Petr Lukes[1], Michal Zabrodsky[1], Jan Plzak[1,2], Martin Chovanec[1,2], Jaroslav Betka[1], Eva Foltynova[1] and Jan Betka[1]

1 Department of Otorhinolaryngology, Head and Neck Surgery, First Faculty of Medicine, Charles University in Prague and University Hospital Motol, Czech Republic

2 Institute of Anatomy, First Faculty of Medicine, Charles University in Prague, Czech Republic

References

[1] Ridge, J. A G. B, Lango, M. N, et al. (2008). Head and Neck Tumors. In: Pazdur R WL, Camphausen KA, Hoskins WJ (ed) Cancer Management: A Multidisciplinary Approach. 11th edn.,

[2] De Boer, M. F, & Pruyn, J. F. van den Borne B, Knegt PP, Ryckman RM, Verwoerd CD (1995). Rehabilitation outcomes of long-term survivors treated for head and neck cancer. Head Neck , 17(6), 503-515.

[3] Fielding, D, Agnew, J, Wright, D, & Hodge, R. (2010). Autofluorescence improves pretreatment mucosal assessment in head and neck cancer patients. Otolaryngol Head Neck Surg 142 (3 Suppl 1):Sdoi:10.1016/j.otohns.2009.12.021, 20-26.

[4] Hughes, O. R, Stone, N, Kraft, M, Arens, C, & Birchall, M. A. (2010). Optical and molecular techniques to identify tumor margins within the larynx. Head Neck , 32(11), 1544-1553.

[5] Muto, M, Nakane, M, Katada, C, Sano, Y, Ohtsu, A, Esumi, H, Ebihara, S, & Yoshida, S. (2004). Squamous cell carcinoma in situ at oropharyngeal and hypopharyngeal mucosal sites. Cancer , 101(6), 1375-1381.

[6] Sano, Y, Kobayashi, M, Hamamoto, Y, & Al, e. (2001). New diagnostic method based on color imaging using narrowband imaging (NBI) endoscopy system for gastrointestinal tract. Gastrointestinal Endoscopy 53 (5):AB125

[7] Watanabe, A, Tsujie, H, Taniguchi, M, Hosokawa, M, Fujita, M, & Sasaki, S. (2006). Laryngoscopic detection of pharyngeal carcinoma in situ with narrowband imaging. Laryngoscope , 116(4), 650-654.

[8] Muto, M, Hironaka, S, Nakane, M, Boku, N, Ohtsu, A, & Yoshida, S. (2002). Association of multiple Lugol-voiding lesions with synchronous and metachronous esophageal squamous cell carcinoma in patients with head and neck cancer. Gastrointest Endosc doi:10.1067/mge.2002.128104, 56(4), 517-521.

[9] Piazza, C, Dessouky, O, Peretti, G, Cocco, D, De Benedetto, L, & Nicolai, P. (2008). Narrow-band imaging: a new tool for evaluation of head and neck squamous cell carcinomas. Review of the literature. Acta Otorhinolaryngol Ital , 28(2), 49-54.

[10] Gono, K. (2007). An introduction to high-resolution endoscopy and narrowband imaging. In: Cohen J (ed) Advanced Digestive Endoscopy: Comprehensive Atlas of High Resolution Endoscopy and Narrowband Imaging. Blackwell Publishing, , 9-22.

[11] Watanabe, A, Taniguchi, M, Tsujie, H, Hosokawa, M, Fujita, M, & Sasaki, S. (2009). The value of narrow band imaging for early detection of laryngeal cancer. Eur Arch Otorhinolaryngol doi:10.1007/s00405-008-0835-1, 266(7), 1017-1023.

[12] Takano, J. H, Yakushiji, T, Kamiyama, I, Nomura, T, Katakura, A, Takano, N, & Shibahara, T. (2010). Detecting early oral cancer: narrowband imaging system observation of the oral mucosa microvasculature. Int J Oral Maxillofac Surg , 39(3), 208-213.

[13] Matsuba, H, Katada, C, Masaki, T, Nakayama, M, Okamoto, T, Hanaoka, N, Tanabe, S, Koizumi, W, Okamoto, M, & Muto, M. (2011). Diagnosis of the extent of advanced oropharyngeal and hypopharyngeal cancers by narrow band imaging with magnifying endoscopy. Laryngoscope doi:10.1002/lary.21553, 121(4), 753-759.

[14] Watanabe, A, Taniguchi, M, Tsujie, H, Fujita, M, & Sasaki, S. (2007). Early detection of recurrent hypopharyngeal cancer after radiotherapy by utilizing narrow-band imaging--report of a case]. Nippon Jibiinkoka Gakkai Kaiho , 110(10), 680-682.

[15] Lin, Y. C, & Wang, W. H. (2011). Narrow-band imaging for detecting early recurrent nasopharyngeal carcinoma. Head Neck doi:10.1002/hed.21310, 33(4), 591-594.

[16] Ni, X. G, He, S, Xu, Z. G, Gao, L, Lu, N, Yuan, Z, Lai, S. Q, Zhang, Y. M, Yi, J. L, Wang, X. L, Zhang, L, Li, X. Y, & Wang, G. Q. (2010). Endoscopic diagnosis of laryngeal cancer and precancerous lesions by narrow band imaging. J Laryngol Otol , 125(3), 288-296.

[17] Piazza, C, Cocco, D, De Benedetto, L, Bon, F. D, Nicolai, P, & Peretti, G. (2010). Role of narrow-band imaging and high-definition television in the surveillance of head and neck squamous cell cancer after chemo- and/or radiotherapy. Eur Arch Otorhinolaryngol doi:10.1007/s00405-010-1236-9, 267(9), 1423-1428.

[18] Peery, A. F, Hoppo, T, Garman, K. S, Dellon, E. S, Daugherty, N, Bream, S, Sanz, A. F, Davison, J, Spacek, M, Connors, D, Faulx, A. L, Chak, A, Luketich, J. D, Shaheen, N. J, & Jobe, B. A. (2012). Feasibility, safety, acceptability, and yield of office-based, screening transnasal esophagoscopy (with video). Gastrointest Endosc e942. doi: 10.1016/j.gie.2012.01.021, 75(5), 945-953.

[19] Sanli, A, Celebi, O, Eken, M, Oktay, A, Aydin, S, & Ayduran, E. (2008). Role of the 30 degrees telescope in evaluation of laryngeal masses during direct laryngoscopy. Journal of voice : official journal of the Voice Foundation doi:10.1016/j.jvoice.2007.02.001, 22(2), 238-244.

[20] Eryilmaz, A, Akmansu, H, Topcu, E, Acar, A, & Korkmaz, H. (2004). The role of 70-degree telescopic examination during direct laryngoscopic evaluation of laryngeal cancers. Eur Arch Otorhinolaryngol doi:10.1007/s00405-003-0674-z, 261(5), 267-269.

[21] Piazza, C, Cocco, D, & De Benedetto, L. Del Bon F, Nicolai P, Peretti G (2009). Narrow band imaging and high definition television in the assessment of laryngeal cancer: a prospective study on 279 patients. Eur Arch Otorhinolaryngol , 267(3), 409-414.

[22] Fujii, S, Yamazaki, M, Muto, M, & Ochiai, A. (2010). Microvascular irregularities are associated with composition of squamous epithelial lesions and correlate with sube-

pithelial invasion of superficial-type pharyngeal squamous cell carcinoma. Histopathology doi:10.1111/j.1365-2559.2010.03512.x, 56(4), 510-522.

[23] Inoue, H, Kaga, M, Yato, Y, Sugaya, S, & Kudo, S. (2007). Magnifying endoscopic diagnosis of tissue atypia and cancer invasion depth in the area of pharyngo-esophageal squamous epithelium by NBI enhanced magnification image: IPCL pattern classification. In: Cohen J (ed) Advanced Digestive Endoscopy: Comprehensive Atlas of High Resolution Endoscopy and Narrowband Imaging. Blackwell Publishing, Malden, Massachusetts, , 49-66.

[24] Lukes, P. (2012). Discrimination of laryngeal papillomas and superficial laryngeal cancer using NBI HDTV magnifying endoscopy. Lecture. Laryngology- Cutting Edge Laryngology for the 21st Century, Kuala Lumpur, Malaysia

[25] Andrea, M, Dias, O, & Santos, A. (1995). Contact endoscopy during microlaryngeal surgery: a new technique for endoscopic examination of the larynx. Ann Otol Rhinol Laryngol , 104(5), 333-339.

[26] Zabrodsky, M, Plzak, J, Betka, J, & Lukes, P. (2011). NBI HDTV Magnifying Endoscopy in Laryngeal Papillomatosis and Laryngeal Spinocellular Cancer. Otolaryngol Head Neck Surg 145 (2 suppl):195

Chapter 6

Therapeutic and Diagnostic Approaches in Rhinology and Allergy

Pongsakorn Tantilipikorn

Additional information is available at the end of the chapter

1. Introduction

1.1. Diagnostic rhinoscopy

1.1.1. Applied anatomy of nose & paranasal sinuses

Nasal cavity is the complex structure. It is divided by the nasal septum into the left and right side. Lateral nasal wall composed of three turbinates and their meati.(figure 1).

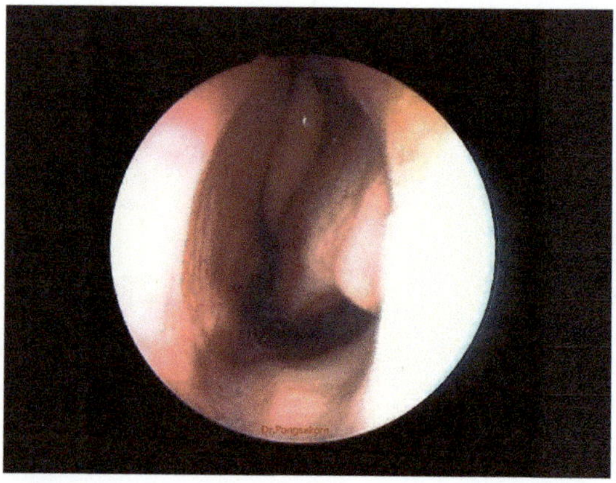

Figure 1. Normal anatomy of left nasal cavity, shows nasal septum, inferior turbinate & meatus, and middle turbinate & meatus.

The anterior group of paranasal sinuses consists of the frontal, maxillary and anterior ethmoid sinus. The posterior group of paranasal sinuses consists of the sphenoid and posterior ethmoid sinus.

By histology, nasal and paranasal sinus mucosa is the psuedostratified ciliated columnar epithelium. The mucous blanket is moved from sinuses through their ostium. The drainage of anterior group of paranasal sinuses is through their ostium and middle meati.The posterior group is drained through the superior meati & sphenoethmoidal recess.

With the concept of 'mucous drainage drain through meatus", the most important structure inside the nose is called "ostiomeatal complex", especially the middle meatus area.[1]

1.1.2. Clinical presentation of common rhinologic condition

The most common disease of nose is the inflammatory conditions – rhinitis. It can be caused by the infectious vs non-infectious causes.The non-infectious rhinitis can be further divided into allergic rhinitis (AR) and non-allergic rhinitis (NAR). When the inflammatory process extended beyond the nasal cavities, the inflammation spread into the paranasal sinuses, leads to be 'rhinosinusitis'.

Besides the mucosal inflammation, some anatomic variations may caused the symptoms resemble to rhinitis. Those anatomic variations are pneumatization of middle turbinate (Concha Bullosa), paradoximal middle turbinate, or deviated nasal septum (DNS), etc. (figure 2).

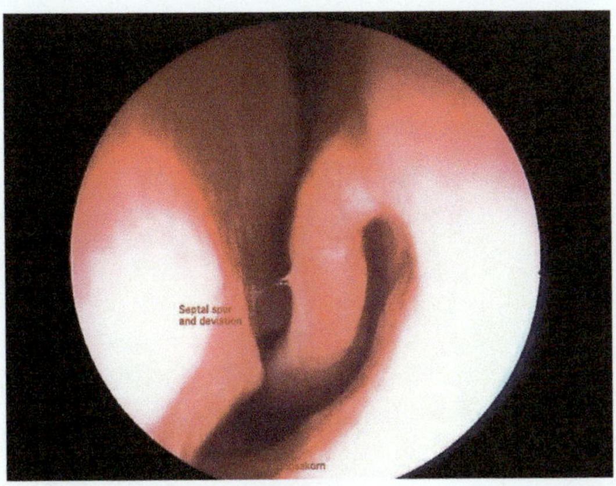

Figure 2. Deviation of nasal septum to the left, with its contact point to the inferior turbinate.

The tumor of nose & paranasal sinuses commonly arises from the maxillary sinuses and lateral nasal wall. Squamous cell carcinoma is the most common malignant type, and Inverted papilloma is the most common benign type. The other tumors are adenocarcinoma, adenoidcysticcarcinom, olfactory neuroblastoma, lymphoma, vascular tumor, etc. (figure 3).

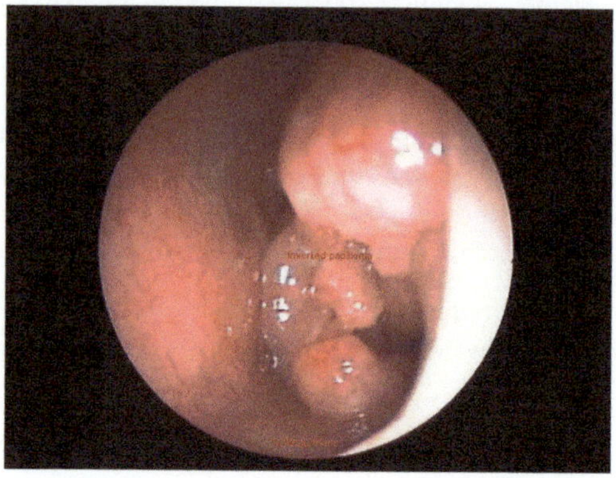

Figure 3. Squamous cell carcinoma of left nasal cavity.

1.1.3. Diagnostic application of endoscopy

Nasal endoscopy can reveal the detail of color of nasal mucosa, the swelling, and the discharge. These detail help rhinologist to differential the various causes of rhinitis.For instances, the turbinate of AR will be in pale color with watery discharge. (figure 4). On the contrary, NAR will be injected and swelling turbinate or atrophic in some conditions.

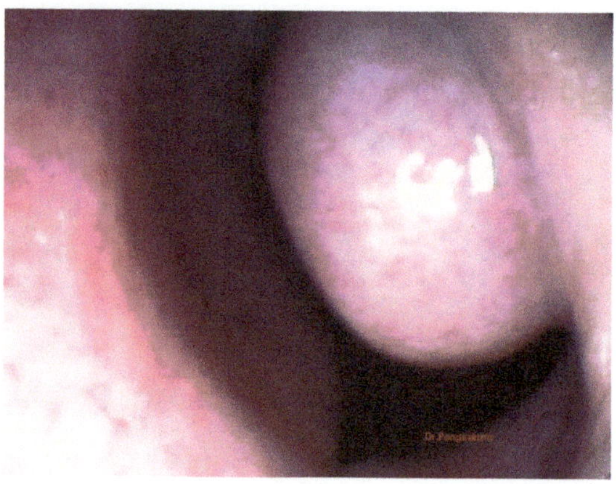

Figure 4. Congest inferior turbinate with pale color.

Because of the tumor of nose&paranasal sinuses usually presents with the subtle symptoms. The early stage may present with minimal nasal congestion or minor nasal bleeding. Nasal endoscopy will be a good armamentarium to exam the detail of deep structure inside the nasal cavities.

According to the most recent guideline – European Position Paper of Sinusitis (EPOS) 2012, the rhinosinusitis is a disease of 'clinical diagnosis'.[2] By using the two symptoms of nasal obstruction and rhinorrhea with the duration longer than 10 days, the diagnosis of acute rhinosinusitis (ARS) is made.[3] But if the initial treatment cannot alleviate the symptoms, nasal endoscopy should be done. Moreover, the chronic rhinosinusitis (CRS) need nasal endoscopy along with the history for diagnosis. The CRS can be subclassified into CRS with nasal polyp (CRS c NP) and CRS without nasal polyp (CRS s NP).

NP can be seen as the pale, semi-translucent mass protruding from the middle meatus. (figure 5).

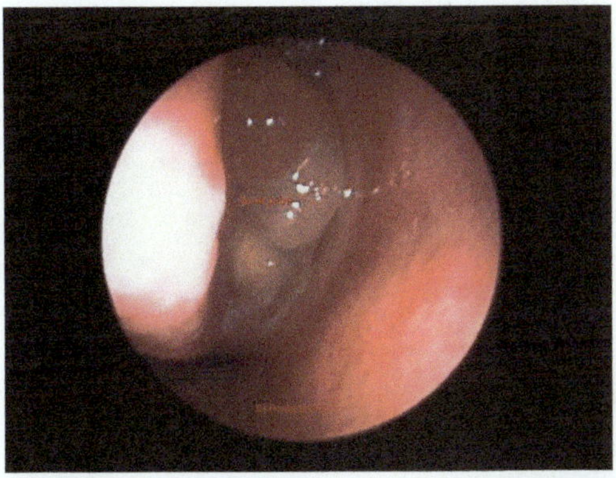

Figure 5. Nasal polyp of the right nasal cavity.

Its etiology remains obscure but related to mucosal inflammation by eosinophilic cell.[4,5] The principle of treatment of CRS, especially CRS c NP, is topical nasal steroid. Oral prednisolone may be used for the short course of large NP 's treatment.Nasal endoscopy is the essential instrument to differentiate CRS c NP from CRS s NP.Due to their different natural course, these conditions should be made since the initial treatment process.

2. Therapeutic options of nasal endoscope

2.1. Rhinologic condition

2.1.1. Rhinosinusitis

Three principle treatments of rhinosinusitis (RS) are the eradication of infectious process, promotion of secretion in sinus cavity and treatment of underlying disease (eg. Allergic inflammation).Endoscopy has its role in the treatment of RS by 1) utilization of endoscope for obtaining responsible organism, and 2) utilization of endoscope as a principle instrument of surgical procedure.

The selection of antibiotic for treatment of infectious RS usually follows the guideline that depends on the prevalence of responsible organism in each community. Three most common organisms of RS are *Streptococcus pneumoniae, Haemophilusinfluenzae and Moraxella catarrhalis*.[6,7]Most of the guidelines suggest the high dose-amoxycillin with/without clavulanic acid as the first –line drug.When there is little (minimal) response of RS patient, the physician may switch to the second-line drug or consider taking the microbiologic culture/sensitivity test.

The gold standard of obtaining RS specimen for culture is the sinus puncture, usually from the maxillary sinus through the inferior meatus. But the so-called maxillary Antral puncture&Irrigation (AI) is considered as an invasive procedure, which can cause the significant pain for RS patient. To avoid this limitation and minimal contamination of non-pathogenic organism in the nasal cavity, endoscopic-guided culture at the ostiomeatal complex (OMC) is the alternation procedure with comparable accuracy to AI.[8] (figure 6)

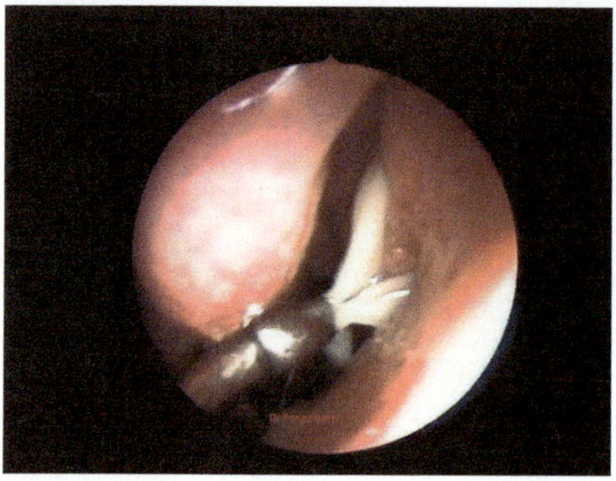

Figure 6. Endoscopic-guide culture from the left middle meatus.

If the RS patient fails to the medical treatment, the surgical procedure is needed. Conventionally, the open-approach sinus surgeries are the Caldwell-Luc (CWL) and the external frontoethmoidectomy (eg. Lynch). Prof Messerklinger proposed the breakthrough principle of mucociliary drainage through OMC in 1975.With this principle and the advancement of surgical instrument (especially the rigid endoscope), Prof Kennedy and Prof Stammberger lead the concept of "Functional Endoscopic Sinus Surgery-FESS" into the acceptable sinus procedure as a standard treatment.[9]

FESS consists of the utilization of rigid nasal endoscope and the cutting forceps to clear the pathology at OMC area. Then, obstructed secretion inside the sinus cavities can be drained out through OMC by the function of respiratory cilia.

Over the 30 years, there are tremendous improvement of surgical instrument and the adjunctive procedure.For instance, the cutting&suction instrument such as the microdebrider helps the surgeon to minimize tissue trauma, which leads to less intraoperative bleeding and better postoperative result.[10] (figure 7). The image-guidance system also helps the rhinologist to operate in the high-risk area, such as the orbit or skull base, or the uncertain anatomy with more accuracy.[11]

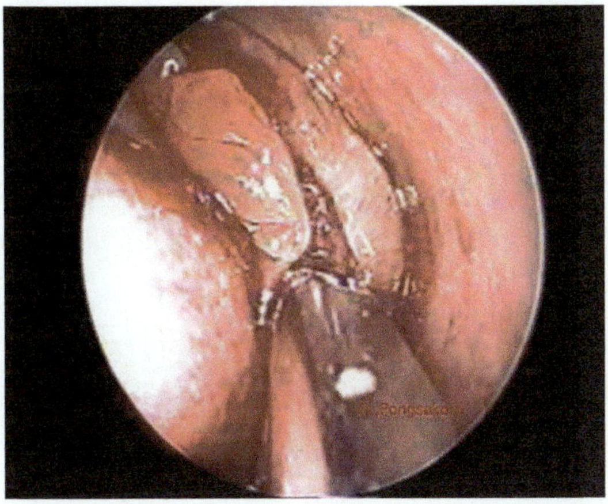

Figure 7. Endoscopic resection of left nasal polyp by microdebrider.

2.1.2. Allergic rhinitis with turbinate hypertrophy

Allergic Rhinitis (AR) is the disease mediated by 'antigen-antibody' reaction. The responsible antigen is the immunoglobulin E (Ig E). This pathomechanism leads to mast cell degranulation and subsequently releasing of various mediators, especially histamine and leukotrienes (LTs). The principle treatments of AR are the avoiding of responsile allergens, anti-allergic medication (eg. Antihistamine, corticosteroid nose spray), and modulation of immune response (eg. Allergen Immunotherapy – AIT).[12]

The most troublesome symptom of AR is nasal blockage/obstruction. Antihistamine (AH) and Intranasal corticosteroid (INCS) have their excellent result in alleviating of nasal obstruction. In some unresponsive AR patients, their inferior turbinates are hypertrophic from the submucous gland/vascular structures.

The original turbinate-reduction procedures are the total/subtotal turbinate resection or the cauterization by chemical agents, electrical instruments. These procedure leads into the losing of mucosal surface and subsequently crusting and dryness of nasal cavities.

More conservative procedures, with the utilization of nasal endoscopy, are done with more physiologic state. The endoscopic submucous resection (either by cutting-forceps or microdebrider) and radiofrequency volumetric tissue reduction (RFVTR) can be done with the excellent accuracy and surgical result.[13] (figure 8).

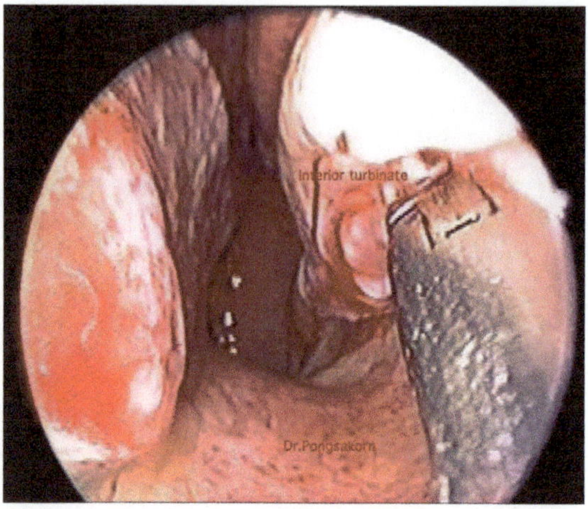

Figure 8. Endoscopic submucous resection of the left inferior turbinate.

2.1.3. Tumor of nose & paranasal sinuses (PNS)

Tumor of nose&PNS can be benign or malignant in-origin.The most common benign tumor is inverted papilloma.Inverted papilloma has its natural course of frequent recurrence due to its histologic character of 'inverted tumor cell into the attachment bony origin. So the principle of surgical treatment is the medial maxillectomy through open-approach such as the lateral rhinotomy or CWL.Nowadays, the medial maxillectomy procedure can be done under endoscope with the help of suction&cutting device (eg. Microdebrider). The endoscopic medial maxillectomy procedure reaches it comparable result as the open procedure.[14]

Another benign lesion that can be benefit from endoscopic procedure is the transnasal pituitary procedure. The hypophysectomy procedure has been done as the microscopic transeptal approach. Rhinologic surgeon can work along with neurosurgeon as a 'four-handed technique' through the nostrils by using endoscope.[15] The sphenoid sinus can be approach and further procedure of hypophysectomy can be done with the same principle of transeptal approach.

Malignant tumors of nose & PNS can be squamous cell carcinoma that commonly originates from the maxillary sinus or lateral nasal wall. Its symptom is subtle and the patient usually comes to visit the otorhinolaryngologist as the advance stage. To obtain the free-margin, the open procedure should be done to provide the good 5-years survival. But for some malignant lesions near skull base, such as olfactory neuroblastoma, the endoscope can help rhinologic surgeon to delineate the surgical margin and precise surgical resection with minimized injury to the vital structure.[16]

2.1.4. Nasal bleeding (epistaxis)

Nasal bleeding (Epistaxis) can be categorized into two groups, anterior or posterior epistaxis. Anterior epistaxis is usually bled from Little's area, which located at anteroinferior part of nasal septum. The mild degree anterior bleeding can be stopped by cold compression or cauterization. The more severe one can be stopped by standard anterior nasal packing.

The location of posterior epistaxis is around the posterior end of middle turbinate, which is supplied by the sphenopalatine artery. The sphenopalatine is the terminal branch of internal maxillary artery. Before the era of nasal endoscopy, the severe posterior epistaxis, which is failed from the posterior nasal packing, can be treated by internal maxillary artery ligation through the CWL approach. Nowadays, the sphenopalatine artery can be directly ligated or clipped by endoscopic approach.[17,18] (figure 9). This procedure requires less operative time and provides less tissue trauma comparing to the CWL approach.

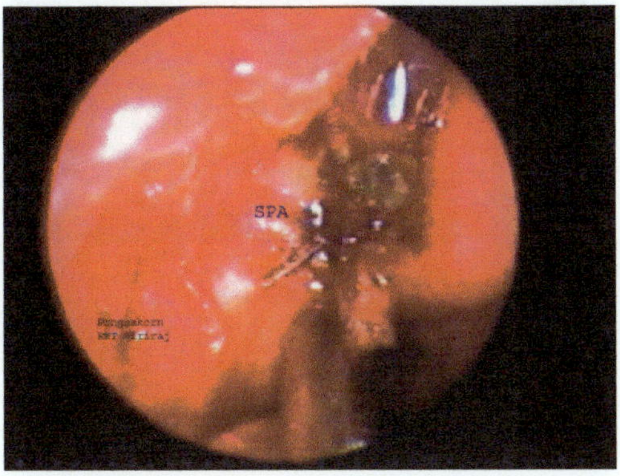

Figure 9. Clipping the right sphenopalatine artery in the posterior epistaxis case.

2.2. Non-rhinologic condition

2.2.1. Obstruction of nasolacrimal system

Lacrimal system consists of the lacrimal punctum, cannaliculus, lacrimal sac and lacrimal duct. The duct drains tear into the inferior meatus. Location of lacrimal drainage obstruction commonly occurs below the level of sac. Dacryocystorhinostomy (DCR) is the procedure for the treatment of obstructive of lacrimal system at that level. DCR can be bone via the incision around the medial canthus region. Then, the cavity of sac is entered. The medial (nasal surface) of sac is drained into the nasal cavity.

By using the endoscope approach, intranasal cavity can be examined and corrected if that particular structure may contribute to the obstruction.The intranasal specific area of lacrimal sac is called "AggerNasi" area is approached. The medial side of sac is entered after the AggerNasi bone work is done by drill or ronguer.(figure 10). The next step is to marsupialise the lac and make the sac stay widely open into the nasal cavity. Endoscopic DCR provides many advantages such as: ability to correct intranasal anatomy, less bony drilling, and no scarring.[19,20]

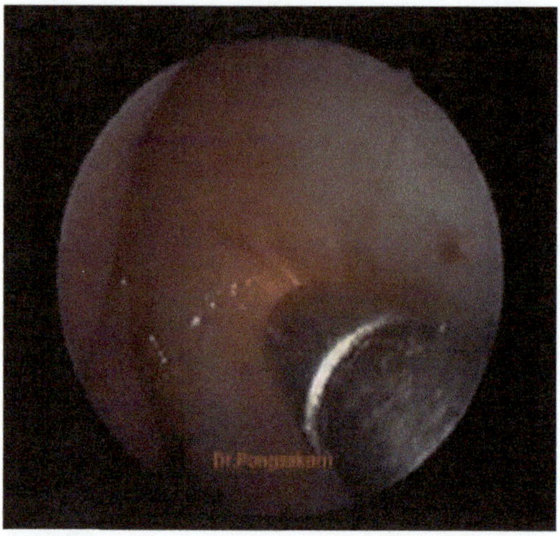

Figure 10. Endoscopic DCR. The transilluminated area is the AggerNasi area.

2.2.2. Cerebrospinal fluid repair

The etiologies of cerebrospinal fluid (CSF) leakage are either traumatic or non-traumatic cause. Most of the traumatic from accidental cause heal spontaneously after a few weeks of conservative treatments.

For the indicated cases of CSF leak, the external approach via bi-coronal incisions with utilization of various materials, such as fascia, can be done with excellent result.[21,22] Endoscopic approach to the anterior skull base is an alternative method, especially for the single-lesion leakage or the same-stage repair with the intranasal resection of tumor.[23] Many choices of repairing material is used, for instance:autologous fat graft, nasal mucosa, cartilage from septum or auricle, and allografts. (figure 11). Metaanalysis study reveals the comparable result with the external approach.[24]

2.2.3. Orbital/optic nerve decompression

Proptosis from thyroid hyperfunction is treated initially by prednisolone and immunosuppressive drugs. Surgical approach reserves for the refractory case, which can be done by removal of the bony wall of orbital. Theoretically, the selective on particular wall can be chosen, depending on the surgeon's preference and the degree of proptosis.

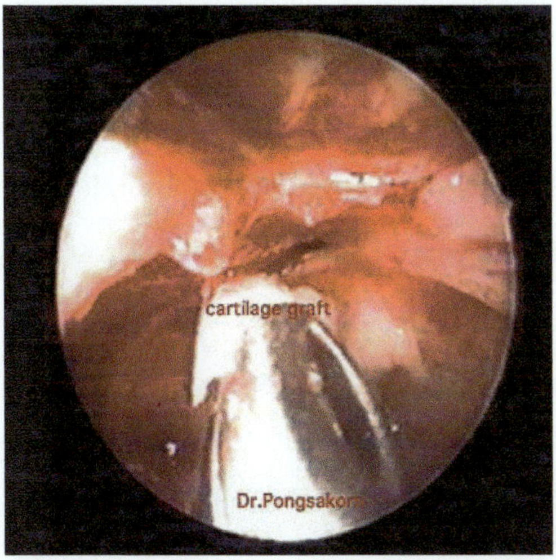

Figure 11. Endoscopic CSF leak repair. The cartilaginous free-graft is inserted to repair the skull base defect.

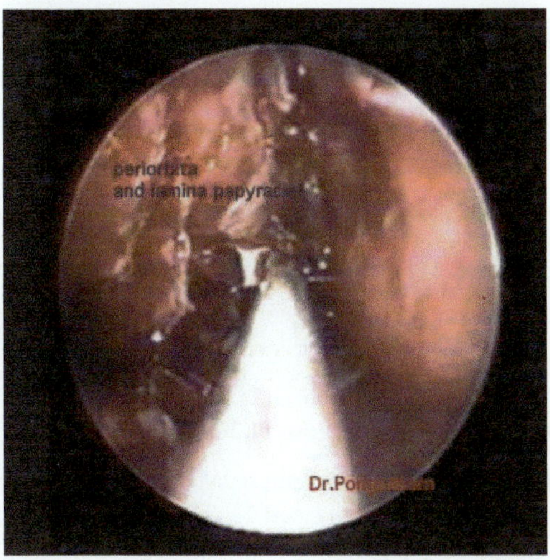

Figure 12. Endoscopic orbital decompression. The lamina papyracea is dissected from the periorbital by curettage.

Endoscopic medial wall decompression is commonly done, allowing the orbital content expands into the ethmoid cavity.[25,26] The first step of medial wall decompression is to do the ethmoidectomy with/without middle meatal antrostomy. Lamina papyracea is exposed and the surgeon can estimate the area of bony area to match with the degree of patient's proptosis. Then, the bony decompression is done with minimally disturbance of orbital content. The hyperplastic orbital content protrudes into the ethmoid cavity (figure 12), which will make the proptosis improves. When more space is needed, the additional inferior orbital wall is performed in the same setting. In this 'infero-medial wall decompression', the orbital content gains more space into the maxillary & ethmoid cavities.

For the blunt traumatic injury of optic nerve, rhinologic surgeon can use the endoscope to decompress the medial&interior wall of orbital apex. This procedure provides more space for the compressed optic nerve.

3. Conclusion

Endoscope can be utilized in various conditions in rhinology&allergy. It provides both diagnostic and therapeutic value.The surgical treatment with endoscopic approach can be done in the inflammatory condition and the others conditions such as tumor resection, CSF leakage repair, DCR, orbital decompression, vascular ligation in epistaxis.

Author details

Pongsakorn Tantilipikorn

Division of Rhinology & Allergy, Faculty of Medicine Siriraj Hospital, Mahidol University, Bangkok, Thailand

References

[1] Kennedy DW ,Zinreich SJ. Endoscopic middle meatalantrostomy: theory, technique, and patency. Laryngoscope. 1987; 97(8 pt 3 Suppl 43): 1-9.

[2] Fokkens WJ, Lund VJ, Mullol J, et al. The European Position Paper on Rhinosinusitis and Nasal Polyps. Rhinology. 2012; Suppl(23): 1-299.

[3] Benninger MS. Adult chronic rhinosinusitis: Definition, diagnosis, epidemiology, and pathophysiology. Otolaryngol Head Neck Surg. 2003; 129(3 Suppl): S1-S32.

[4] Tan BK, SchleimerRP , Kern RC. Perspectives on the etiology of chronic rhinosinusitis. CurrOpinOtolaryngol Head Neck Surg. 2010; 18(1): 21-6.

[5] Shin SH, Lee SH, JeongHS , Kita H. The effect of nasal polyp epithelial cells on eosinophil activation. Laryngoscope. 2003; 113(8): 1374-7.

[6] Tantilipikorn P, Bunnag C, Srifuengfung S, et al. A Surveilance Study of Bacteriologic Profile in Rhinosinusitis. Siriraj Med J. 2007; 59: 117-80.

[7] Brook I. Microbiology and management of sinusitis. J Otolaryngol. 1996; 25(4): 249-56.

[8] Ozcan M, Unal A, Aksaray S, Yalcin F, Akdeniz T. Correlation of middle meatus and ethmoid sinus microbiology in patients with chronic sinusitis. Rhinology. 2002; 40(1): 24-7.

[9] Stammberger H. Functional endoscopic sinus surgery: concept, indications and results of the Messerklinger technique. Eur Arch Otorhinolaryngol. 1990; 247: 63-76.

[10] SetliffRC , Parsons DS. The "hummer": new instrumentation for functional endoscopic sinus surgery. Am J Rhinol. 1994; 8: 275-8.

[11] Tantilipikorn P, Metheetrairut C, Lumyongsatien J, Bedavanija A, Assanasen P. Image-guided Surgery in Rhinology. Siriraj Med J. 2010; 62(203-6).

[12] Bousquet J, Khaltaev N, Cruz AA, et al. Allergic Rhinitis and its Impact on Asthma (ARIA) 2008. Allergy. 2008; 63(Suppl 86): 8-160.

[13] Banhiran W, Tantilipikorn P, Metheetrairut C, Assanasen P, Bunnag C. Quality of Life in Patients with Chronic Rhinitis after Radiofrequency Inferior Turbinate Reduction. J Med Assoc Thai. 2010; 93(8): 950-60.

[14] Sham CL, Woo JK , van Hasselt CA. Endoscopic resection of inverted papilloma of the nose and paranasal sinuses. J Laryngol Otol. 1998; 112(8): 758-64.

[15] Briner HR, Simmen D, Jones N. Endoscopic sinus surgery: advantages of the bimanual technique. Am J Rhinol. 2005; 19: 269-73.

[16] Harvey RJ, Winder M, Parmar P, Lund V. Endoscopic skull base surgery for sinonasal malignancy. OtolaryngolClin North Am. 44(5): 1081-140.

[17] Agreda B, Urpegui A, Ignacio Alfonso J, Valles H. Ligation of the sphenopalatine artery in posterior epistaxis. Retrospective study of 50 patients]. ActaOtorrinolaringol Esp. 62(3): 194-8.

[18] Howe DJ , Skinner DW. Outcomes of endoscopic sphenopalatine artery ligation for epistaxis: a five-year series from a single institution. Ear Nose Throat J. 91(2): 70-2.

[19] Al-Qahtani AS. Primary endoscopic dacryocystorhinostomy with or without silicone tubing: A prospective randomized study. Am J Rhinol Allergy. 26(4): 332-4.

[20] Feng YF, Cai JQ, Zhang JY , Han XH. A meta-analysis of primary dacryocystorhinostomy with and without silicone intubation. Can J Ophthalmol. 46(6): 521-7.

[21] McCormack B, Cooper PR ,Persky M. Extrncranial repair of cerebrospinal fluid fistulas: technique and results in 37 patients. Neurosurgery. 1990; 27: 412-7.

[22] Persky MS, Rothstein SG , Breda SD. Extracranial repair of cerebrospinal fluid otorhinorrhea. Laryngoscope. 1991; 101: 7-15.

[23] Lanza D, O'Brien D , Kennedy D. Endoscopic repair of cerebrospinal fluid fistulae and encephaloceles. Laryngoscope. 1996; 106: 1119-25.

[24] Hegazy H, Carrau R ,Snyderman C. Transnasal endoscopic repair of cerebrospinal fluid rhinorrhea: a meta-analysis. Laryngoscope. 2000; 110: 1166-72.

[25] Sheng H, Cai C, Cheng Y, et al. Endoscopic orbital decompression for thyroid-associated ophthalmopathy. Lin Chung Er Bi Yan HouTou Jing WaiKeZaZhi. 26(1): 27-9.

[26] Boboridis KG, Bunce C. Surgical orbital decompression for thyroid eye disease. Cochrane Database Syst Rev. 2011; (12): CD007630.

Chapter 7

Role of Endoscopic Sinus Surgery in Pediatric Acute Complicated Sinusitis

Timothy P. McEvoy, Charles A. Elmaraghy and Kris R. Jatana

Additional information is available at the end of the chapter

1. Introduction

Sinus surgery was initially done transnasally or by a transmaxillary approach with the use of external lighting (often a headlight) and the surgeon's direct vision. Endoscopic techniques for intranasal surgery were first pioneered for adult applications and were gradually applied to pediatric sinus surgery as endoscope technology improved and smaller diameter endoscopes became available. Techniques that were developed in Europe were championed by Kennedy in the United States, with an emphasis on targeted removal of diseased tissue and preservation of normal mucosa [1, 2].

In 1989, Gross *et al.* published one of the first case series documenting functional endoscopic sinus surgery in the pediatric population. They noted that all 57 children in the series tolerated the procedure well and that there were no major complications [3]. Since that time, endoscopic intranasal surgical techniques in children have become commonplace for applications ranging from chronic sinusitis and nasal polyposis to the treatment of complications of acute sinusitis as well as approaches to the skull base.

2. Equipment

2.1. Camera and monitors

Initially, endoscopic sinus surgery was performed with the surgeon looking directly through the optical telescope. As digital cameras improved, the images could be magnified and viewed on a monitor allowing the surgeon better visualization as well as improving their working room and ability to operate. In recent years, improvements in the size and reasonable cost of high-definition monitors and cameras have allowed these to become commonplace in many operating rooms and clinics.

2.2. Endoscopes

There are a variety of endoscopes that can be used for pediatric sinus surgery. Depending on the size of the patient, the 4.0 mm diameter endoscope (used for adult sinus procedures) provides the best field of view and resolution. If the child's anatomy is too small to accommodate the 4.0 mm endoscope, a 2.7 mm diameter endoscope can be used. However, the 2.7 mm telescope is more fragile and can be easily broken if too much pressure is placed on the shaft.

Depending on the surgical application, different angled endoscopes are available to provide optimal visualization into the sinuses. The 0 degree endoscope is one of the easiest endoscopes to use as it provides a straight-on view. Scopes with angled tips that allow for views of 30, 45 and 70 degrees are frequently used for endoscopic sinus surgery. During a particular procedure, the surgeon may switch endoscopes frequently depending on which portion of the anatomy they would like to view and operate upon. The 0 degree scope is most commonly used for visualizing the ethmoid and sphenoid sinuses, however angled scopes are most commonly used for viewing the maxillary and frontal sinuses. The angle of most scopes is fixed, however the scope can be turned to visualize in any direction. A scope is now available, which is a heavier than others, that allows for adjustment of the angle on a single scope. The stem of scope, which is where the light cord attaches, can be turned to facilitate looking in other directions. In order to avoid interference of instruments used, scopes that have the light cord coming off the same side or opposite side that the scope is directed are available. Both the standard and reverse-post scopes are an important component of a surgeon's armamentarium.

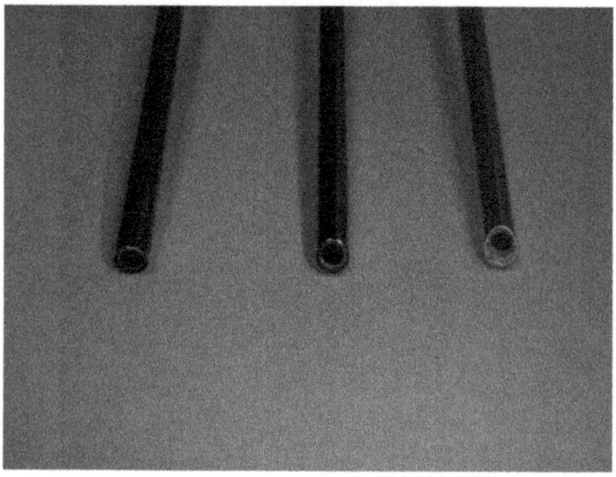

Figure 1. Telescopes, from left to right, 0, 30, 70 degree respectively.

2.3. Endoscopic surgical instruments

Miniaturized versions of adult sinus surgery instruments are available from several instrument manufacturers. These instruments allow surgeons to open particular sinuses while avoiding disturbing normal mucosa.

Another important instrument for endoscopic sinus surgery is the microdebrider. Several manufacturers have produced powered devices that can remove tissue during endoscopic sinus surgery. For example, a 4.0 and a 2.9 mm microdebrider blade can be used depending on the size of the patient. The smaller powered instruments do tend to get clogged with bone chips more frequently. In addition, endoscopic drills exist which can precisely remove bone.

3. Pertinent sinonasal embryology

During fetal development the nasal placode is noted at around four and a half weeks. The nasal cavity is then formed due to the fusion of the medial and lateral nasal processes. The turbinates develop shortly thereafter at around 40 days [4]. Ethmoid budding is noted around 11 to 12 weeks and maxillary budding is noted around 14 to 15 weeks of development [5].

The progression of sinus development was initially documented via cadaver studies, and a recent large-scale imaging study helped re-confirm these findings through non-invasive MRI scanning to evaluate the volume of the paranasal sinuses of patients with healthy sinuses undergoing scans for other reasons. It was found that initial pneumatization was noted for the maxillary and ethomid sinuses at birth, for the sphenoid sinus at 9 months, and for the frontal sinus after 5 years of age. Additionally the development of the paranasal sinuses was noted to be ongoing until at least the late teen years [5].

The fact the sinuses are continuing to develop as children grow becomes important in considering the possible acute complications of sinusitis that will be discussed later in this chapter. The peak time for development of the frontal sinus and the diploic venous system is in adolescence [6], which partially explains why adolescents are the most common age group afflicted by intracranial complications of sinusitis.

4. Clinical presentation of pediatric acute complicated sinusitis

Due the relative rarity of cases of acute complicated sinusitis in children, the exact incidence is unclear. The most frequent complications of sinusitis in children are extracranial and include periorbital/orbital cellulitis and subperiosteal/orbital abscess. These two complications comprise up to 90 percent of complications of sinusitis in children [7]. Opthalmological evaluation is critical in these cases to thoroughly assess the status of the eye. However, in the subset of patients who require inpatient admission for treatment, the incidence of intracranial complications has been estimated to be around 3% based on a large review of patients admitted with sinusitis [8]. Interestingly, male patients account for 60-70% of the cases of complications of acute sinusitis [9].

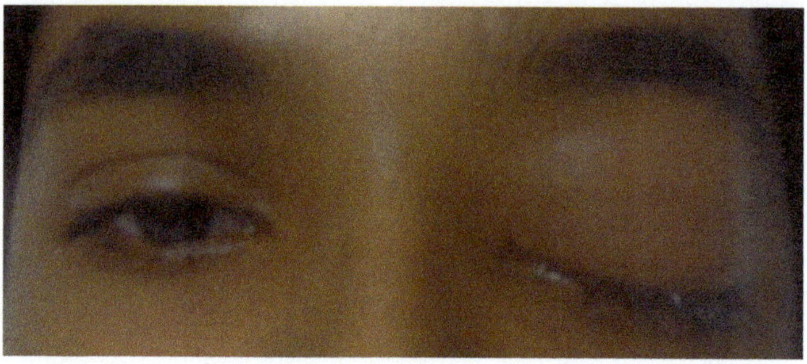

Figure 2. Left periorbital cellulitis with associated subperiosteal abscess

Orbital complications and intracranial complications can present somewhat differently, but at times they can have overlapping symptoms. In addition to systemic symptoms of fever and change in energy level and nasal symptoms of congestion and purulent drainage, patients with orbital complications such as cellulitis and abscess typically develop erythema and edema of the eyelid as well as proptosis [10]. Decreased ocular motility is also a frequent sign of orbital cellulitis and abscess with a reported incidence of approximately 35% and 80% respectively [7]. Visual acuity can be worsened, and in severe cases nonreactive pupils are noted. Complete opthalmological evaluation is an important part of the management of these patients with orbital complications.

Intracranial complications can present in a somewhat non-specific manner with the most frequent symptoms being fever in about 75% and headache in 67-92% of children [11-13]. Other systemic symptoms include nausea and vomiting and lethargy. Some patients with intracranial pathology can present with extracranial complications at the same time, such as orbital cellulitis and forehead abscesses [11]. A significant number patients with intracranial complications of sinusitis (38-59%) will present with *normal* neurological exams [11, 13], which makes diagnosis more difficult and emphasizes the importance of proper imaging studies in the evaluation of these patients. Patients that present with central neurologic signs and symptoms can present with an altered level of consciousness, cranial nerve palsies, hemiparesis, new onset seizures, visual disturbances, slurred speech, and meningeal signs [7, 11-13].

Of note, patients with intracranial complications of sinusitis have a high incidence of seizures and anticonvulsant therapy as prophylaxis should be considered for all patients with intracranial complications [13].

5. Role of imaging in pediatric acute complicated sinusitis

5.1. Computed Tomography (CT)

CT scanning is the gold standard for imaging of the paranasal sinuses. Unlike for patients with chronic sinusitis for whom non-contast studies may be sufficient, children with possible complications of acute sinusitis require contrast-enhanced studies. One drawback of CT scanning is that it does lack specificity due to mucosal changes that may be considered incidental and due to the slow resolution of edema after infections [10, 14]. Although there is a priority to avoid the radiation of a CT scan in children, it remains a crucial imaging modality for diagnosis and management of acute complicated sinusitis. CT can often miss intracranial involvement in cases of acute complicated sinusitis up to 50% of the time. Patients 7 years and older with orbital infections have been shown to have about a 10% incidence of concomitant intracranial involvement [15].

5.2. Magnetic Resonance Imaging (MRI)

Contrast-enhanced MRI scans are necessary for patients who are suspected of having intracranial complications of sinusitis. MRI is superior to CT in that it is able to delineate early cerebritis changes as well as provide further detail regarding the meninges, marrow spaces as well as the orbital apex and cavernous sinus [10, 14].

5.3. Intraoperative surgical guidance

Image guidance systems are used widely by both otolaryngologists and neurosurgeons for adult applications. Data regarding the utility of image guidance in children is not as abundant. However, literature reviews of the indications and safety of image guidance in pediatric sinus and skull base surgery supports its use for complex cases and cases with distorted anatomy which includes cases of acute complicated sinusitis. Additionally, there were no complications that were reported in either retrospective studies[16, 17]. Image guidance can include CT and/or MRI, however, for cases of acute complicated sinusitis, CT is the most useful for defining bony landmarks within the sinonasal cavity. MRI can certainly assist with soft tissue landmarks when needed in complex cases.

6. Role of medical management

Medical management of children with acute complicated sinusitis is mainly centered around the administration of IV antibiotics. Broad-spectrum antibiotics are chosen until culture-directed therapy can be provided. Adjunctive therapy to help reduce mucosal edema includes systemic steroids and decongestants, and topical decongestants (oxymetazaline) and topical steroids. However, there is not much literature to support the use of these agents in the setting of acute complicated sinusitis, but there is no definitive evidence that these would be harmful. Additionally, nasal saline irrigation or nasal saline spray can be helpful to clear secretions in the sinonasal cavity. However, the utility of topical therapies depend on the age and developmental level of each child.

7. Complications of acute sinusitis

7.1. Periorbital and orbital cellulitis

About 60 to 85% of orbital and periorbital infections are attributed to the paranasal sinuses [14]. Periorbital cellulitis is the most frequent complication of sinusitis in the pediatric population. Fortunately, most cases of periorbital cellulitis will respond to medical management with nasal decongestants and systemic antibiotics. For all cases of orbital cellulitis the involvement an ophthalmologist is crucial for full assessment of the eye.

It is important to distinguish pre-septal periorbital cellulitis from post-septal (orbital) cellulitis. The orbital septum is an important landmark. It is a continuation of the orbital periosteum that extends to the tarsal plate.

Garrett *et al.* examined CT scans of 100 consecutive patients with periorbital cellulitis and noted that children with a dehiscence of the lamina papyracea have a higher incidence of requiring endoscopic sinus surgery to address periorbital infection [18]. Jatana *et al.* reported a rare case of recurrent periorbital sinusitis in a young child which ultimately required endoscopic surgical management; this patient had an abnormal lateralized uncinate and a dehiscence of the lamina papyracea. Congenital anatomical abnormalities may contribute to the pathophysiology of this complication of sinusitis; this highlights the importance of imaging studies including high-resolution CT and consideration of early surgical intervention particularily in the event of recurrence [19].

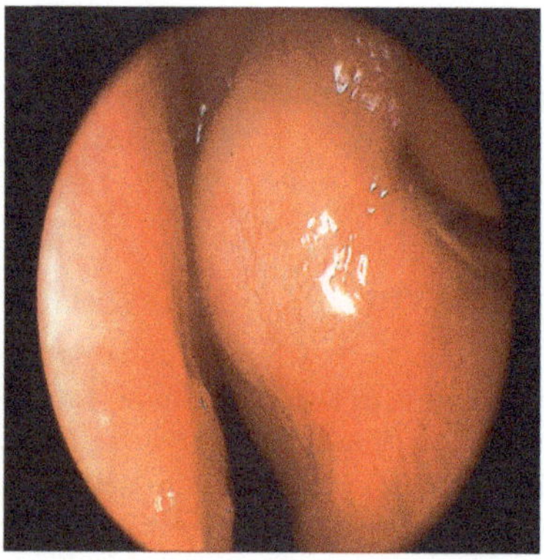

Figure 3. Endoscopic view with a 0 degree telescope demonstrating scarring of left middle meatus imparing sinus drainage and causing periorbital cellulitis.

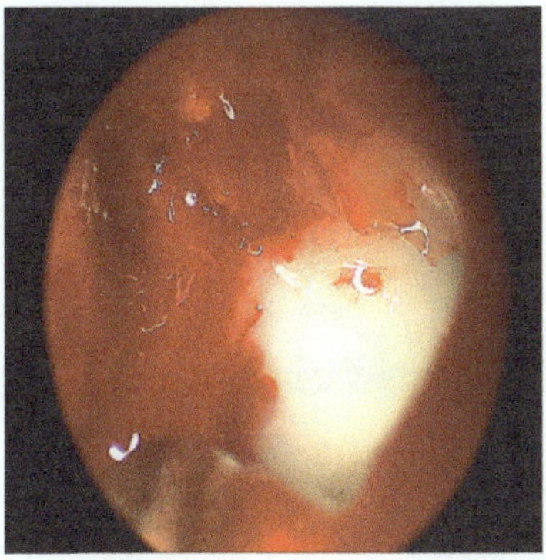

Figure 4. Endoscopic view of the left maxillary sinus with a 30 degree telescope showing frank purulence after a maxillary antrostomy was created.

7.2. Subperiosteal abscess

The concept of the orbital septum as a continuation of the periosteum becomes important to understand the development of a subperiosteal abscess. The periosteum of the medial orbit lies next to the lamina papyracea; the lamina papyracea is very thin and porous and a potential space can be dissected by an infectious process. The spread of infection from the ethmoid sinuses can lead to phlegmon and abscess between the bone and the orbital periosteum. In rare cases, subperiosteal abscess can also be caused by frontal or maxillary sinusitis [14, 20]. Oxford and McClay suggested guidelines to help determine if surgical treatment is warranted for subperiosteal abscesses. They recommend medical management with frequent re-evaluation of the eye if the following criteria are met: normal vison, pupil, and retina, no ophthalmoplegia, IOP<20mmHg, proptosis<5mm, and an abscess width of < 4 mm [21].

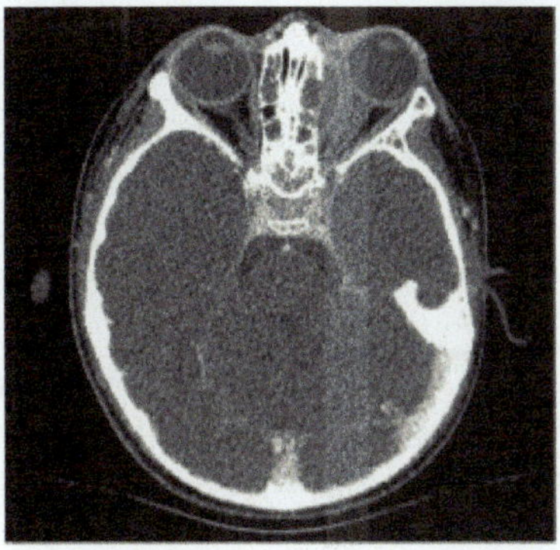

Figure 5. CT scan with contrast, axial, with demonstration of left subperiosteal abscess (enhancing rim).

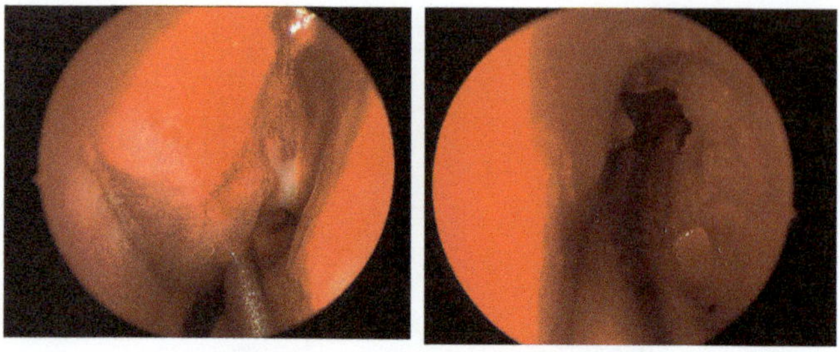

Figure 6. Left-Endoscopic view of left middle meatus with 0 degree telescope, purulence encountered in the ethmoid sinuses; Right-After endoscopic surgical removal of a portion of the lamina papyracea for drainage of the subperiosteal abscess, a blunt probe was placed through the defect. The left periorbita is immediately medial to the tip of the probe.

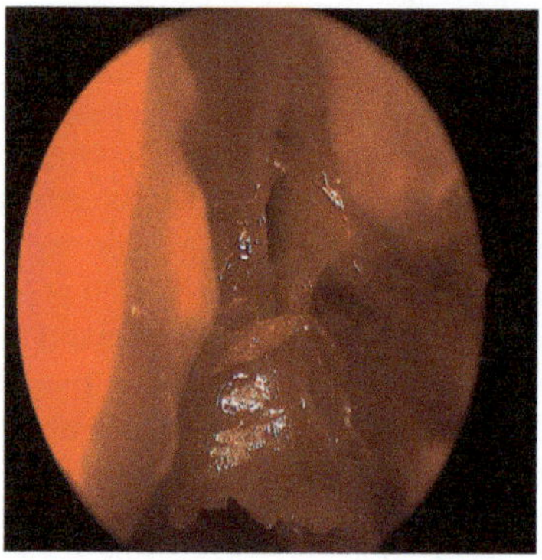

Figure 7. Endoscopic view with a 0 degree telescope of left lamina papyracea and periorbita, the instrument is on the periorbita after removal of a portion of the lamina papyracea. Using endoscopic visualization, an incison through the periorbita (parallel to the medial rectus muscle) could be made if orbital decompression was needed; this is an important consideration in cases of orbital cellulitis/abscess.

The recent trend in treatment for subperiosteal abscesses along the lamina has been to proceed with endoscopic treatment with external approaches reserved for treatment failures and abscess that are not accessible via the lamina [22]. Some authors suggest that patients who fail to improve 24 hours after endoscopic drainage could undergo re-imaging to see if they would benefit from an additinal drainage procedure [20]

7.3. Orbital abscess

When a post-septal infection organizes, an orbital abscess can occur. Orbital abscesses are accessible endoscopically by making an incision in the periorbita. Some orbital abscesses require an orbitotomy, which is an external incision to approach the intraorbital contents. Endoscopic treatment of the sinuses is important in addition to drainage of the abscess. Orbital abscesses are true emergencies as they are often associated with acute vision changes secondary to pressure on the optic nerve or vasospasm of the retinal artery.

7.4. Meningitis

Meinigitis can be seen in conjunction with other suppurative complications of sinusitis. Enhancement of the meninges is seen on CT or MRI if performed with contrast [14]. Meningitis as the sole complication of sinusitis does not always need to be treated with endoscopic surgery. Patients can be started on broad-spectrum antibiotics that cross the blood brain barrier and their clinical progress can be watched closely for 48 hours [23]. Any patient with bacterial meningitis needs to have a close follow-up with audiological testing as significant hearing loss can occur.

7.5. Epidural abscess

Epidural abscess is a collection of purulence external to the dural layer. For children with epidural abscesses due to paranasal sinus infections, there is some controversy as to the appropriate treatment. Some neurosurgeons feel that if the sinuses are addressed surgically and antibiotics are used, some patients may be able to avoid craniotomy, but this belief is not shared by all in the specialty [24]. Regardless of the exact surgical treatment modality (endoscopic treatment alone or in conjunction with craniotomy), it is important to treat patients with a multidisciplinary team that includes infectious disease, otolaryngology, and neurosurgery specialists.

7.6. Subdural empyema

Subdural empyema is a collection of purulence between the dura and arachnoid layers. It is considered to be a surgical emergency. Coordination between the neurosurgery and otolaryngology teams is paramount to address the collection via a craniotomy and to address the sinus disease that was causative via endoscopic sinus surgery [6, 25].

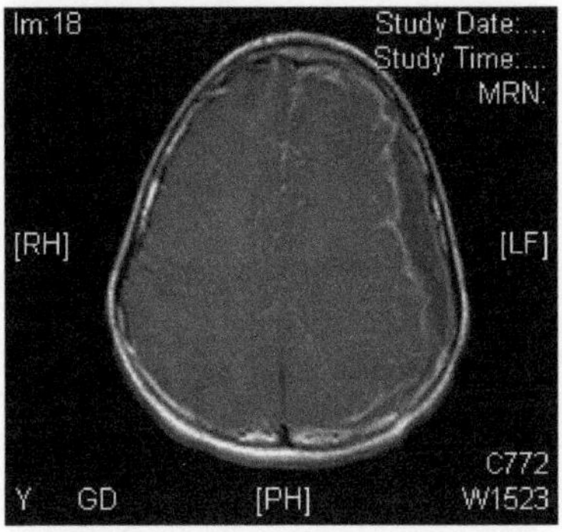

Figure 8. T1 contrast enhanced MRI showing large subdural empyema in left temporal-parietal region in a 9 year-old with mental status changes and paresis.

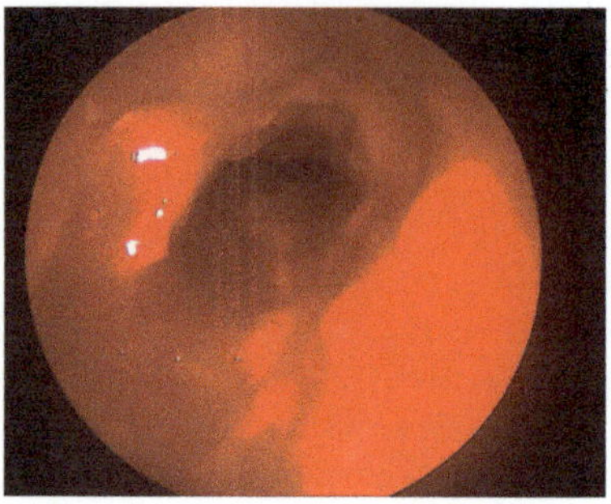

Figure 9. Endoscopic view of the right frontal recess using a 70 degree telescope, purulence was drained from the frontal sinus after craniotomy in this 9 year-old patient.

7.7. Intracerebral abcess

Cerebritis can be considered a pre-cursor of actual abscess within the brain parynchema. Cerebritis can be suggested on contrast-enhanced CT and also on MRI with ill-defined enhancement. Actual abscesses within the brain are best diagnosed with MRI and are at times difficult to distinguish from cystic tumors [14]. Intracerebral abscesses are most frequent in the frontal lobe adjacent to the frontal sinus [10]. In general, neurosurgical drainage of the intracranial abscess and endoscopic sinus surgery for any associated intranasal pathology are of the utmost importance.

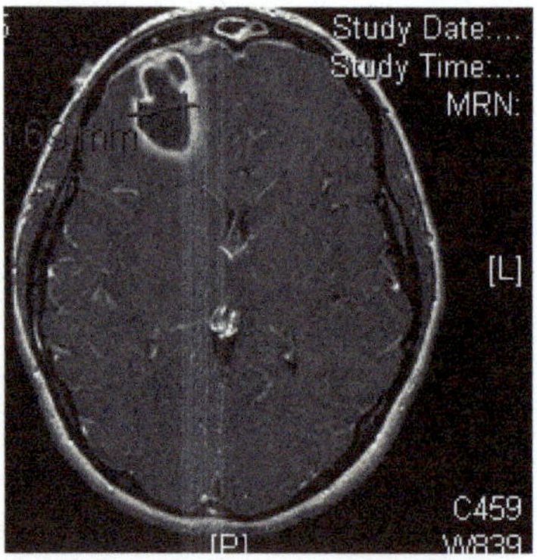

Figure 10. MRI with contrast, showing enhancing abscess within right frontal lobe.

7.8. Pott's Puffy/osteomyelitis

Pott's puffy "tumor" is an infectious complication of sinusitis involving frontal bone osteomyelitis with an associated frontal subperiosteal abscess that creates swelling of the forehead [26]. It can also be associated with intracranial abscesses in some cases. The etiology can be infection from sinus disease or due to trauma to the frontal bone resulting in a conduit for spread of infection. Medical management of sinus disease is a component of treatment, but surgical intervention is paramount. The approach to treat Pott's puffy tumor can be endoscopic with a frontal sinusotomy and anterior ethomidectomy, but a combined approach with an external incision may be required depending on the size of the subperiosteal abscess and whether or not there are associated intracranial complications. Following surgical treatment, patients will require prolonged courses of IV antibiotics until the osteomyelitis has resolved [27].

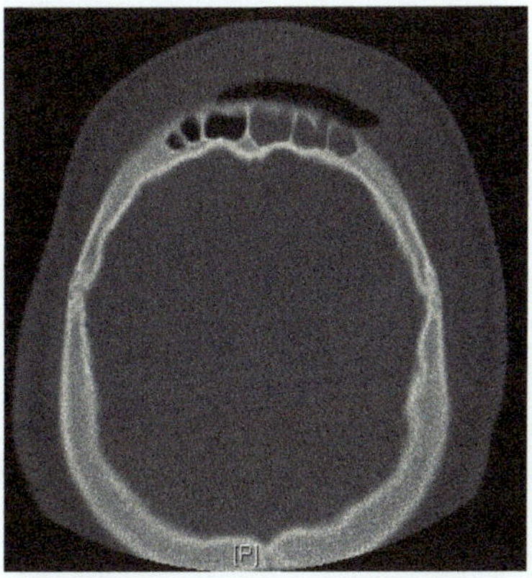

Figure 11. Axial CT showing left frontal sinus opacification and connection to scalp, consistent with Pott's Puffy. Approximately 80 mL of purulence was drained from the scalp abscess.

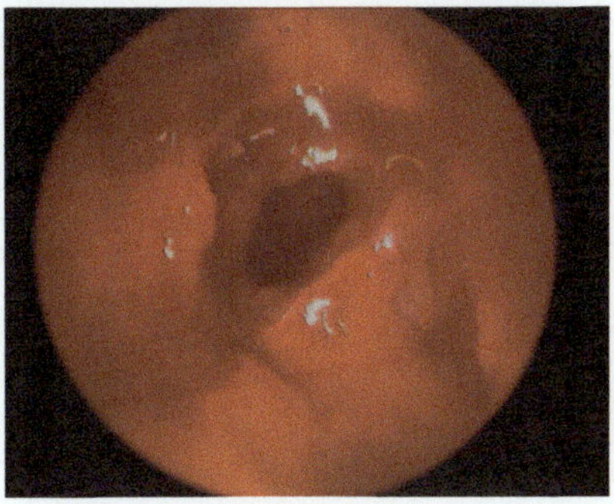

Figure 12. Endoscopic view of the left frontal sinus with a 70 degree telescope.

7.9. Cavernous sinus thrombosis

Cavernous sinus thrombosis can occur due to the spread of infection from the middle third of the face or from the sinuses and orbit due to the valveless venous system in the anatomical region [28]. Emergent drainage of any paranasal sinus or orbital infection is important in conjunction with intravenous antibiotics. Systemic anticoagulation is considered in all of these cases. Despite aggressive treatment, cavernous sinus thrombosis remains a life-threatening illness (in addition to causing to cranial neuropathy and blindness) that requires multidisciplinary care in an intensive care unit setting.

8. Complications of endoscopic sinus surgery

Major complications after endoscopic sinus surgery include CSF leak, orbital injury and hemorrhage. A recent retrospective study by Ramakrishnan *et al.* looked at overall rates of major complications after endoscopic sinus surgery. The overall rate of major complications across all age groups was 1%. This was divided among patients with CSF leak (0.17%), patients with orbital injuries (0.07%), and patients with significant hemorrhage that required blood transfusion (0.76%). This data represents significant improvement from previous retrospective analyses. When the complications were stratified by age, they found that CSF leak was less likely to occur in children, but orbital injury was more likely in the pediatric population. This likely stems from smaller maxillary sinuses and lower orbital floors in young children.

Concerns have been raised that sinus surgery in children could affect facial growth. An animal study looking at facial growth in piglets that underwent endoscopic sinus surgery revealed decreased facial growth on the operative side. This same study investigated the types of bone that were removed from pediatric patients who underwent endoscopic sinus surgery and noted that children less than 9 years old had immature bone in contrast to children over 9 years old and older who had more mature bone in their specimens [29].

A quantitative study in pediatric patients was performed by Senior *et al.* in order to evaluate facial growth using CT scan images and volumetric analysis. Their study looked at patients who underwent sinus surgery due to orbital cellulitis and abscess and re-evaluated the patients 4 to 10 years later. There was no statistically significant difference in sinus volume from the operated side to the non-operated side. However, a small difference in orbital volume was noted from the operated side to the non-operated side. Overall, they concluded that sinus surgery in children has minimal impact on sinus and facial growth [30].

9. Post-operative management

9.1. Inpatient

Patients with acute complicated sinusitis will require close monitoring after surgical intervention. Patients with intracranial involvement may require intensive care unit management until they show clinical improvement. These patients generally need multidisciplinary involvement including the surgical teams of neurosurgery, otolaryngology and ophthalmology as well as an infectious disease specialist. Serial opthalmological examinations are important to optimize visual outcomes when the orbit is involved. Given the consequences of persistent or recurrent infection, the threshold for repeat imaging and possible return to the operating room must remain low. Antibiotic therapy can be tailored to the particular culture results when available. Adjunctive therapy such as topical and systemic decongestants and nasal saline spray or irrigation are also of importance during this period.

9.2. Outpatient

Primary outpatient management of complicated acute sinusitis is not the standard of care. Once patients are stabilized clinically, they can often be treated with outpatient antibiotic regimens via PICC lines or in some cases be transitioned to an oral regimen. From the otolaryngologist's perspective, some children who have endoscopic sinus surgery may need to return to the operating room for debridement during the healing process. During the early years of endoscopic sinus surgery, taking children back to the operating room two to three weeks after surgery for debridement was the standard of care [31]. However, after further evaluation, this approach was found to have no benefit in terms of nasal obstruction, drainage or cough [32]. A secondary procedure in the operating room should be considered for select patients depending on how well they are able to irrigate as well as how easily they tolerate endoscopic exam and gentle debridement in the clinic. The threshold for return to the operating room for patients who underwent major dissections should be lower than for those who had more limited procedures [33]. Parents must be informed at the time of the initial surgery that multiple surgical procedures may be required. Surveillance of scar tissue formation, which is more common in the setting of acute infection, can be performed endoscopically in the office. If there is concern that the sinuses are not draining properly, revision surgery should be performed to prevent return of the previous complication.

10. Open surgical approaches

10.1. Lynch incision

Although intranasal approaches are frequently the preferred route for accessing the paranasal sinuses and the medial orbit, patients and their families should be counseled that external approaches to the anterior ethmoid region may be required. The Lynch approach leaves a scar that courses from the medial brow along the side of the nose but may be required in cases where the medial orbit cannot be accessed endoscopically due to severe edema or inflammatory tissues that interfere with endoscopic visualization.

10.2. Trephination

Trephination is another adjunctive external approach that is particularly helpful to access the frontal sinus. It requires a small external incision but can help minimize operating room time in patients that are clinically unstable. Additionally, a case series reported the use of mini-trephination of the frontal sinus with drain placement as a possible adjunct for patients with sinusitis complicated with intracranial infection [34]. An endoscope can also be used for improved visualization of the frontal sinus through the trephination and has been described by Jatana *et al.* to assist in repair of a subclinical CSF leak from an isolated posterior table frontal sinus fracture that caused recurrent meningitis in a pediatric patient [35].

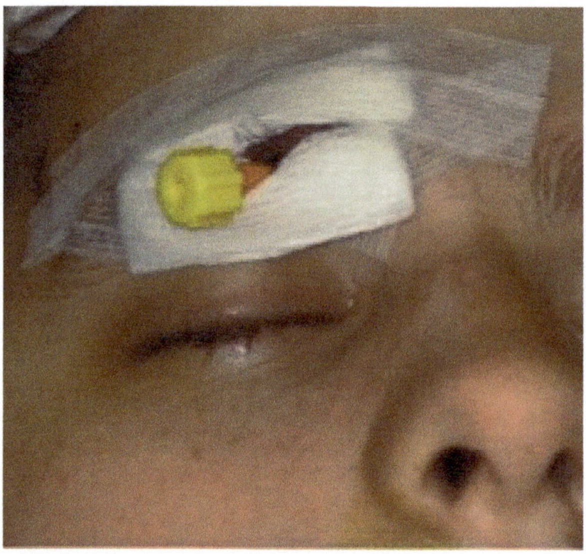

Figure 13. Right frontal sinus trephination performed in conjuction with an endoscopic approach and a drain for irrigation was placed into the right frontal sinus.

10.3. Transcaruncular

Another external approach that does not have the drawback of visible scarring is the transcaruncular approach. This approach is performed by making a transconjunctival incision just lateral or medial to the lacrimal caruncle and then dissecting to the anterior medial orbital wall. Dissection then continues by elevating the periorbita from the lamina until the abscess is accessed. This approach can be used in conjunction with endoscopic drainage of a subperiosteal abscess to ensure that the entire cavity is adequately drained and reduce the risk of recurrence [36].

11. Conclusion

Endoscopic surgical techniques are an important component of treatment for acute complicated sinusitis in the pediatric population. Given the diverse nature or presenting signs and symptoms, a high index of suspicion for complications of sinusitis must be maintained for patients presenting with complaints previously described. Using endoscopic approaches to the sinuses, the otolaryngologist is an important member of the multidisciplinary team that cares for patients with complications of sinusitis.

Author details

Timothy P. McEvoy[1], Charles A. Elmaraghy[1,2] and Kris R. Jatana[1,2]

*Address all correspondence to: Kris.Jatana@nationwidechildrens.org

1 Department of Pediatric Otolaryngology-Head and Neck Surgery, Nationwide Children's Hospital, Columbus, Ohio, USA

2 Department of Otolaryngology-Head and Neck Surgery, Wexner Medical Center at The Ohio State University, Columbus, Ohio, USA

References

[1] Kennedy DW.Functional endoscopic sinus surgery. Technique. Arch Otolaryngol. (1985). Epub 1985/10/01., 111(10), 643-9.

[2] Kennedy DW, Zinreich SJ, Rosenbaum AE, Johns ME.Functional endoscopic sinus surgery. Theory and diagnostic evaluation. Arch Otolaryngol. (1985). Epub 1985/09/01., 111(9), 576-82.

[3] Gross CW, Gurucharri MJ, Lazar RH, Long TE.Functional endonasal sinus surgery (FESS) in the pediatric age group. The Laryngoscope(1989). Epub 1989/03/01., 99(3), 272-5.

[4] al, R., & , . Embryology and Anatomy of the Paranasal Sinuses. 4th ed(2003).

[5] Adibelli, Z. H., Songu, M., & Adibelli, H. Paranasal sinus development in children: A magnetic resonance imaging analysis. American journal of rhinology & allergy. (2011). Epub 2011/06/30., 25(1), 30-5.

[6] Yucel, O. T., & Ogretmenoglu, O. Subdural empyema and blindness due to cavernous sinus thrombosis in acute frontal sinusitis. International journal of pediatric otorhinolaryngology(1998). Epub 1999/04/06., 121 EOF-5 EOF.

[7] Oxford, L. E., & Mc Clay, J. Complications of acute sinusitis in children. Otolaryngology--head and neck surgery : official journal of American Academy of Otolaryngology-Head and Neck Surgery(2005). Epub 2005/07/19., 133(1), 32-7.

[8] Lerner DN, Choi SS, Zalzal GH, Johnson DL.Intracranial complications of sinusitis in childhood. The Annals of otologyrhinology, and laryngology. (1995). Pt 1):Epub 1995/04/01., 288 EOF-93 EOF.

[9] DeMuri GP, Wald ER.Complications of acute bacterial sinusitis in children. The Pediatric infectious disease journal(2011). Epub 2011/07/14., 30(8), 701-2.

[10] Vazquez, E., Creixell, S., Carreno, J. C., Castellote, A., Figueras, C., Pumarola, F., et al. Complicated acute pediatric bacterial sinusitis: Imaging updated approach. Current problems in diagnostic radiology(2004). Epub 2004/06/25., 33(3), 127-45.

[11] Germiller JA, Monin DL, Sparano AM, Tom LW.Intracranial complications of sinusitis in children and adolescents and their outcomes. Archives of otolaryngology--head & neck surgery(2006). Epub 2006/09/20., 132(9), 969-76.

[12] Kombogiorgas, D., Seth, R., Athwal, R., Modha, J., & Singh, J. Suppurative intracranial complications of sinusitis in adolescence. Single institute experience and review of literature. British journal of neurosurgery(2007). Epub 2007/12/12., 21(6), 603-9.

[13] Hicks, C. W., Weber, J. G., Reid, J. R., & Moodley, M. Identifying and managing intracranial complications of sinusitis in children: a retrospective series. The Pediatric infectious disease journal(2011). Epub 2011/03/19., 30(3), 222-6.

[14] Reid JR.Complications of pediatric paranasal sinusitis. Pediatric radiology(2004). Epub 2004/07/28., 34(12), 933-42.

[15] Herrmann BW, Forsen JW, Jr.Simultaneous intracranial and orbital complications of acute rhinosinusitis in children. International journal of pediatric otorhinolaryngology(2004). Epub 2004/04/15., 68(5), 619-25.

[16] Parikh, S. R., Cuellar, H., Sadoughi, B., Aroniadis, O., & Fried, M. P. Indications for image-guidance in pediatric sinonasal surgery. International journal of pediatric otorhinolaryngology(2009). Epub 2009/01/23., 73(3), 351-6.

[17] Benoit, Silvera. V. M., Nichollas, R., Jones, D., Mc Gill, T., & Rahbar, R. Image guidance systems for minimally invasive sinus and skull base surgery in children. International journal of pediatric otorhinolaryngology(2009). Epub 2009/08/22., 73(10), 1452-7.

[18] Garrett, M. G. J., & Elmaraghy, Jatana. K. R. Radiographic findings in pediatric periorbital cellulitis. American Society of Pediatric Otolaryngology (ASPO); San Diego, California(2012).

[19] Jatana KR, Grischkan JM, Skomorowski MJ, Elmaraghy CA.Recurrent unilateral periorbital cellulitis in a pediatric patient--an anatomic abnormalit. y. International journal of pediatric otorhinolaryngology(2008). Epub 2008/08/16., 72(10), 1577-80.

[20] Noordzij JP, Harrison SE, Mason JC, Hashisaki GT, Reibel JF, Gross CW.Pitfalls in the endoscopic drainage of subperiosteal orbital abscesses secondary to sinusitis. American journal of rhinology(2002). Epub 2002/05/28., 16(2), 97-101.

[21] Oxford, L. E., & Mc Clay, J. Medical and surgical management of subperiosteal orbital abscess secondary to acute sinusitis in children. International journal of pediatric otorhinolaryngology(2006). Epub 2006/08/15., 70(11), 1853-61.

[22] Soon VT.Pediatric subperiosteal orbital abscess secondary to acute sinusitis: a 5-year review. American journal of otolaryngology. (2011). Epub 2009/12/25., 32(1), 62-8.

[23] Younis, R. T., Anand, V. K., & Childress, C. Sinusitis complicated by meningitis: current management. The Laryngoscope(2001). Epub 2001/09/25., 111(8), 1338-42.

[24] Heran, N. S., Steinbok, P., & Cochrane, D. D. Conservative neurosurgical management of intracranial epidural abscesses in children. Neurosurgery(2003). discussion 7-8. Epub 2003/10/02., 53(4), 893-7.

[25] Waseem, M., Khan, S., & Bomann, S. Subdural empyema complicating sinusitis. The Journal of emergency medicine(2008). Epub 2007/12/25., 35(3), 277-81.

[26] Blumfield, E., Misra, M., Pott's, puffy., tumor, intracranial., orbital, complications., the, initial., presentation, of., sinusitis, in., healthy, adolescents. a., & case, series. Emergency radiology(2011). Epub 2011/03/08., 18(3), 203-10.

[27] Parida, P. K., Surianarayanan, G., Ganeshan, S., & Saxena, S. K. Pott's puffy tumor in pediatric age group: A retrospective study. International journal of pediatric otorhinolaryngology(2012). Epub 2012/06/19.

[28] Cannon ML, Antonio BL, McCloskey JJ, Hines MH, Tobin JR, Shetty AK.Cavernous sinus thrombosis complicating sinusitis. Pediatric critical care medicine : a journal of the Society of Critical Care Medicine and the World Federation of Pediatric Intensive and Critical Care Societies(2004). Epub 2003/12/31., 5(1), 86-8.

[29] Mair EA, Bolger WE, Breisch EA.Sinus and facial growth after pediatric endoscopic sinus surgery. Archives of otolaryngology--head & neck surgery(1995). Epub 1995/05/01., 121(5), 547-52.

[30] Senior, B., Wirtschafter, A., Mai, C., Becker, C., & Belenky, W. Quantitative impact of pediatric sinus surgery on facial growth. The Laryngoscope(2000). Epub 2000/11/18., 110(11), 1866-70.

[31] Mair EA.Pediatric functional endoscopic sinus surgery: postoperative care. Otolaryngologic clinics of North America(1996). Epub 1996/02/01., 29(1), 207-19.

[32] Mitchell RB, Pereira KD, Younis RT, Lazar RH.Pediatric functional endoscopic sinus surgery: is a second look necessary? The Laryngoscope. (1997). Epub 1997/09/18., 107(9), 1267-9.

[33] Cable BB, Mair EA.Pediatric functional endoscopic sinus surgery: frequently asked questions. The Annals of otologyrhinology, and laryngology. (2006). Epub 2006/10/19., 115(9), 643-57.

[34] Mc Intosh, D. L., & Mahadevan, M. Frontal sinus mini-trephination for acute sinusitis complicated by intracranial infection. International journal of pediatric otorhinolaryngology(2007). Epub 2007/07/14., 71(10), 1573-7.

[35] Jatana, K. R., Ryoo, C., Skomorowski, M., Butler, N., & Kang, D. R. Minimally invasive repair of an isolated posterior table frontal sinus fracture in a pediatric patient. Otolaryngology--head and neck surgery : official journal of American Academy of Otolaryngology-Head and Neck Surgery. (2008). Epub 2008/05/28., 138(6), 809-11.

[36] Pelton RW, Smith ME, Patel BC, Kelly SM.Cosmetic considerations in surgery for orbital subperiosteal abscess in children: experience with a combined transcaruncular and transnasal endoscopic approach. Archives of otolaryngology--head & neck surgery(2003). Epub 2003/06/18., 129(6), 652-5.

Chapter 8

Endoscopy - An Advancement in Sinus and Skull Base Surgery

Rickul Varshney, Faisal Zawawi, Marc A Tewfik and Saul Frenkiel

Additional information is available at the end of the chapter

1. Introduction

Skull base and sinus surgery has evolved dramatically throughout the past century. It is not long ago that the maxillary sinus would principally be reached via an anterior approach through the gingivobuccal sulcus of the oral cavity. The earliest days of endoscopy date back to the early 1900s, when Hirschmann used a modified cystoscope to examine the sinuses. Thereafter, modern endoscopy has seen advances not only in the types of endoscopes available, but also the types of interventions amenable to the endoscopic approach.

However, even in this modern era of refined endoscopic instrumentation and technique, opinion remains split regarding the optimal approach to certain areas of the skull base. For example, areas such as the anterior cranial fossa and the infratemporal fossa are often approached through external transcutaneous approaches despite the development of adequate and safe transnasal endoscopic pathway.

The current chapter aims to provide a complete comparison of endoscopic versus open approaches of routinely performed sinus and skull base surgical procedures. It will also emphasize the advantages of endoscopy versus traditional approaches for sinus and skull base surgery, including management of tumors, infectious processes, congenital anomalies and traumatic injuries.

2. Evolution of endoscopic sinus surgery

2.1. History of the emergence of endoscopes

The historical evolution of endoscopic sinus surgery is quite fascinating. Hippocrates can be considered one of the first practitioners of rhinology. He was one of the first to document treatment of nasal polyps using snares or sponges on a string.[1] Thereafter, there were many ancient rhinology physicians that contributed to the evolution of rhinology, however we will focus on the evolution of endoscopic sinus surgery in this chapter.

The first reports of endoscopic visualization of the sinuses date back to 1901 when Hirschman used a small cystoscope with an electric bulb to examine the maxillary sinus through an oroantral fistula.[2] Thereafter, in 1902, Reichert performed the first known endoscopic sinus surgery, performing maxillary sinus manipulation through an oroantral fistula.[3] Continuing this trend, in 1922, Spielberg employed antroscopes to access the maxillary sinus via the inferior meatus.[2] The term "sinuscopy" was later popularized by Maltz in 1925.[2]

At that time, these endoscopes were not surprisingly restricted in terms of optical quality, field of view and illumination, relying on flame or electric bulbs.[2] In the 1960s, Hopkins developed the rod optic endoscope. Hopkins, also known for the development of the fiber optic gastroscope and zoom lens for cameras, revolutionized the optical quality available to surgeons.[3] Thereafter, Karl Storz in Germany created angled endoscopes ranging from 0 to 120 degrees, thus allowing visualization of a field of view never previously imagined.[2]

In the 1970s, this new and exciting armamentarium of endoscopic tools allowed surgeons such as Messerklinger, Stammberger, Draf and Wigand to transition sinus surgery from a radical operation to a minimally invasive procedure.[2,3] In 1978, Messerklinger published the landmark reference "Endoscopy of the nose", due to large part from this remarkable evolution in endoscopic sinus surgery tools. He thoroughly examined the mucociliary clearance pattern and endoscopic changes of the osteomeatal complex,[3] thus further understanding sinus disease.

At that time, Draf published his own work on the sinuses and it was his experience that made frontal sinus access more realistic and safe.[4] Stammberger was also enthusiastic and prominent in the field of endoscopic surgery and popularized Messerklinger's ideas worldwide. The immense work of these pioneers remodeled sinus surgery. The principle of treating sinus disease from a functional point of view at the site of obstruction replaced the traditional mucosal stripping approach to treat inflammatory disease.[3] This work led to the term "functional endoscopic sinus surgery," which was coined by Kennedy in 1985.[2] In the same year, the first two established courses in North America on endoscopic sinus surgery were given at the Johns Hopkins Hospital.[3]

Furthermore, more contemporary surgeons, following the work of the pioneers of rhinology, expanded the limits to which nasal endoscopy could treat disease. Areas of the skull base were also accessed and different types of procedures amenable to this approach revolutionized the field of rhinology. The first description of trans-sphenoidal approach to the sellar region dates back to 1907, perfored by Schloffer.[4,5] Another prominent surgeon, Cushing, performed this procedure for many years, but abandoned this approach in 1927 due to the high complication rate. The procedure rapidly lost popularity until Dott, a disciple of Cushing, created a lighted speculum as an aid for trans-sphenoidal visualization.[6] In the 1960s, Guiot, a disciple of Dott, popularised this approach.[4] He was the first neurosurgeon to perform transsphenoidal surgery.[6]

In 1967, Jules Hardy reported the use of the surgical microscope for transsphenoidal surgery.[5]He is credited for developing the fundamental principles of pituitary surgery upto this day.[5] Jankowski published the first series on endoscopic pituitary surgery procedures in 1992.[7] The term "functional endoscopic pituitary surgery" was coined by Cappabianca and de Divitiis.[6]

However, the endoscopic approach to the skull base didn't end at the sella region. Weiss, in 1987, was the first to publish about extending the transsphenoidal approach to access suprasellar lesions.[5] Thereafter, the first report of endoscopic transsphenoidal approach for resection of a large clivus chordoma was published in 1996 by Jho.[8] More contemporary surgeons have continued this endoscopic advacement towards the skull base with new approaches to areas such as the infratemporal fossa and the anterior cranial fossa.

With the evolution of endoscopes, also came an evolution in surgical instruments used in sinus surgery. Early endoscopic surgery was performed using grasping forceps, which often stripped mucosa and denuded bone. At first, this was considered ideal as the theory of removing all the diseased mucosa was preached. However, with endoscopes, surgeons were able to visualize the sinuses on post-operative follow-ups and discover the osteitis, scarring and osteoneogenesis that their surgery had caused. Thus, there was a movement to create new endoscopic fine-cutting instruments, originally developped for orthopedic cartilage work, to perform minimally invasive "functional" surgery. Later, an evolutionary descendent of the through cutting instruments, was the emergence of the microdebrider, also originally used in orthopedics. Setliff and Parsons introduced the microdebrider to sinonasal surgery.[3]

It is important to emphasize the work of pioneers such as Messerklinger, Draf, Wigand and others as a focal transition point in the medical community's understanding of sinus disease. In fact, before their reports, sinus disease treatment was based on an invasive exenterative approach of removing all the inflammed mucosa of the sinuses. The main focus of treatment was to obliterate and remove all the sinonasal regions of disease. However, the work of these legendary surgeons allowed physicians to understand the functional aspect of sinus anatomy. They demonstrated that a large amount of sinus disease was based on an impairment of adequate drainage and that resolution of the latter obstruction would allow symptomatic relief.

This concept of mucosal preservation still applies today and is the basis of a large portion of rhinology practice. In fact, rhinologists are careful to avoid mucosal stripping that can potentially cause impaired mucociliary clearance or neo-osteogenesis.[9] This has motivated the development of precise instrumentation including sharp through-cutters and microdebriders that mimise trauma to adjacent healthy tissue.

2.2. Endoscopes of the 21ST century

Endoscopes today have offered sinus surgeons the ability to increase the potential applications of endoscopic sinus surgery. There is a strong movement by manufacturers to improve optical quality of their endoscopes. One such improvement is the use of the xenon light, which was an upgrade to the halogen light source, with advantages such as durability, diminished heat production and energy consumption. Another improvement is the diameter of the endoscopes with some available as small as 2 mm. The most common scopes currently employed in sinus and skull base surgery are 4 mm in diameter by 20 cm long; 2.7 mm diameter scopes are commonly reserved for pediatric cases. These scopes are available in various angles ranging from 0 to 30, 45, and 70 degrees and provide high quality imaging.[9]

Furthermore, there have been improvements in the processing camera used for endocopic surgery. Modern cameras have gone from 1 silicone chip to 3 silicone chip cameras in order to process the three primary colors [red, blue and green] as a means to enhance contrast and balance of the projected image.[2] High definition cameras have replaced traditional cameras, working through a progressive scanning mechanism instead of an interlaced scanning manner. This refers to the way each frame is scanned by the camera, and results in an upgrade of 60 frames per second being seen by the high definition cameras instead of 30 frames per second provided by the older generation. The previously used interlaced scanning provided a significant amount of flickering, which was compensated by image blurring.

Finally, as the image viewed is dependent on the resolution of the monitor, even the latter has evolved dramatically. With the advent of high definition monitors, 16:9 aspect ratio has replaced the traditional 4:3 aspect ratio provided by standard definition monitors, translating in an increase in pixel density from 640x480 to 1929x1080.[2] What this means for the surgeon is better color, contrast, resolution and peripheral visualization of the surgical field.

3. Endoscopic surgery versus open traditional approach

Sinus surgery traditionally was performed via open approaches, be it a Caldwell-Luc procedure for the maxillary sinus or an osteoplastic flap approach to the frontal sinus. With the advent of the endoscopes, these traditional invasive extenterative methods have largely been replaced by functional endoscopic sinus surgery. In this section, we examine the different sinuses and contrast these approaches.

3.1. Frontal sinus

The first report of frontal sinus surgery was by Rimge in 1750, where he used an external approach to obliterate the sinus.[10] In 1884, Ogston and Luck described an anterior wall perforation technique using a trephine to create a drainage pathway into the anterior ethmoid cells.[10,11] Thereafter, in 1891, Kuhnt proposed anterior wall ablation.[11] Similarly, in 1893, Jansen published his procedure where he removed the floor of the frontal sinus and collapsed the anterior table against the posterior wall.[10] The latter procedure was elaborated by Reidel-Schenke who promoted breaking down the anterior and inferior walls of the sinus and collapsing the skin of the forehead against the posterior wall.

	Traditional Approach	New Approach
Frontal Sinus	Osteoplastic flap	Frontal Drillout
Maxillary Sinus	Caldwell-Luc	Endoscopic Antrostomy
Ethmoid Sinus	External ethmoidectomy	Endoscopic ethmoidectomy
Sphenoid Sinus	Transantral approach	Endoscopic sphenoidotomy

Table 1. Comparison of traditional and new approaches to the paranasal sinuses.

Later in that decade, Schonborn and Brieger performed frontal osteoplastic flaps. As one can imagine, these were associated with poor cosmetic results. Thus, in the early 1900s, transorbital approaches were attempted to access the frontal sinus. Knapp was a pioneer in this access way, performing one of the first external frontoethmoidectomies through the medial orbital wall, resecting the frontal sinus floor and preserving the frontal duct. The latter was made famous by Lynch in 1921.[10]

At that time, intranasal access was also attempted, but the poor visual field caused a large amount of intracranial complications and deaths. It was thus abandoned for other approaches until the emergence of endoscopes. In 1991, Draf published his experience with transnasal frontoethmoidal surgery using a microscope.[12] He published variations on the dissection of the frontal recess and floor, known today as the Draf 1, 2 or 3 procedures. With his descriptions and the advent of the endoscope, the often disfiguring open approaches were largely replaced by transnasal minimally invasive accesses. Today, angled telescopes and angled instruments produce success rates equal to the traditional morbid procedures with decreased morbidity.[12]

Along with better cosmesis, endoscopy is associated with decreased morbidity, preservation of mucociliary drainage and decreased hospital stay.[10] The disadvantages include potential difficulties in managing complications such as severe bleeding and in achieving margins for malignant lesions. Also, large lesions affecting the fronto-ethmoidal region may need to be managed by an osteoplastic flap technique, lateral rhinotomy or anterior direct approach.[11,13]

Open surgery has the advantage of a wide field of view, better management of complications and an increased ease of obtaining adequate margins for malignant lesions. The disadvantages are longer hospital stay, increased morbidity including possible injury to the superior branches of the facial nerve. However, although endoscopic sinus surgery of the frontal sinus is often highly effective, certain select cases nevertheless still require open approaches with osteoplasties.

3.2. Maxillary sinus

The first descriptions of open approaches to the maxillary sinus date back to the early 1700s. Over a century later, in 1893, in the United States, Caldwell described an anterior approach via an incision in the gingivobuccal sulcus coupled with an inferior antrostomy. This procedure was almost simultaneously popularized in Europe by Luc, and was later coined the Caldwell-Luc procedure.[14] A century after that, Stammberger and then Kennedy introduced the middle meatus antrostomy in the 1980s.[15] At that time, inferior and middle meatal antrostomies were being performed by different group of surgeons. When compared, middle meatal antrostomies demonstrate better resolution of symptoms and longer patency rates.[14] The reason for this is believed to be the fact that the normal mucociliary clearance patterns of the maxillary sinus tend to move secretions toward the natural ostium in the midle meatus, and not toward the inferior meatal antrostomy.

With the emergence of endoscopes, especially angled telescopes to look within the maxillary sinus, as well as the development of the coronal bone view on CT scans in 1987, the approach to the maxillary sinus changed dramatically. A study performed by Penttila et al. demonstrated that patients undergoing surgery for chronic maxillary sinusitis reported improvement in 50.7% of the Caldwell-Luc group and in 76.7% of the endoscopic sinus surgery group.[16] Also, higher complication rates have been described in patients undergoing the Caldwell-Luc procedure.[17] These include pain, facial swelling and numbness, dental numbness, persistent oroantral fistulas, wound dehiscence, dacrocystitis, tooth decay, persistent symptoms and bleeding.[15]

Although endoscopic surgery has largely replaced Caldwell-Luc procedures, there is still a role for the latter in certain cases. Cutler et al. performed the procedure in 37 patients who had failed endoscopic sinus surgery for refractory sinusitis and reported a 92% response based on follow-up endoscopic examination or computed tomography scan imaging.[18] Other possible indications include the removal of dentigerous cyst and benign tumors located within the maxillary sinus.

3.3. Ethmoid sinus

The management of ethmoid sinus disease has been the source of a lot of controversy in the past. Many surgical methods for ethmoidectomies have been described, ranging from intranasal, transantral, external approaches employing a headlight, to endoscopic approaches.

In 1912, Mosher described intranasal extirpation of the ethmoid labyrinth.[19] He promoted the complete resection of the middle turbinate along with the ethmoid sinuses, which was debated by opposing surgeons, including Pratt. The latter preached the importance of the middle turbinate as a landmark to reduce operative morbidity.

In 1929, Mosher and Smith, a well-known rhinologist, promoted a transition towards an external approach as means to reduce complications.[19] At the same time, other surgeons promoted a transantral approach, originally described by Jansen in the 1800s. All these approaches were being practiced without any consensus as to the optimal technique.

The transnasal approach, which was popularized by Mosher, consisted of progressive exenteration of the ethmoid air calls in antero-posterior direction. As mentioned, certain surgeons removed the middle turbinate as well. Along with the ethmoidectomy, the nasofrontal duct was also unroofed. In this method, the procedure was performed through a nasal speculum with a headlight. Magnification was provided by loupes or insertion of lenses onto the headlight. Certain surgeons, namely Dixon and Heermann, advocated the use of microscopes during the transnasal approach to the ethmoids.[19] However, the high incidence of complications and the availability of the transantral and external approaches, caused this method to fall in popularity over the next few decades.[19]

These procedures have all been replaced by endoscopic sinus surgery. The latter permits controlled removal of the diseased tissue and obstructing bony partitions in a stepwise fashion, with decreased complications. Ethmoidectomies are also commonly performed in conjunction with other procedures, thus a vast access with the endoscope is essential.

3.4. Sphenoid sinus

The history, indications and approaches to the sphenoid sinus will be discussed in details in the skull base section. The open, microscopic approach versus the endoscopic approach to sphenoid sinus surgery and access to the skull base will be contrasted.

4. Septoplasty

Apart from the sinuses, the nasal septum is also amenable to open or endoscopic surgery. In 1842, Langenbeck first described the entities of septal crests and spurs.[1] Thereafter, in the early 1900s, Freer published about the removal of thickened portions of the septal cartilage. He invented a number of instruments to perform this procedure. Simultaneously, Killian further developed many of the techniques of septal surgery.[1]

Cottle first described septoplasty in 1947 to treat nasal obstruction.[20] It is only in 1991 that the endoscopic technique to treat septal deformities was first popularized by Lanza et al. and Stammberger.[21] Thereafter, Lanza described isolated septal spur surgery using endoscopic access.[21,22]

Advantages over the open technique include targeted approach to the septal deformity, limited mucosal flap dissection, superior magnification of the field and less physical distortion as there is no need of a nasal speculum. Finally, it is a superior teaching tool as trainees can visualize the surgery on a screen in real-time.[23] Furthermore, endoscopic visualization allows assessment of deformities in the nasal valve region and posterior septum.[21]

Proponents of endoscopic surgery advocate the minimally invasive aspect of this approach as only the mucosa overlying the deviated segment is elevated through a Killian incision.

This may explain why authors have reported higher degrees of septal tears with the open technique.[23] This is particularly useful in revision cases, where fibrosis adheres the septal mucosa in areas previously operated. Other advantages of the endoscopic approach include shorter operative time, decreased bleeding, decreased pain[24,25] and decreased synechiae formation.[20]

Rotenberg's group recently demonstrated that there was no difference in post-operative outcomes in terms of nasal obstruction between both groups,[23] in support of previous surgeons' findings.[25] However, other authors have stated significant differences in nasal symptoms with endoscopic groups doing better in follow-up assessments.[20,24]

The endoscopic septoplasty has gained popularity in recent years. Nevertheless, certain cases still require an open approach. The relative contraindications to endoscopic septoplasty are when the deformity involves a deflection of the caudal septal cartilage, and when external nasal deformities require a concomitant open rhinoplasty.[20,21]

5. Skull base

Through the years, the work of Messerklinger and other pioneers in nasal endoscopy helped to develop functional endoscopic sinus surgery as a means to treat sinus disease from a mechanical point of view. However, contemporary surgeons have expanded the limits to which nasal endoscopy can treat disease. In fact, the areas of the skull base accessible and the types of procedures amenable to this approach have revolutionized the field of rhinology.

Traditional methods required external skin incisions, translocation of the cranium or maxillofacial skeleton and retraction of the brain.[26] Endoscopic access is based on modular anatomical approaches in the sagittal planes, for anterior cranial fossa, pituitary, and transclival posterior cranial fossa surgery; and coronal planes, for pterygopalatine fossa and infratemporal fossa surgery.[27]

Endoscopic endonasal approaches have improved visualization and decreased collateral trauma to the craniofacial tissues. They provide faster healing and recovery time, decreased neurovascular injuries, complete oncologic resections and better endocrinologic outcomes. Potential limitations of the endoscopic approach include location, extent and nature of the disease and importantly surgeon expertise and available equipment, including image guidance.[26]

There are multiple approaches available to the skull base depending on the location of the disease, namely the transcribriform, transsellar, transplanum [drilling the planumsphenoidale and the tuberculum sellae, transclival and the transodontoid approaches.[6] The latter apply to sagittal plane. In terms of coronal plane, the skull base can be divided into medial petrous apex, petroclival region, Meckel's cave, cavernous sinus and infratemporal fossa.[6]

In this section, we explore endoscopic surgery as it relates to the pituitary gland, the anterior cranial fossa, the clivus and the infratemporal fossa.

	Traditional Approach	New Approach
Sella	Open microscope	Endoscopic transsphenoid
Anterior cranial fossa/ Suprasellar area	Craniofacial approach	Endonasal endoscopic approach
Clivus	Traditional clival approach	Endoscopic transclival approach
Infratemporal fossa	Transtemporal/Transmaxillary approach	Endoscopic transmaxillary approach

Table 2. Comparison of traditional and new approaches to the skull base.

5.1. Pituitary surgery

Sir Victor Horsley performed the first transcranial pituitary operation in 1889.[5] It is only in the next century that the first description of trans-sphenoidal approach to the sellar region was made, dating back to 1907, performed by Schloffer.[4,5] Another prominent surgeon, Cushing, performed this procedure for many years, using a sublabial approach, but abandoned this approach in 1927 due to the high complication rate and difficult nature of the surgery.

Simultaneously, Hirsch, an Otolaryngologist in Vienna, introduced the technique that is the basis of today's surgical practice. He made a submucosal resection of the nasal septum, then opened the sphenoid sinus and resected the sphenoid septum. He then perforated the floor of the sella and the dura.[5] After Cushing abandoned the transsphenoidal technique, it rapidly lost popularity until Dott, a disciple of Cushing, created a lighted speculum as an aid for trans-sphenoidal visualization.[6] In the 1960s, Guiot, a French surgeon and a disciple of Dott, gave new life to this approach.[4] He was the first neurosurgeon to perform transsphenoidal surgery.[6]

The use of the surgical microscope by Jules Hardy in 1967 was a major step in transsphenoidal surgery.[5] It allowed better illumination, provided magnification and stereoscopic visualization. His contribution credits him with developing the fundamental principles of pituitary surgery upto this day.[5] In 1992, Jankowski published the first series on endoscopic pituitary surgery procedures.[7] Later, Jho standardized the procedure.[4] Thereafter, Cappabianca and de Divitiis coined the term "functional endoscopic pituitary surgery" and developed improved instrumentation.[6]

Endoscopic access is considered by many to be superior to traditional neurosurgical access.[28] Currently, the technique involves posterior septectomy, followed by bilateral anterior sphenoidotomies, sellar floor resection and dural incision. This provides improved field of view around the tumor, as well as better magnification.[4] Some authors promote that tumor resection using the endoscope is superior to the microscope because of the improved view resulting from the magnification, illumination and angled views that modern telescopes provide.[29,30] Moreover, Graham and colleagues demonstrated significant superior rhinology-specific quality of life after the endoscopic approach.[29]

With the increasing popularity of trans-sphenoidal sellar surgery, the concept of approaching parasellar regions through this pathway gained massive enthusiasm. Weiss, in 1987, was the first to publish about extending the transsphenoidal approach to access suprasellar lesions.[5] Therefore, anterior cranial fossa lesions, for example craniopharyngiomas, can be well managed through endoscopic routes.[31]

Compared to traditional approaches, transsphenoidal approaches for craniopharyngiomas and Rathke's cyst of the anterior cranial fossa demonstrate lower recurrence rate and decreased complications.[4,32] Couldwell and colleagues published about 105 patients undergoing extended transsphenoidal approaches to the cavernous sinus, suprasellar region and clival region. They concluded this approach to be a safe alternative to cranial approaches.[33] This approach has the advantage of less operative time, less brain manipulation and thus, decreased infarction and decreased neurovascular risk.

Exclusive endoscopic transsphenoidal technique, without an accompanying microscope, was described in the 1990s.[34] Jho and Carrau, considered the pioneers of the pure endoscopic endonasal approach, published a series of patients in 1997.[5,34] An advantage of the improved visualization with the endoscope over the microscope includes the decreased need of fluoroscopy intraoperatively, as vital structures are more easily identified.

5.2. Anterior cranial fossa

Among the most recent advances in skull base surgery is the fully endoscopic approach for lesions of the anterior cranial fossa. These include esthesioneuroblastomas, olfactory groove meningiomas, and select sinonasal malignancies with extension to the skull base. Devaiah and colleagues published a meta-analysis of articles with patients undergoing resection of esthesioneuroblastomas.[35] They found that there was a significantly greater survival rate for endoscopic resections versus open surgery. However, patients undergoing open resections had higher tumor stage thus biasing results to a certain degree.[35] This, however, is secondary to the mentality of a number of surgeons who believe that larger tumors should be resected via an open approach. Komotar and colleagues similarly demonstrated better resection of tumors in the endoscopic group.[36] They also demonstrated better results in terms of post-operative CSF leaks and recurrence rates.

The concern of adequacy of piecemeal resections of neoplasms obtained via the endoscopic approach has been a motivating factor for many surgeons to prefer an open approach for certain tumors. However, Wellman and colleagues presented cases of malignancies of the paranasal sinuses that either underwent en-bloc resection or piecemeal resection through an anterior craniofacial approach.[37] They demonstrated less complication and improved survival in the piecemeal group with an average follow-up of over four years. Thus, given the recent experience of surgeons with these tumors, the current practice for esthesioneuroblastoma is to obtain negative margins, regardless of which approach is utilized.[36,38]

Cushing was one of the first to report the resection of olfactory groove meningiomas through a unilateral frontal craniotomy.[39] Thereafter, other approaches such as a wide bifrontal craniotomy, a pterional approach and more recently the endoscopic pathway have been described.

The advantages of the open approaches, consisting of the bifrontal or unilateral frontal craniotomy, include wide exposure for large tumor resection. Other than the risk to neurovascular structures such as the optic nerves, the disadvantages are the need to retract the brain, thus a potential for cerebral infarction[40] and brain edema resulting in brain herniation into the craniotomy window. The latter may even sometimes necessitate a partial frontal lobectomy.[39] Furthermore the open approach limits access to the sellar, suprasellar and retrochiasmal regions.[40]

The pterional approach is a more recent approach that doesn't require frontal sinus transections and thus the risk of CSF leaks. However, it does not provide a good field of view due to its narrow pathway and may require a lot of brain retraction.[39]

The endoscopic 2-surgeon technique has replaced the open approach to anterior cranial fossa meningiomas in certain cases. In their review, Komotar and colleagues found that meningiomas were the most challenging in terms of isolated endoscopic approach, thus demonstrating a need for more research and technical innovation. Wormald's group published a large series on endoscopic resections of anterior cranial fossa meningiomas.[40] They demonstrated complete resections in over 90% of cases. Other then the obvious cosmetic benefit of the endoscopic approach, another advantage is the avoidance of brain retraction. Furthermore, this access allows the surgeon to identify the dural attachment of the meningioma early in the procedure and thus minimise bleeding.[40] Another major benefit is that the main site of recurrence, namely the anterior cranial fossa bone floor, is adequately resected in order to visualize the mass.[39] It is known that recurrence of these tumors is thought to be prevented by proper resection of surrounding bone and dura, which is more easily performed by endoscopic access. Also, similarly to other skull base resections, the angled endoscopes allow superior visualization of the tumor and the surrounding vital structures.

In terms of CSF leak post-endoscopic resections, Wormald's group demonstrated a decrease in incidence with use of the vascularized pedicled septal flap.[40] Cases where the endoscopic approach may not be suitable include those with major optic canal extension or encasement of the internal carotid or anterior communicating arteries.[40]

5.3. Clivus

Traditionally, clival lesions were treated through an anterior approach, necessitating large facial incisions and significant brain retraction. In fact, clivus region lesions often necessitated extensive dissections such as transfacial maxillotomy, lateral transcranial skull base approaches, transoral approaches and petrosal approaches.[41,42] However, despite these wide facelifts, the view of this region was still limited.

The use of endonasal microscopic transsphenoidal approach has also been described.[43] However, the narrow field of view doesn't expose the petrous apex, optic canal, parasellar region, lower clivus, and ventral craniocervical junction adequately.[44] Furthermore, the close proximity of vital structures such as the carotid arteries, the basilar arteries, the brainstem and the cavernous sinuses make resection even more difficult and dangerous.

Despite the obvious cosmetic complications of these open approaches, there was also significant risk of neurovascular injury, cerebral infarction, carotid artery and optic nerve injury.[44] Furthermore, the transoral approach involved splitting the palate, with the potential for velopharyngeal insufficiency.

Considering the above, endoscopic techniques were tried with improved illumination, magnification, as well as wider field of view which are essential in the narrow space of work. The first report of endoscopic transsphenoidal approach for resection of a large chordoma was published in 1996 by Jho.[8] Thereafter, this technique has been reported by several surgeons for the clivus.[42,45]

Another advantage of the endoscopic technique relates to the theory of surgical seeding of chordoma tumor cells during dissection. Thus, it is not surprising that traditional methods with extensive tissue dissection have conferred a high recurrence rate.[44] In order to avoid the latter, dissection should be limited to the shortest distance possible. This is provided through a transnasal route, as the floor of the nasal cavity is at the level of the inferior border of the clivus.[42] Finally, some may feel that the endonasal route may lead to increased intracranial infections. However, authors have shown that the incidence of meningitis did not increase after endonasal approach with antibiotics.[46]

The experience of our institution with endoscopic endonasal approaches to this region has been quite positive. This has been echoed by other authors who have demonstrated that regions such as the clivus[27] and petrous apex[27,47] are well accessible endoscopically. However, in our experience, certain cases may require a combined approach with a craniotomy, such as tumors with a large intradural component. Thus, careful pre-operative planning with imaging is essential in these cases with the two key components of decision making being safety and adequate resection of the tumor.

5.4. Infratemporal fossa

Authors have described the Caldwell-Luc procedure[48], a trans-facial access[49,50] and trans-oral approach[51] to access the infratemporal fossa abscesses. For tumors of this region, peri-auricular, transtemporal and transmaxillary approaches have been described.[52,53] However, these approaches are associated with significant complications such as facial nerve dysfunction, facial deformities, conductive hearing loss and dental malocclusion.[54]

With the rising use of endonasal approaches to the skull base, many surgeons have started to perform adequate resections of ITF tumors through the nasal cavity. There are multiple variations described to achieve access to the ITF such as the transseptal approach[54], the use of Denker's approach and different degrees of turbinate resection.[55] The indications for endoscopic approach to the ITF are evolving, however there no established contraindications.

At our institution, our method consists of performing a medial maxillectomy with a tailored resection of the nasal turbinates. We also prefer the 2-surgeon transseptal technique for tumor resection, achieved using a contralateral Killian incision and an ipsilateral horizontal mucosal incision after removal of a window of cartilage. The transseptal technique was reinforced by Robinson et al. who described that a key aspect of endoscopic removal of disease in the ITF is the ability of a second surgeon to apply traction to the tumor.[54]

6. Future

During the past three decades, the world has witnessed an immense evolution in rhinological practice. However, there is a lot more developments that are being trialed even today. In fact, there are multiple researchers and surgeons attempting to innovate the field of rhinology through various new tools and procedures. In this section, we focus on 3-dimensional endoscopes and robotics.

Similar to our colleagues in urology and head and neck oncology, rhinologists have attempted to use new tools to ameliorate our approach to the skull base. Many innovators have attempted to develop adequate three-dimensional endoscopic technology but no commercially-viable technology has been created. Attempted techniques include two channel endoscopes, image splitters and electronically generated three-dimensional displays.[3] Amongst other issues, difficulties with camera orientation and surgeon annoyance and fatigue have challenged the adoption of 3-dimensional endoscopes.

Another growing field of endonasal surgery is robotics. The latter confers proper three-dimensional visualization and increased ability to accomplish two-handed surgery through small openings.[4,56] Some authors have published feasibility studies using robotic surgery to access the skull base. O'Malley et al. used transoral combined with a transcervical approach with robotic surgery to access infratemporal fossa.[57] Similarly, Hanna et al. employed robotic surgery using Caldwell-Luc antrostomies with maxillary antrostomies to access the midline skull base.[58] However, application of robotic surgery in rhinology is still at the animal model stage. It will require technical and feasibility assessments prior to its incorporation in patient care.

7. Conclusion

Endoscopic sinus and skull base surgery has an extensive evolutionary history. It is evident that we have come a long way from the traditional treatment modalities of sinus disease, thanks to pioneers in the field of rhinology. Endoscopic surgeons today are enthusiastic about the innovations that are being employed to our current endoscopic armentarium. At this rate of evolution, it is imaginable that in a few short decades, our current endoscopic techniques will be historical.

Author details

Rickul Varshney, Faisal Zawawi, Marc A Tewfik and Saul Frenkiel

*Address all correspondence to: sfrenkie@jgh.mcgill.ca

McGill University, Jewish General Hospital, 3755 Chemin de la Cote-Sainte-Catherine, Montreal, Quebec, Canada

References

[1] Frenkiel, S., & Wright, E. D. (2001). The specialty of rhinology, part 1: a historical glimpse. J Otolaryngol. 30[Suppl 1]: , 26-31.

[2] Chandra, R. K., Conley, D. B., & Kern, R. C. (2009). Evolution of the Endoscope and Endoscopic Sinus Surgery. OtolaryngolClin N Am , 42, 747-752.

[3] Govindaraj, S., Adappa, N. D., & Kennedy, D. W. (2010). Endoscopic sinus surgery: evolution and technical innovations. The Journal of Laryngology & Otology , 124, 242-250.

[4] Castelnuovo, P., Dallan, I., Battaglia, P., & Bignami, M. (2010). Endoscopic endonasal skull base surgery: past, present and future. Eur Arch Otorhinolaryngol , 267, 649-663.

[5] Gandhi, C. D., Christiano, L. D., Eloy, J. A., Prestigiacomo, C. J., & Post, K. D. (2009). The historical evolution of transsphenoidal surgery: facilitation by technological advances. Neurosurg Focus 27[3]: , E8 EOF.

[6] Prevedello, D. M., Kassam, A. B., Snyderman, C., Carrau, R. L., Mintz, A. H., Thomas, A., Gardner, P., & Horowitz, M. (2007). Endoscopic cranial base surgery: ready for prime time? ClinNeurosurg , 54, 48-57.

[7] Jankowski, R., Auque, J., Simon, C., Marchal, J. C., Hepner, H., & Wayoff, M. (1992). Endoscopic pituitary tumor surgery. Laryngoscope , 102, 198-202.

[8] Jho, H. D., Carrau, R. L., Mc Laughlin, M. R., & Somaza, S. C. (1996). Endoscopic transsphenoidal resection of a large chordoma in the posterior fossa. Neurosurg Focus 1[1]:e3.

[9] Wright, E. D., & Frenkiel, S. (2005). Advances in the surgical management of chronic rhinosinusitis. Allergy Asthma ClinImmunol. 1[1]: , 21-27.

[10] Chiu, A. G. (2006). Frontal sinus surgery: its evolution, present standard of care, and recommendations for current use.." Ann OtolRhinolLaryngolSuppl , 196, 13-19.

[11] Castelnuovo, P., Giovannetti, F., Bignami, M., Ungari, C., & Iannetti, G. (2009). Open Surgery Versus Endoscopic Surgery in Benign Neoplasm Involving the Frontal Sinus. The Journal of Craniofacial Surgery, 180-3.

[12] Draf, W. (1991). Endonasal micro-endoscopic frontal sinus surgery: the Fulda concept.."OperTechnOtolaryngol Head Neck Surg , 2, 234-240.

[13] Constantinidis, J., Weber, R., Brune, M., et al. (2000). Cranialization of the frontal sinus. Indications, technique and results.." HNO , 48, 361-366.

[14] Lund, V. (2002). The Evolution of Surgery on the Maxillary Sinus for Chronic Rhinosinusitis. Laryngoscope 112[3]:, 415-9.

[15] Kim, E., & Duncavage, J. A. (2010). Prevention and management of complications in maxillary sinus surgery. OtolaryngolClin North Am 43[4]: , 865-873.

[16] Penttila, M. A., Rautiainen, M. E. P., Pukander, J. S., & Karma, P. H. (1994). Endoscopic versus Caldwell-Luc approach in chronic maxillary sinusitis: comparison of symptoms at one-year follow up.." Rhinology , 32, 161-165.

[17] Närkiö-Mäkelä, M., & Qvarnberg, Y. (1997). Endoscopic sinus surgery or Caldwell-Luc operation in the treatment of chronic and recurrent maxillary sinusitis." ActaOtolaryngolSuppl , 529, 177-180.

[18] Cutler, J. L., Duncavage, J. A., Matheny, K., Cross, J. L., Miman, M. C., & Oh, C. K. (2003). Results of Caldwell-Luc after failed endoscopic middle meatus antrostomy in patients with chronic sinusitis." Laryngoscope 113[12]: , 2148-2150.

[19] Lawson, W. (1994). The Intranasal Ethmoidectomy: Evolution and an Assessment of the Procedure." Laryngoscope 104[6 Pt 2]:, 1-49.

[20] Jain, L., Jain, M., Chouhan, A. N., & Harshwardhan, R. (2011). Conventional Septoplasty verses Endoscopic Septoplasty: A Comparative Study." People's Journal of Scientific Research 4[2]: , 24-28.

[21] Hwang, P. H., Mc Laughlin, R. B., Lanza, D. C., & Kennedy, D. W. (1999). Endoscopic septoplasty: indications, technique, and results." Otolaryngol Head Neck Surg 120[5]: , 678-682.

[22] Lanza, D. C., Rosin, D. F., & Kennedy, D. W. (1993). Endoscopic septal spur resection.." Am J Rhinol , 7, 213-216.

[23] Paradis, J., & Rotenberg, B. W. (2011). Open versus endoscopic septoplasty: a single-blinded, randomized, controlled trial." J Otolaryngol Head Neck Surg. 40 [S1]: S, 28-33.

[24] Nayak, D. R. B. R., & Murty, K. MurtyKD[1998-1] [(1998). An Endoscopic approach to the deviated nasal septum- a preliminary study.." The Journal of Laryngology and Otology, , 112, 934-939.

[25] Bothra, R., & Mathur, N. N. (2009). Comparative evaluation of conventional versus endoscopic septoplasty for limited septal deviation and spur." J Laryngol Otol. 2009 Jul; 123[7]: , 737-741.

[26] Kasemsiri, P., Carrau, R. L., Prevedello, D. M., Ditzel, Filho. L. F. S., de Lara, D., Otto, B. A., & Kassam, A. B. (2012). Indications and Limitations of Endoscopic Skull Base Surgery." MEDSCAPE.

[27] Kassam, A. B., Gardner, P., Snyderman, C., Mintz, A. A., & Carrau, R. (2005). Expanded endonasal approach: a fully endoscopic, completely transnasal approach to the middle third of the clivus, petrous bone, middle cranial fossa and infratemporal fossa." Neurosurg Focus 19[1]: E6.

[28] Sethi, D. S., & Leong, J. L. (2006). Endoscopic pituitary surgery." OtolaryngolClin N Am , 39, 563-583.

[29] Graham, S. M., Iseli, T. A., Karnell, L. H., Clinger, J. D., Hitchon, P. W., & Greenlee, J. D. (2009). Endoscopic approach for pituitary surgery improves rhinologic outcomes." Ann OtolRhinolLaryngol 118[9]: , 630-635.

[30] Zada, G., Kelly, D. F., Cohan, P., Wang, C., & Swerdloff, R. (2003). Endonasaltranssphenoidal approach for pituitary adenomas and other sellar lesions: an assessment of efficacy, safety, and patient impressions." J Neurosurg , 98, 350-358.

[31] Stamm, A. C., Vellutini, E., Harvey, R. J., Nogeira, J. F., & Herman, D. R. (2008). Endoscopic transnasal craniotomy and the resection of craniopharyngioma." Laryngoscope , 118, 1142-1148.

[32] Landolt, A. M., & Zachmann, M. (1991). Results of transsphenoidal extirpation of craniopharyngiomas and Rathke's cysts.." Neurosurgery , 28, 410-415.

[33] Couldwell, W. T., Weiss, M., Rabb, C., Liu, J., Apfelbaum, R., & Fukushima, T. (2004). Variations on the standard transsphenoidal approach to the sellar region, with emphasis on the extended approaches and parasellar approaches: surgical experience in 105 cases." Neurosurgery , 55, 539-550.

[34] Jho, H. D., & Carrau, R. (1997). Endoscopic pituitary surgery: an early experience." SurgNeurol , 47, 213-223.

[35] Devaiah, A. K., & Andreoli, M. T. (2009). Treatment of esthesioneuroblastoma: a year meta-analysis of 361 patients." Laryngoscope 119[7]: 1412-1416., 16.

[36] Komotar, R. J., Starke, R. M., Raper, D. M., Anand, V. K., & Schwartz, T. H. (2012). Endoscopic skull base surgery: a comprehensive comparison with open transcranial approaches." Br J Neurosurg.Epub.

[37] Wellman, B. J., Traynelis, V. C., Mc Culloch, T. M., Funk, G. F., Menezes, A. H., & Hoffman, H. T. (1999). Midline anterior craniofacial approach for malignancy: results of en bloc versus piecemeal resections." Skull Base Surg 9[1]:, 41-6.

[38] Soler, Z. M., & Smith, T. L. [. (2012). Endoscopic versus open craniofacial resection of esthesioneuroblastoma: what is the evidence?" Laryngoscope 122[2]: , 244-245.

[39] Adappa, N. D., Lee, J. Y., Chiu, A. G., & Palmer, J. N. (2011). Olfactory groove meningioma." OtolaryngolClin North Am 44[4]: , 965-980.

[40] Padhye, V., Naidoo, Y., Alexander, H., Floreani, S., Robinson, S., Santoreneos, S., Wickremesekera, A., Brophy, B., Harding, M., Vrodos, N., & Wormald, P. J. (2012). Endoscopic Endonasal Resection of Anterior Skull Base Meningiomas." Otolaryngol Head Neck Surg.Epub.

[41] Al-Mefty, O., & Borba, L. A. B. (1997). Skull base chordomas: a management challenge.." J Neurosurg 86[2]:, 182-9.

[42] Holzmann, D., Reisch, R., Krayenbühl, N., Hug, E., & Bernays, R. L. (2010). The transnasaltransclival approach for clivuschordoma." Minim Invasive Neurosurg. 53[5]: , 211-217.

[43] Cooke, R. S., & Jones, R. A. (1994). Experience with the direct transnasaltranssphenoidal approach to the pituitary fossa." Br J Neurosurg 8[2]:, 193-6.

[44] Hong, Jiang. W., Ping, Zhao. S., Hai, Xie. Z., Zhang, H., Zhang, J., & Yun, Xiao. J. (2009). Endoscopic resection of chordomas in different clival regions." ActaOtolaryngol 129[1]: , 71-83.

[45] Jho, H., , D., & Ha-G, H. (2004). Endoscopic endonasal skull base surgery: Part The clivus and posterior fossa." Minim InvasNeurosurg 47[1]:16-23., 3.

[46] Brown, S. M., Anand, V. K., Tabaee, A., & Schwartz, T. H. (2007). Role of perioperative antibiotics in endoscopic skull base surgery." Laryngoscope 117[9]:, 1528-32.

[47] Snyderman, C. H., Kassam, A. B., Carrau, R. L., & Mintz, A. (2006). Endoscopic approaches to the petrous apex." Op Tech Otolaryngol , 17, 168-173.

[48] Weiss, B. R. (1977). Infratemporal fossa abscess unusual complication of maxillary sinus fracture." Laryngoscope. 87[7]: , 1130-1133.

[49] Diacono, M. S., & Wass, A. R. (1998). Infratemporal and temporal fossa abscess complicating dental extraction.." J AccidEmerg Med 15[1]: , 59-61.

[50] Kamath, M. P., Bhojwani, K. M., Mahale, A., et al. (2009). Infratemporalfossaabscess: a diagnostic dilemma." EarNoseThroat J 88[5]: E23.

[51] Akst, L. M., Albani, B. J., & Strome, M. (2005). Subacuteinfratemporal fossa cellulitis with subsequent abscess formation in an immunocompromisedpatient " Am J. Otolaryngol , 26, 35-38.

[52] Fisch, U., Fagan, P., & Valavanis, A. (1984). The infratemporal fossa approach for the lateral skull base." OtolaryngolClin North Am , 17, 513-552.

[53] Mansour, O. I., Carrau, R. L., Syderman, C. H., et al. (2004). Preauricularinfratemporal fossa surgical approach: modifications of the technique and surgicalindication. Skull Base 2004;Skull Base 14: 143-151., 14, 143-151.

[54] Robinson, S., Patel, N., & Wormald, P. J. (2005). Endoscopic management of benign tumors extending into the infratemporal fossa: a two-surgeon transnasal approach." Laryngoscope 115[10]: , 1818-1822.

[55] James, D., & Crockard, H. A. (1991). Surgical access to the base of the skull and upper cervical spine by extended maxillotomy." Neurosurgery , 29, 411-416.

[56] Virgin, F. W., Bleier, B. S., & Woodworth, B. A. (2010). Evolving materials and techniques for endoscopic sinus surgery." OtolaryngolClin North Am 43[3]: , 653-672.

[57] O'Malley, B. W. J., & Weinstein, G. S. [. (2007). Robotic anterior and midline skull base surgery: preclinical investigations.."Int J RadiatOncolBiolPhys 69[Supplement 2]: S, 125-128.

[58] Hanna, E. Y., Holsinger, C., De Monte, F., et al. (2007). Robotic endoscopic surgery of the skull base: a novel surgical approach.." Arch Otolaryngol Head Neck Surg 133[12]: , 1209-1214.

Section 3

Respiratory Tract

Chapter 9

Bronchology – A Well Branched Tree

Mihai Olteanu, Costin Teodor Streba,
Bogdan Oprea, Raluca Marinas, Mimi Floarea Nitu,
Emilia Crisan and Tudorel Ciurea

Additional information is available at the end of the chapter

1. Introduction

1.1. Lung cancer – Stadialization

Lung cancer is responsible for 1.3 million deaths worldwide annually, and it is the most common cause of cancer-related death in men and the second most common in women. Lung cancer staging is the assessment of the degree to which a lung cancer has spread from its original source. As with most cancers, for lung cancer staging is of paramount importance for the treatment planning process and prognosis. Two primary methods of lung cancer staging are available: clinical staging and pathologic staging. In clinical staging, information is provided by noninvasive or minimally invasive techniques, such as physical examination, radiologic examination, endoscopic ultrasound, bronchoscopy, mediastinoscopy, and thoracoscopy. In pathologic staging, information obtained from clinical staging is combined with findings from both the invasive surgical procedure and the pathologic evaluation of excised tissue. Clinical staging is important and can help to determine the next appropriate step in therapy, such as the decision to proceed with pathologic staging, which remains the reference standard because the overall level of agreement between the two systems only ranges from 35% to 55% [1].

Definition of the stage is an essential part of the approach to patients with lung cancer, and it has led to the development of a universally accepted stage classification systems for most tumors. The Union Internationale Contre le Cancer (UICC) and the American Joint Committee on Cancer (AJCC) periodically define, review, and refine the stage classification systems. Nearly half of all patients with lung cancer have mediastinal disease at diagnosis, and this implies metastases to ipsilateral or subcarinal nodes (N2) that are classified as stage IIIA disease. Management of stage IIIA disease is more controversial, but many centers treat it with radiation and chemotherapy, with surgery performed under investigational protocols. Direct mediastinal invasion (T4) or metastasis to contralateral mediastinal nodes (N3) is classified as stage IIIB disease. The 5-year survival rate in this case is at best 5%, and patients are generally offered treatment with chemoradiotherapy without surgery.

The previous tumor, node, and metastasis (TNM) classification, the sixth edition of the TNM Classification of Malignant Tumors, was published in 2002. The last revision of the staging system for lung cancer has been presented by Dr. Clifton Mountain in 1997 [2], after his proposal had been adopted in 1973 by the AJCC in the same year and by the UICC in 1974, and this revision remained unaltered on the 2002 manual [3]. The 1973 original system was based on a database of 2,155 patients from the MD Anderson Cancer Center in Houston, TX. Subsequent revisions of the TNM staging system continued to be based on this database, which grew to include 5,319 cases at the time the lung cancer staging system was revised in 1997 and it was also validated by Dr. Naruke from Japan in 2001. Mountain's revision was based on a relatively small population of patients who underwent surgical treatment in a single geographic area, and no validation was presented to justify the individual descriptors [4]. In order to overcome the limitations of the sixth TNM classification, the International Association for the Study of Lung Cancer (IASLC) launched the Lung Cancer Staging Project in 1996, and in 1998 created an International Staging Committee (ISC) of multidisciplinary members to conduct revisions [5]. Changes to the sixth edition were proposed by the IASLC based on an international collection and review of 100,869 patients from 46 sources of 20 countries. Data were drawn from lung cancer cases treated by all modalities between 1990 and 2000. After exclusion of ineligible cases, 81,015 patients (67,725 NSCLC and 13,290 SCLC) remained for investigation [6]. Proposals for revision were submitted to the AJCC and UICC for consideration in the new edition of the staging manual, the 7th, and both accepted the recommendations. In the last months of 2009, the Seventh Edition of the TNM Classification of Malignant Tumors was published, with a new lung cancer staging system. The new edition took effect on January 1, 2010 [7].

The changes recommended by the IASLC for the 7th edition of TNM classification for lung cancer were based on differences in survival [8], and the results of the data analysis were internally and externally validated [9]. These changes include new T and M definitions and consequent new stage groupings, a new lymph node map, a novel definition on pleural invasion, as well as recommendations to apply the TNM system to broncho-pulmonary carcinoid tumors and SCLC.

The success story of EBUS-TBNA starts in 2003 with a publication in Thorax by Mark Krasnik and Peter Vilmann from Gentofte University Hospital, Denmark [10]. This article gave the first description of the principle of EBUS-TBNA. In the same journal, in 2006, the same group, together with a group from the Thoraxklinik in Heidelberg and Harvad Medical School's Beth Israel Deaconess MC, published their study on 502 patients that showed that EBUS-TBNA resulted in 93% diagnostic yield, a sensitivity of 94%, specificity of 100% and accuracy 94%, with PPV at 100% and NPV at 11% [11]. In 2006, an international EBUS-TBNA focus group was formed by Felix J.F. Herth (Copenhagen), Kazuhiro Yasufuku (Chiba), Robert Rintoul (Cambridge) and Armin Ernst (Boston) that published in the Journal of Bronchology a description of how to do an EBUS-TBNA thus offering a detailed description of local lymph node position and orientation within the mediastinum [12]. EBUS-TBNA has been studied and compared also in relation with existing modalities like EUS –FNA (by Vilmann et al. in 2005 on 33 pts. and by Herth et al. in 2005 on 160 pts.), PET-CT (by Yasufuku et al. in 2006 on 102 pts.), classical TBNA and EUS-FNA (by Wallace et al. in 2008 on 138 pts.).

EBUS-TBNA was proven in 2007 by Wong and Yasufuku et al. on 65 patients to be a safe method allowing a high yield also for the diagnosis of sarcoidosis [13].

It soon became widely accepted that EBUS-TBNA is a reliable diagnostic tool for enlarged lymph nodes in patients with NSCLC and that lymph nodes below the one centimeter range could also be sampled. This led to a study with 100 patients published in 2006 in European Respiratory Journal [14] that showed that every sixth patient with no evidence of mediastinal disease on CT was diagnosed positive using EBUS-TBNA. Thus, EBUS-TBNA showed potential to avoid unnecessary exploratory thoracoscopies. Following the same idea, in 2008 Hwangbo et al. showed that in cases with both CT- and PET-negative and –positive scans, EBUS-TBNA is an excellent tool for detecting mediastinal metastasis, thereby confirming that EBUS-TBNA is an effective invasive method following CT and PET scanning [15].

In the same year, Armin Ernst et al. showed in Journal of Thoracic Oncology on 66 patients that EBUS-TBNA can have a superior yield compared to cervical mediastinoscopy, which intuitively suggested that mediastinoscopy is not necessarily of additional diagnostic benefit in evaluating negative EBUS-TBNA staged lymph nodes [16]. However, mediastinoscopy has an important role especially in operable patients with non-enlarged lymph nodes for assessing local mediastinal invasion and the exclusion of metastatic disease.

Herth et al. evaluated EBUS-TBNA for re-staging in 124 patients with tissue-proven IIIA-N2 disease after induction chemotherapy (Journal of Clinical Oncology 2008) and concluded that EBUS-TBNA is a valuable and practical tool for re-staging with a sensitivity of 76%, specificity of 100%, PPV of 100%, NPV of 20% and diagnostic accuracy of 77% [17]. These results imply that a negative EBUS-TBNA for re-staging should be surgically re-staged.

In 2006, the compatibility between EBUS-TBNA and the Aloka Prosound alpha5 ultrasound processor made additional Doppler modes available, and this led to a consecutive study by Herth et al. on 89 patients that described changes in flow resistance parameters (resistance index by Pourcelot) in malignant lymph nodes [18].

Yasufuku et al. from Chiba University have shown great dedication to evaluating the benefits of EBUS-TBNA samples for immunohistochemical analysis and reported encouraging results with cell cycle-related proteins in chemotherapy patients in Thorax 2008, and a year earlier in Chest the same group showed that epidermal growth factor receptor (EGFR) mutation can be easily detected in metastatic lymph node samples for EBUS-TBNA and so the samples gained by EBUS-TBNA allowed genetic evaluations of tumour cells from lymph nodes [19, 20].

In 2009 Tournoy et al. provided a detailed analysis of endosonographic landmarks (where available), describing the anatomic borders of the lymph node stations as defined in the 7th edition of the IASLC's TNM-staging nomenclature, which is relevant for correctly staging patients with lung cancer [21].

Building on the strong results of combined EUS-FNA and EBUS-TBNA procedures – a study published by Vilman et al. in 2005 had already indicated their complementary nature – Annema et al. challenged in 2010 the pre-dominant surgical staging algorithm by comparing the combined EBUS-TBNA and EUS-TNA with surgical staging alone [22] and showed that combining endosonographic and surgical staging resulted in greater sensitivity for mediastinal nodal metastases and fewer unnecessary thoracotomies. These results indicated that the combination of both procedures may be able to replace surgical stages as the primary staging method for patients with lung cancer.

Instead of using different scopes for EBUS-TBNA and EUS-TNA, two separate studies published in Chest in 2010 by Hwangbo et al. and Herth et al. [23] used only one bronchoscope for both procedures, starting via the trachea and continuing via the oesophageal route. They came to the conclusion that EBUS-TBNA and EUS-TNA are complementary methods and showed that both procedures can be performed with a single EBUS echoendoscope in one sitting by one operator. A further study in 2011, "Nonsurgical staging of the mediastinum: EBUS and EUS" conducted by Herth, stated that the combination of both procedures achieves a complete and accurate mediastinal staging. Therefore it can be expected that the implementation of combined EBUS-TBNA and EUS-FNA will reduce the need for surgical staging of lung cancer significantly [24].

The summary of scientific studies on EBUS-TBNA provided about clearly shows the procedure's power in helping to improve mediastinal staging of lung cancer during the past 10 years. The technological development of less invasive staging and sampling devices continues endoscopists using endosonography, we can expect further exciting developments in clinical practice in the years to come.

Endobronchial ultrasound with real-time-guided transbronchial fine-needle aspiration (EBUS-TBNA) is a minimally invasive outpatient procedure by which mediastinal [25] and hilar lymph nodes [26] as well as centrally located primary lung lesions [27] can be visualised and sampled under ultrasound guidance. In a systematic review, EBUS-TBNA has shown a pooled sensitivity of 93% in the staging of non-small-cell lung cancer. In a direct comparison with surgical staging, EBUS-TBNA even showed to be superior [28]. Therefore, EBUS-TBNA has been adopted in the most recent lung cancer staging guidelines as a minimally invasive alternative to surgical staging [29]

EBUS-TBNA is an accurate, minimally invasive and safe staging procedure and can be considered the procedure of choice for patients with extrathoracic malignancies in whom hilar or mediastinal lesions are observed. In patients with (concurrent or previously treated) extrathoracic malignancy, EBUS-TBNA has a sensitivity of 85% to demonstrate metastatic spread. Implementation of EBUS-TBNA in these patients obviates invasive surgical diagnostic procedures in 61%. [30, 31]

The development and introduction of the new convex probe endobronchial ultrasound (CP-EBUS) that performs endobronchial ultrasound-guided transbronchial needle aspiration has changed the practice of bronchoscopic biopsy of the mediastinum in respiratory diseases. In particular, the role of EBUS-TBNA in the diagnosis and mediastinal lymph node staging of lung cancer, the leading cause of death from malignant disease worldwide [32], is becoming an interest to pulmonologists as well as thoracic surgeons. The newest CP-EBUS now being used in clinical practice is a hybrid bronchofibervideoscope which features a unique optical system that exploits both video and fiber-optic technologies (BFUC160F- OL8, Olympus, Tokyo, Japan). This CP-EBUS is a linear curved array transducer that scans parallel to the insertion direction of the bronchoscope. Images can be obtained by directly contacting the probe or by attaching a balloon on the tip and inflating with saline (Figure 1). The outer diameter of the insertion tube of the CP-EBUS is 6.2 mm, and that of the tip is 6.9 mm. The angle of view is 80º and the direction of view is 35º forward oblique [33].

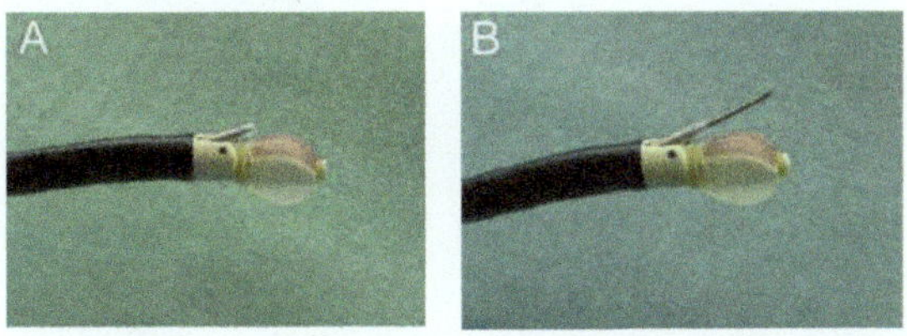

Figure 1. Tip of the new convex probe endobronchial ultrasound (CP-EBUS, BF-UC160FOL8, Olympus, Tokyo, Japan). The outer diameter of the insertion tube of the flexible bronchoscope is 6.2 mm. CP-EBUS has a linear curved array ultrasonic transducer of 7.5 MHz. The balloon attached to the tip of the bronchoscope is inflated with normal saline (A). The dedicated TBNA needle is inserted through the working channel (B) [33].

The built-in CCD in the control section allows sharp images similar to those of regular videoscopes and allows a slimmer insertion tube of 6.2 mm. The ultrasound images can be frozen and the size of lesions can be measured in two dimensions by the placement of cursors. It is also equipped with the Color Power Doppler mode. The display range covers 2–24 cm (Figure 2).

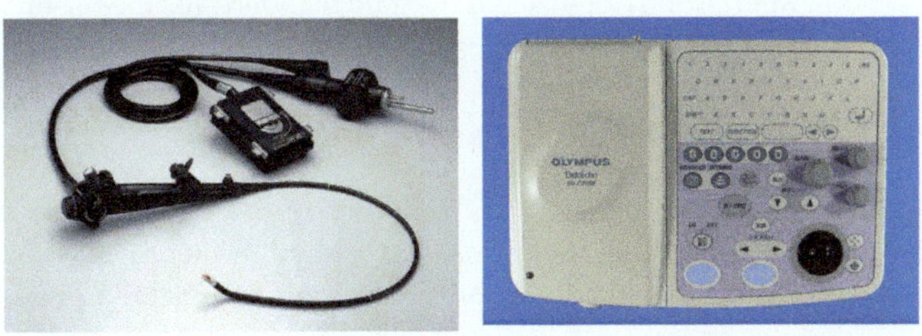

Figure 2. The convex probe endobronchial ultrasound (CP-EBUS, BF-UC160F-OL8, Olympus, Tokyo, Japan) and The dedicated ultrasound processor (EU-C60/EU-C2000, Olympus, Tokyo, Japan) [33].

The dedicated 22-gauge needle is used for EBUS-TBNA (Figure 3). The needle is a single use aspiration needle with echogenic dimpled tip design to improve visibility on ultrasound images. This needle has various adjuster knobs which work as a safety device to prevent damage to the channel. The maximum extruding stroke is 40 mm and to prevent excessive protrusion, a safety mechanism stops the needle at the stroke of 20 mm. The needle is attached onto the working channel of the bronchoscope which allows the operator to actually perform EBUS-TBNA. The needle is also equipped with an internal sheath which is withdrawn after passing the bronchial wall, avoiding contamination during TBNA. This internal sheath is also used to clear out the tip of the needle after passing the bronchial wall. The use of this sheath has significantly increased the yield of EBUS-TBNA. The exit of the needle is at 20° with respect to the outer covering of the insertion tube. The needle can be visualized through the optics and on the ultrasound image [33].

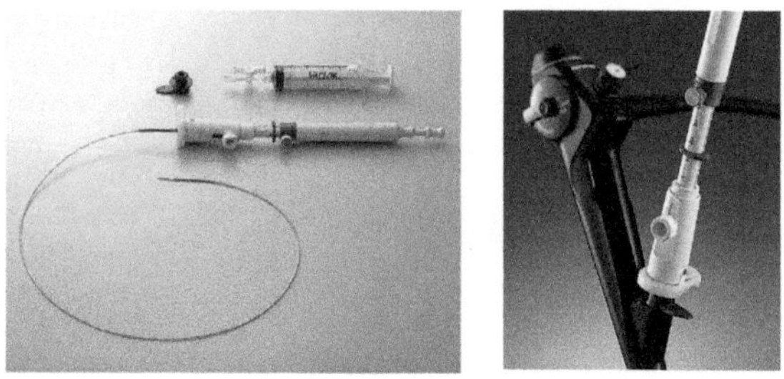

Figure 3. A Dedicated 22-gauge needle (NA-201SX-4022, Olympus, Tokyo, Japan) and the Vaclok syringe used to create negative pressure. B The needle attached to the working channel of the EBUS-TBNA bronchoscope. The maximum extruding stroke is 40 mm and to prevent excessive protrusion, a safety mechanism stops the needle at the stroke of 20 mm [33].

Mediastinal staging can be divided into noninvasive staging (imaging) and invasive (sampling) staging. Computed tomography (CT), magnetic resonance imaging (MRI), positron emission tomography (PET) and PET-CT are used for noninvasive imaging [34]. Other imaging modalities include the use of transesophageal ultrasonography (EUS) and endobronchial ultrasound (EBUS) using a radial probe for detecting even small mediastinal lymph nodes [35-36]. Mediastinoscopy is still the gold standard for mediastinal lymph node staging [37]. However, it requires general anesthesia and complications cannot be ignored.

1.2. Changes to T descriptors [38-39]

Rami-Porta R et al. evaluated in 2007 for the 7th Edition of the TNM Classification of Malignant Tumors only patients without metastasis and, although there was information about different aspects of the T component, they only could analyze in detail tumor size, existence of accompanying nodules and pleural dissemination.

The prognostic value of the tumor size was studied in patients with completely resected pathological T1 and T2 N0 M0 tumors who had not received adjuvant therapy. The statistical calculations determined three cut-points at 2, 5 and 7cm, which, in addition to the 3cm, the border between T1 and T2, gave rise to 5 groups of tumors with significantly worse survival with larger tumor diameters. The groups and their 5-year survival rates were: T1≤2cm, 77%; T1>2cm and ≤3cm, 71%; T2>3cm and ≤5cm, 58%; T2>5cm and ≤7cm, 49%, and T2>7cm, 35%. This prognostic gradation was maintained when less selective patient populations were evaluated: clinical staging, incomplete resection and different lymph node affectation. With such arguments, it was decided to subdivide the T1 tumors into T1a (≤2cm) and T1b (>2cm and ≤3cm), and T2 tumors into T2a (>3cm and ≤5cm) and T2b (>5cm and ≤7cm). Likewise, the 5-year survival was compared between patients with T2>7cm tumors and T3 tumors. Similar results were found in the different populations, except in the N0 cases with complete resection, in which it was verified that the survival was even higher in the T3 (41%) than in the T2>7cm (35%), therefore it was decided to reclassify the latter as T3. When they analyzed the tumors that, with pathological staging, presented additional nodules, it was observed that: (a) the 5-year survival of the T3 (31%) was similar to the T4 classified as such due to the existence of an additional nodule or nodules in the same lobe as the primary tumor (28%); (b) the T4 due to other factors had the same survival as those classified as M1 due to an additional nodule(s) in a different homolateral lobe than the primary tumor (22%); and (c) the T4 due to pleural dissemination had a clearly worse prognosis (11% 5-year survival). For the new classification, it was therefore recommended to consider as T3 those tumors with additional nodule(s) in the same lobe as the primary tumor, to consider as T4 those tumors with additional nodule(s) in a homolateral lobe other than that of the primary tumor, and to include in the M category those tumors with pleural dissemination (Table 1).

T descriptor		**6th ed.**	**7th ed.**
T size	Tumors = 2 cm	T1	T1a
	Tumors > 2 cm and = 3 cm	T1	T1b
	Tumors > 3cm and = 5cm	T2	T2a
	Tumors > 5 cm and = 7 cm	T2	T2b
	Tumors > 7 cm	T2	T3
Separate nodule(s) in the primary lobe.		T4	T3
Separate nodule(s) in a different ipsilateral lobe.		M1	T4
Malignant pericardial effusion.		T4	M1a
Pleural dissemination.		T4	M1a

Table 1. T descriptor changes: comparison between 6th and 7th edition of the TNM Classification of Malignant Tumors [38]

1. *Tumor size cut points at 2, 3, 5, and 7 cm:*

   • T1 subclassified:

   - T1a: tumors = 2 cm

   - T1b: tumors: > 2 cm and = 3 cm

   • T2 subclassified:

   - T2a: > 3cm and = 5cm

   - T2b: > 5 cm and = 7 cm

   • T2 reclassified:

   - T2 > 7 cm became T3.

2. *Multicentric tumors of similar histology:*

   - Separate nodule(s) in the primary lobe: became T3 from T4.

   - Separate nodule(s) in a different ipsilateral lobe: became T4 from M1.

3. *T4 descriptors:*

   - Pleural dissemination (pleural nodules or malignant effusion): became M1a from T4.

   - Malignant pericardial effusion: became M1a from T4.

In the *AJCC Cancer Staging Manual* and *UICC TNM Classification of Malignant Tumors* the T factor is divided into four descriptors (T1-4) depending on size, site, number, and local extent of the primary tumor: the size and non-size based descriptors [40].

1.2.1. Size-based T descriptors

The value of tumor size in NSCLC prognosis is supported by large clinical evidence [41-45]. The tumor size threshold of 3 cm was set-up on the 2nd edition of the TNM classification of malignant tumors in 1974.[46], and despite the advances in surgical procedures, adjuvant treatment, and mostly in imaging technology, this measure remained unchanged for 35 years. The 7th edition of the TNM for lung cancer confers more importance to the size-based T descriptors and divides them as seen earlier. These modifications have been validated by recent studies that showed better survival stratification and prognosis estimation with the new T definitions [47-49].

Table 2a describes lower survival rates as the T factor increases [50-51].; survival rates are improved with the new system due to reclassification (up- and down-staging) of patients when compared to series reporting survival rates with the previous TNM, showed in Table 2b [52-53].

T component	5-year survival (%)	
	Kameyama et al [25]	Li et al [24]
T1a	82.6	75.49
T1b	73.3	74.58
T2a	63.5	60.87
T2b	50.1	55.63
T3	40.6	46.15
T4	34.6	NS

T component	5-year survival (%)	
	Mountain CF [26]	Naruke et al. [27]
T1	67	68.9
T2	57	42.5
T3	38	31.9
T4	7 (cT)	18.9

Table 2. a. Five year survival by pT classification with the 7th edition. **b.** Five year survival by pT classification with the 6th edition [40].

1.2.2. Non–size-based T descriptors

1.2.2.1. Multiple nodules

The existence of multiple primary cancers (MPC) was initially reported by Warren and Gates in 1932 [54], but in spite of these past 80 years, to date accurate diagnosis of MPC is not yet clearly established due to a lack of consensus on definition and diagnostic criteria [55]

In 1975, Martini and Melamed were the first to propose clinical and histopathologic criteria for the differential diagnosis of second lung cancers [56]. MPLCs are defined synchronous, if detected simultaneously, or metachronous, if tumors are separated in time [57-58]. Synchronous nodules may represent a MPLC (second primary), a metastasis, or an extension from the primary (satellite nodule) [59] (Table 3).

Deslauriers et al. described in 1989 intrapulmonary nodular metastasis in patients with NSCLC as satellite nodules, and the 5- year survival rates for these patients with satellite nodules were 21.6% compared to 44% for patients without satellite nodules. They concluded that patients with satellite nodules should be classified as stage IIIA [60].

Type		Definition
Satellite nodule		Same histology And same lobe as primary cancer And no systemic metastasis
MPLCs	Same histology, anatomically separated	Tumors in different lobes And no N2-3 involvement And no systemic metastasis
	Same histology, temporally separated	=4-yr interval between tumors And no systemic metastasis from either tumor
	Different histology	Or different molecular genetic features Or arising separately from foci of CIS
Metastasis	Same histology	With multiple systemic metastasis
	Same histology, in different lobes	And presence of N2-3 involvement Or < 2-yr interval

Table 3. Definitions of second primary, satellite nodules and metastasis [61-62].

The concept of satellite nodules was not considered in NSCLC staging system until 1992 by the AJCC and in 1993 by the UICC [63-64].

Prior to this, all nodules were classified as M1.

The T4 descriptor includes diverse tumors with different evolution and prognosis:

- invasion of the mediastinum, heart, great vessels, trachea, esophagus, vertebral body, and carina;
- tumor with a malignant pleural or pericardial effusion, or with satellite tumor nodule(s) within the ipsilateral primary-tumor lobe of the lung.

The IASLC lung cancer staging project committee has acknowledged the multiple reports showing better survival for primary tumors with satellite nodules than other T4 tumors and this is the reason why they downstaged them accordingly [38,65].

Later studies found that the new T descriptor for satellite nodules proposed by the IASLC reflects better the outcomes of that group of patients, which showed superior survival rates, and now these patients are to be considered for surgery [66-67].

1.2.2.2. Pleural dissemination and pericardial effusion

According to the TNM staging manual, pleural dissemination is defined as the presence of ipsilateral malignant pleural effusion (MPE) or pleural nodules [68]. Pleural nodules are defined as pleural tumor foci separated from direct pleural invasion by the primary tumor, classified as T4 [69]. These pleural tumors must be differentiated from direct tumor invasion to the visceral (T2) or parietal pleura (T3) (Table 4).

PL category	Definition	T status	
PL0	Tumor within the subpleural parenchyma or, invading superficially into the pleural connective tissue below the elastic layer.	PL0 is not a T descriptor and the T component should be assigned on other features.	
PL1	Tumor invades beyond the elastic layer.	**pT2**	**Indicates VPI**
PL2	Tumor invades to visceral pleural surface.		
PL3	Tumor invades the parietal pleura.	pT3	

Table 4. Classification of visceral pleural invasion (VPI): Proposed modification of Hammar Classification [70]

Introduction of a new accurate definition of visceral pleural invasion (VPI); VPI is a pT2 descriptor (Table 4). The abbreviation PL is used instead of P which is also used for designation of pTNM in distinction from cTNM. The IASLC also recommends the use of elastic stains to distinguish between PL0 and PL1 when hematoxylin and eosin (H&E) sections are not helpful [71].

In TNM staging, either pleural fluid cytology or clinical judgment are valid to establish the diagnosis of a MPE and consider it as a T4 factor [72], in the absence of relevant conventional or guided pleural biopsy. Malignant pericardial effusions are classified according to the same rules. Pleural dissemination and pericardial effusion are T4 descriptors, grouped into stage IIIB in absence of distant metastasis. The MPE is considered to be a sign of advanced disease, and almost every cancer can involve the pleura [73-74]. However, most MPE's are due to NSCLC's and encompass the worst prognosis [75-77], even worse than in the presence of satellite nodules or mediastinal invasion; only a few patients survive beyond 12 months, regardless of treatment modality, surgery or not, according to studies by Osaki et al., Sugiura et al., Mott et al. and Kameyama et al. [78-81]

Ipsilateral MPE is a locally advanced disease that precludes surgical treatment in lung cancer [82-83]. Unlike other malignant effusions, those caused by NSCLC have low sensitivity to chemo- and radiotherapy [84-86]; therefore these patients are candidates for palliative therapy. In a similar way, NSCLC is the most frequent cause of malignant pericardial effusion, which has a grim prognosis too [87-89].

The IASLC reclassified pleural dissemination from T4 to M1a based on the magnitude of evidence demonstrating that postoperative survival rates of patients with stage IIIB due to MPE are no different from those with stage IV disease and significantly lower than in patients with no pleural effusion and even with non-malignant pleural effusion [90-95].

Status at thoracotomy	5-year survival (%)
No pleural effusion	45.4
Non-MPE	42.5
MPE	15.9
Pathologic stage IV	11.2

Table 5. Postoperative survival rates of NSCLC with malignant pleural effusion (MPE): no significant difference with stage IV disease. (Data from Naruke et al [96])

1.3. Changes to N descriptors [97-98]

The accurate assessment of lymph node involvement is an important part of the management of lung cancer. Lymph node "maps" have been used to describe the location of nodal metastases. However, there are discrepancies in nomenclature among maps used by Asian and Western countries. The IASLC proposed a new lymph node map that reduces these differences among currently used maps, and provides precise anatomic definitions for all lymph node stations. It has also been proposed a new method of grouping lymph node stations together into "zones" for the sake of future survival analyses [99].

Milestones:

1. No changes were made to N descriptors. Analysis from the international database of the IASLC showed that current N descriptors provide good survival stratification, and therefore considered appropriate to maintain them without modifications [100].

2. New International Lymph Node Map: The IASLC has developed a new lymph node chart to resolve disagreements in nomenclature between Naruke's (The Japan Lung Cancer Society) and Mountain-Dresler's maps (American Thoracic Society). Although the nomenclature has changed, the general concept remains the same. Patients without nodal metastatic disease are designated as N0. Patients with N1 disease are defined as having metastatic involvement of lymph nodes in the ipsilateral peripheral or hilar zones. The N2 designation signifies metastatic extension to lymph nodes in the ipsilateral mediastinal (upper, aorticopulmonary, lower) or subcarinal lymph node zones. The N3 nodal designation includes metastatic involvement of any nodes in the supraclavicular lymph node zone or nodes in contralateral mediastinal, hilar–interlobar, or peripheral zone.

3. New classification of lymph nodes by grouping stations into seven "Nodal Zones" for prognostic analysis: supraclavicular, upper, aorticopulmonary, subcarinal, lower, hilar–interlobar, and peripheral (Table 6 and Figure 4); this proposal needs to be validated with prospective studies and it is not yet effective in the new TNM system.

Nodal Zone	Lymph node station
Upper zone	Low cervical, supraclavicular, sternal notch (1R – 1L)
	Upper paratracheal (2R – 2L)
	Prevascular (3a) and retrotracheal (3p)
	Lower paratracheal (4R – 4L)
Aortopulmonary zone	Subaortic (aortopulmonary window - 5)
	Para-aortic (ascending aorta or phrenic nerve - 6)
Subcarinal zone	Subcarinal (7)
Lower zone	Paraesophageal (8)
	Pulmonary ligament (9)
Hilar zone	Hilar (10)
	Interlobar superior (11s) and inferior (11i)
Peripheral zone	Lobar (12)
	Segmental (13)
	Subsegmental (14)

Table 6. Grouping of lymph node stations into "zones".

Survival differences were also calculated on the basis of the number of lymph node zones involved in any single nodal designation. For instance, in pathologically staged patients with any T and M0, those with nodal metastases to a single N1 zone had a median survival of 52 months whereas those with metastatic spread to nodes in multiple N1 zones had a median survival of only 31 months. Similar decreases in survival were also seen in patients with multiple N2 nodal zone involvement (median survival 19 months) compared with those with disease in a single N2 nodal zone (median survival 35 months) [65]. These results showed improved survival in patients with a single N2 zone involved compared with those with multiple N1 zones involved. These findings were validated by an external study [102], and raising the possibility of subdividing the N1 and N2 classifications into N1a (single-zone N1), N1b (multiple-zone N1), N2a (single-zone N2), and N2b (multiple-zone N2).

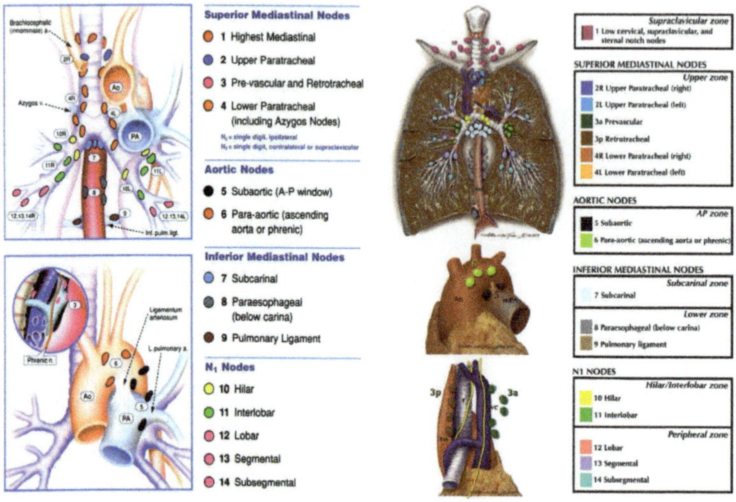

Figure 4. A parallel between previous Mountain-Dresler modified lymph node map originally proposed by the American Thoracic Society and the proposed grouping of lymph node stations into "zones" for the purposes of prognostic analyses from Rusch VW et al. [100].

4. Given the continuous ascension of endoscopic ultrasound techniques such as EBUS (endobronchial ultrasound) and EUS (endocopic ultrasound) guided transbronchial (TBNA) and transesophageal (FNA) fine needle aspiration for the sampling of mediastinal lymph nodes, the borders between lymph node stations have been reconsidered, limiting as much as possible the subjectivism and trying to better standardize and define nodal stations.

As Tournoy et al. showed in this graphic representation, the reach of EUS-FNA and EBUS-TBNA is partly overlapping and partly complementary. EBUS-TBNA follows the large airways, whereas EUS-FNA is excellent for the left, posterior and lower mediastinal and paraoesophageal stations. When both techniques are available, many of the mediastinal and hilar lymph nodes can be reached for fine-needle aspiration. In addition, with EUS-FNA, the left liver lobe, celiac trunk nodes, and the left adrenal gland can be assessed. With EUS, lymph nodes can be identified if they are located in the vicinity of the esophagus. The nodes to be identified with EUS are described in relation to vascular structures (including the aorta, the azygos vein, the left atrium, and the pulmonary artery) and the diaphragm [103-104]. With EBUS, the ultrasound window angle is much smaller, when compared with EUS (50–60 degree angle versus 150– 180 degree angle), which makes the visualization and identification of large vessels or ultrasound landmarks easier with the latter (Figure 5). EUS helps in the identification of structures and landmarks through movements of backward, forward and rotation of the scope. In contrast to EUS, EBUS has the advantage of having a real-time bronchoscopic view into the airways during procedures, which helps with a more accurate identification of the lymph node stations [12].

In general, the lymph nodes are characterized based on EBUS imaging as follows:

a. Size (in short axis): less or more than 1 cm.

b. Shape: oval or round; when the ratio of short vs. long axis of lymph nodes is smaller than 1.5, the lymph node is defined as round; if the ratio is bigger than 1.5, it is oval.

c. Margin: indistinct or distinct; if the majority of the margin (>50%) is clearly visualized with a high echoic border, the lymph nodes are determined as distinct. If the margin is unclear, they are determined as indistinct.

d. Echogenecity: homogeneous or heterogeneous

e. The presence or absence of central hilar structure (CHS); CHS defined as a linear, flat, hyperechoic area in the center of the lymph node.

f. The presence or absence of coagulation necrosis sign (CNS). CNS is a hypoechoic area within the lymph node without blood flow. Typical coagulation necrosis sign represents a low echoic area within the lymph node and that sometimes occupy the majority of the lymph node. The presence of CNS had the highest specificity (92.6%) and the highest hazard ratio (5.6) for prediction of metastatic lymph nodes [106]

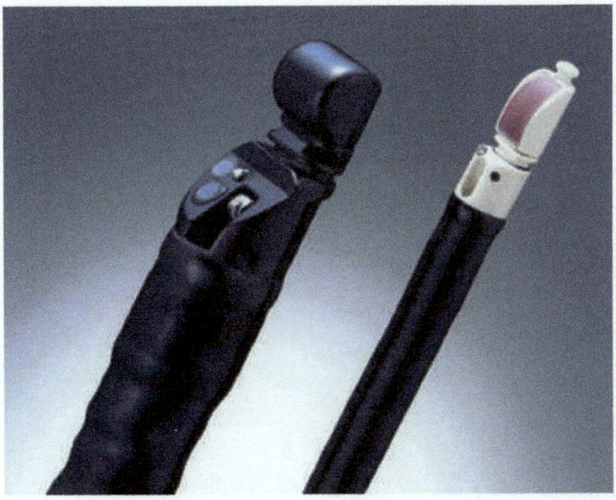

Figure 5. Devices used in endoscopic and endobronchial ultrasound. Endoscopic ultrasound probe (left) and endobronchial ultrasound scope (right) [105].

Since we consider that in the light of the latest TNM classification the knowledge of lymph node stations and their borders is of absolute importance, we will debate about it on a larger scale in this chapter. This, according to our opinion, is going to help especially the EUS-EBUS practitioners, since we are going to correlate from literature the schematics with CT's and ultrasound in every lymph node station, in order to have a detailed mental image of the mediastinum. (Figure 6).

Station 1 lymph nodes (Figure 7) are located caudal to the inferior margin of the cricoid but cranial to the incisura jugularis of the sternum and cranial to the clavicles bilaterally. Therefore, the supraclavicular nodes are also part of station 1. The latter can be felt by a clinical examination when enlarged; however, external ultrasound has shown to be useful for their localization, identification, and puncture.21–24 21 [107-110].

Although the paratracheal part of station 1 can be reached by EBUS-TBNA (1R/L; bilateral–the midline of the trachea serves as the border) or EUS-FNA (1L; left), the proposed anatomic borders cannot be recognized with endoscopic ultrasound. Because these nodes are localized extrathoracic, an endoscopic approach is very unpractical. The endoscopes are not stable for these very proximal stations making interpretation and sampling technically difficult and uncomfortable for the patient. Therefore, endoscopic ultrasound is of limited value for identification, delineation, and sampling of the paratracheally located station 1 nodes [21].

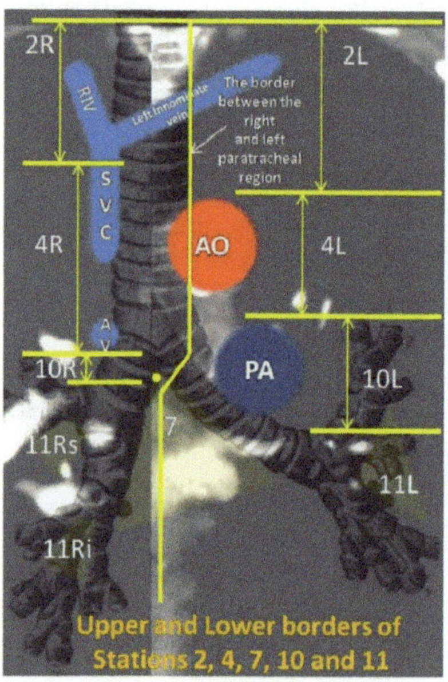

AV	Azygous vein
AO	Aorta
LN	Lymph node
PA	Pulmonary artery
SVC	Superior vena cava
RC1	Primary right carina
RIV	Right innominate vein
RUL	Right upper lobe
RLL	Right lower lobe
LCA	Left carotid artery
LC2	Secondary left carina
LUL	Left upper lobe

Figure 6. General view: CT-WLB-EBUS correlations for regional lymph nodes by IASLC system [106]

Station 2. The inferior border of station 2L is the transverse plane through the superior border of the aortic arch. For 2R, the inferior border is then the intersection of the caudal margin of the brachiocephalic vein with the right-sided border of the trachea. The sagittal plane tangent to the left tracheal wall now makes the difference between right and left. For endoscop-

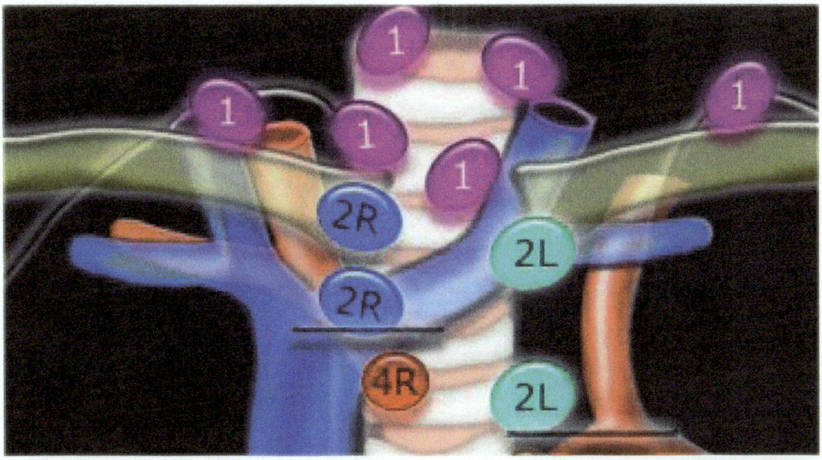

Figure 7. Supraclavicular nodes. These include low cervical, supraclavicular and sternal notch nodes. Upper border: lower margin of cricoid. Lower border: clavicles and upper border of manubrium. The midline of the trachea serves as border between 1R and 1L. 2R. Right Upper Paratracheal. 2R nodes extend to the left lateral border of the trachea. Upper border: upper border of manubrium. Lower border: intersection of caudal margin of innominate (left brachiocephalic) vein with the trachea. 2L. Left Upper Paratracheal. Upper border: upper border of manubrium. Lower border: superior border of aortic arch. [111] Courtesy of Septimiu Murgu, MD and Henri Colt,MD; Bronchoscopy International www.bronchoscopy.org

ic ultrasound node identification and delineation, these revised definitions are important. Ultrasonographic discrimination between stations 2 and 4 is evident, especially on the left side because the apex of the aortic arch can readily be visualized by either EUS-FNA or EBUS-TBNA. For the right-sided nodes, the margin simply follows this transverse plane, which can serve as a surrogate for the intersection of the trachea and brachiocephalic vein (Figure 8).

Discriminating left and right-sided nodes has clinical implications (N2 versus N3). In most of the cases, there is no discussion about the position because the presence and the size of the nodes as seen and measured on the CT scan also help the endoscopist in the identification (Figure 9). However, it can be that similarly enlarged nodes are found in this region and that attention is needed for making the difference between N2 and N3. As a general rule, it can be said that EUS-FNA can only reach the left paratracheal lymph node stations. With EBUS-TBNA, both stations can be approached while no clear endoscopic or ultrasonographic landmarks are available to discriminate left and right. Although the bronchoscopic image helps during EBUS-TBNA, the left side of the trachea never identifies as a straight plane. The large arteries (subclavian artery or the aortic arch) cannot help much because their position relative to that sagittal plane is variable. In addition, the smaller ultrasonography window of EBUS-TBNA also makes the visualization of the anatomic ultrasound landmarks is more limited [21].

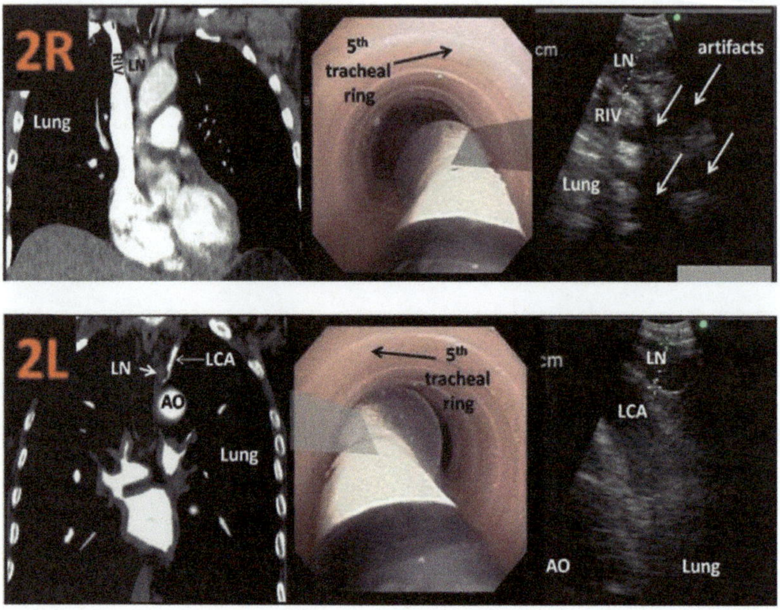

Figure 8. Station 2 visualized by EBUS at the 5th tracheal ring [106]. Courtesy of Septimiu Murgu, MD and Henri Colt,MD; Bronchoscopy International www.bronchoscopy.org

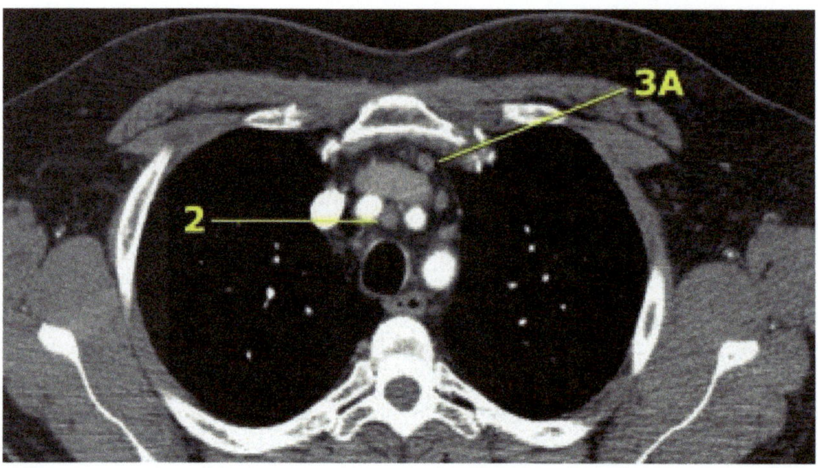

Figure 9. Station 2 node in front of the trachea, i.e. a 2R-node. There is also a small prevascular node, i.e. a station 3A node.

Station 3 lymph nodes are defined with an anterior part being the prevascular nodes and a posterior part being the retrotracheal nodes. The craniocaudal extent goes for both from the sternal notch down to the main carina. Although the prevascular station 3A can be visualized with EBUS as lying ventrally from the large vessels, there are no anatomic ultrasound landmarks to recognize the superior border of this lymph node station. Sampling station 3A by endoscopic ultrasound is impossible because of the interposition of the large vessels. This contrasts with station 3P, which is situated in between the pars membranacea of the trachea and the vertebrae (Figure 11). It can be seen and sampled by both EUS-FNA and EBUS-TBNA. Although there is no ultrasound landmark for the superior margin of 3P either the inferior margin being the main carina level corresponds with the level of the main stem or left pulmonary artery during EUS and can be seen as an anatomic structure during EBUS. The margin between 3P and 2/4L is the left posterior tracheal corner, which is identifiable by EUS-FNA or EBUS-TBNA. The margin between 3P and 2/4R is the right posterior tracheal corner that can be identified during EBUS-TBNA.

Station 4 lymph nodes are located paratracheally but situated caudal to the transverse aortic arch plane (Figure 12). The sagittal plane on the left side of the trachea is the margin between left and right, just like in station 2 nodes. By consequence, EUS-FNA in general cannot approach a right paratracheal node. The comments made to discriminate between 4R and 4L with EBUS-TBNA are identical to those for stations 2. However, what can be helpful for the endoscopist is that 4R nodes are situated posterior to the superior vena cava and/or ascending aorta, both presenting as large vessels with a vertical course, which can be readily visualized by EBUS-TBNA. The inferior margins of station 4 nodes have been redefined with important clinical implications, also for endoscopic ultrasound. The pleural reflection no longer serves as the border between stations 4 and 10. Station 4L has now an inferior border defined by the superior rim of the left main pulmonary artery and a lateral margin defined by the aortopulmonary ligament (Figures 12 – 14). With both EUS-FNA and EBUS-TBNA, the cranial rim of the left main pulmonary artery can be visualized. The aortopulmonary ligament is invisible for ultrasound. Station 4R's inferior border has now been redefined as the inferior border of the azygos vein. This new definition is better because the anatomic margin being the pleural fold is invisible for conventional or endoscopic imaging, whereas the azygos vein is always visible. During EBUS-TBNA, it typically presents in the right tracheobronchial corner as a kidney-shaped vessel (Figures 12, 13). By consequence, EBUS-TBNA now can be used more confidently to discriminate between mediastinal 4R and hilar 10R nodes. The 4R nodes are by consequence characterized by their position just dorsally from the superior caval vein and/or aorta and medially but not distally to the azygos vein.

4R. Right Lower Paratracheal

- Upper border: intersection of caudal margin of innominate (left brachiocephalic) vein with the trachea.
- Lower border:lower border of azygos vein.

4R nodes extend to the left lateral border of the trachea.

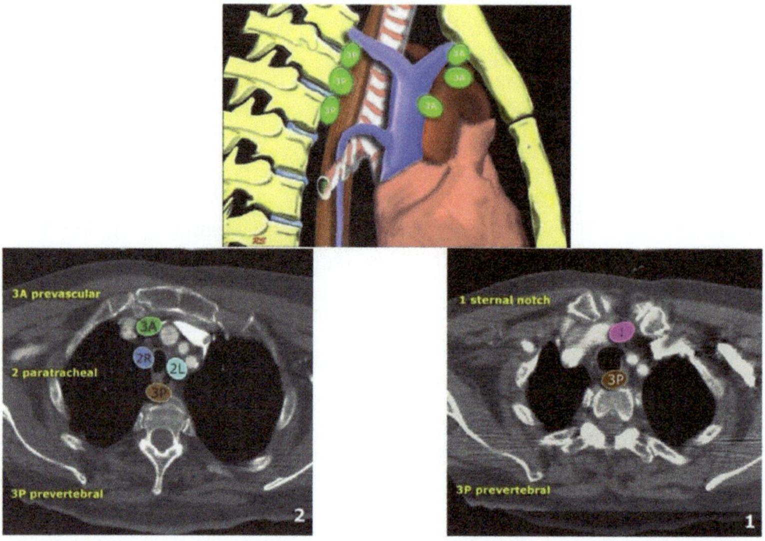

Figure 10. Prevascular and Prevertabral nodes. Station 3 nodes are not adjacent to the trachea like station 2 nodes. They are either: 3A anterior to the vessels or 3P behind the esophagus, which lies prevertebrally. Station 3 nodes are not accessible with mediastinoscopy. 3P nodes can be accessible with endoscopic ultrasound (EUS) [111].

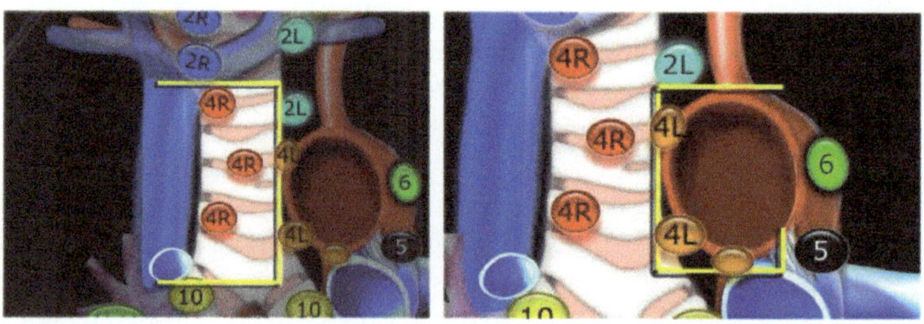

Figure 11. Lymph nodes station 4 and their borders

4L. Left Lower Paratracheal

4L nodes are lower paratracheal nodes that are located to the left of the left tracheal border, between a horizontal line drawn tangentially to the upper margin of the aortic arch and a line extending across the left main bronchus at the level of the upper margin of the left upper lobe bronchus. These include paratracheal nodes that are located medially to the ligamentum arteriosum.

Station 5 (AP-window) nodes are located laterally to the ligamentum arteriosum [111].

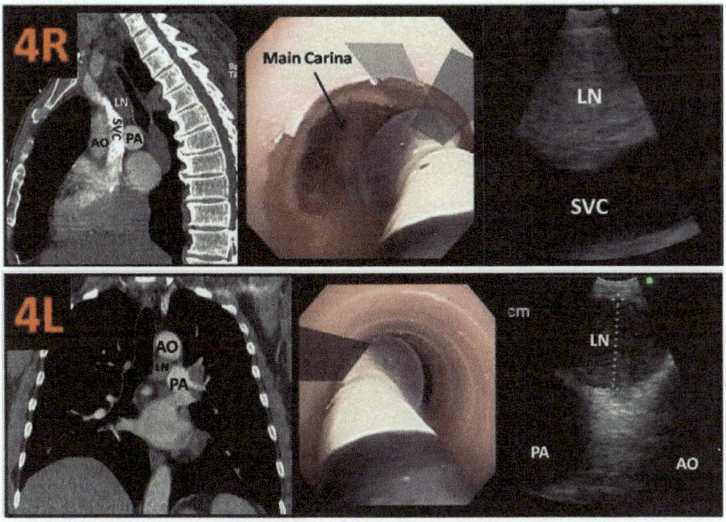

Figure 12. Sagital CT, bronchoscopic image and EBUS image of station 4R and 4L lymph node stations [106]. Courtesy of Septimiu Murgu, MD and Henri Colt,MD; Bronchoscopy International www.bronchoscopy.org

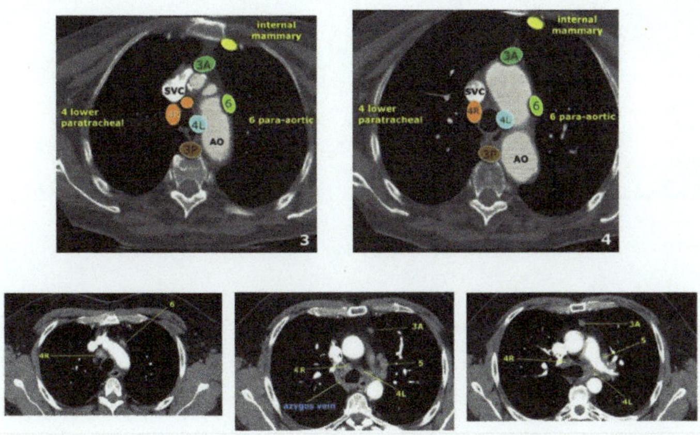

Figure 13. Examples of mediastinal lymph nodes and their anatomic relations with described borders [111].

Station 5 lymph nodes are situated laterally to station 4L nodes with the ligamentum arteriosum as anatomic border (Figures 11, 13). The inferior edge is similar for both, whereas the cranial edge is not. Although 4L nodes are situated caudal to the superior border of the aortic arch, station 5 nodes are located caudal to the inferior border of the aortic arch (Figure 19).

Because the ligamentum arteriosum cannot be discerned by means of ultrasound, the differentiation between 4L and 5 can be difficult, especially when both stations contain suspect lymph nodes. Station 5 nodes can be identified by EUS-FNA and EBUS-TBNA although the latter is often more demanding. Because of the interposition of aortic arch or pulmonary artery, station 5 can only be punctured in selected patients with enlarged nodes.

Station 6 mediastinal lymph nodes are located lateral to the ascending aorta and aortic arch, in between the transverse planes at the superior and inferior border of the aortic arch. (Figures 13, 14) These nodes can most often be identified by means of EUS-FNA, whereas this is not always possible with EBUS-TBNA. The nodes in station 6 can only be punctured by a transaortal approach, but extended mediastinoscopy is advised instead [21, 112].

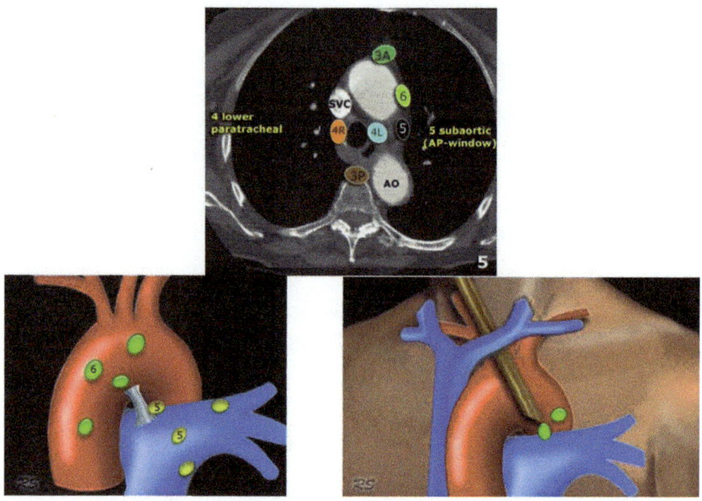

Figure 14. Lymph nodes stations 5 and 6 and their relation with the great vessels [111].

Station 5. Subaortic nodes: Subaortic or aorto-pulmonary window nodes are lateral to the ligamentum arteriosum or the aorta or left pulmonary artery and proximal to the first branch of the left pulmonary artery and lie within the mediastinal pleural envelope.

Station 6. Para-aortic nodes: Para-aortic (ascending aorta or phrenic) nodes are located anteriorly and laterally to the ascending aorta and the aortic arch from the upper margin to the lower margin of the aortic arch [111].

Station 7 lymph nodes have an inferior border that is redefined. (Figure 15).On the left side, this is the superior border of the lower lobe bronchus, and on the right side, this is the inferior border of the intermediate bronchus. (Figure 16) The lymph nodes in this station can be seen and biopsied by both EUS-FNA and EBUS-TBNA. Formerly, an anterior and posterior part of this node was recognized. This was meaningful because a cervical mediastinoscopy cannot reach the posterior part of this station. With EUS-FNA and EBUS-TBNA, the entire subcarinal area can be approached. Although identification of the nodes in this station is easy for both EUS-FNA (the nodes lay just dorsally to the origin of the left pulmonary artery and cranial to the left atrium) and EBUS-TBNA (by means of the endoscopic view), the delineation of the inferior border by means of endoscopic ultrasound is, however, not easy. With EUS-FNA, the left atrium is generally seen as the anatomic border above which the subcarinal nodes are situated, although this is with the new definition probably too restrictive. The relation of the left atrium or pulmonary artery to the bronchus intermedius and the left lower lobe bronchus, the latter being the newly defined inferior borders of station 7, can be variable. With EBUS-TBNA, the delineation of the inferior border is possible because this investigation allows a simultaneous bronchoscopic view of the bronchial tree although there are no distinct corresponding ultrasound landmarks.

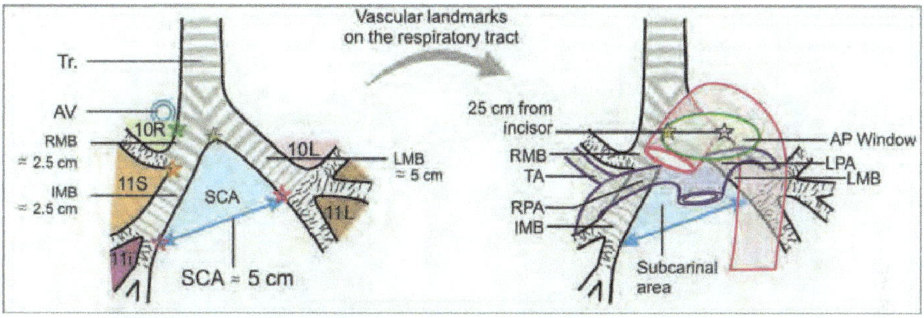

Figure 15. Virtual borders between lymph node stations and their relation with the great vessels of mediastinum [113].

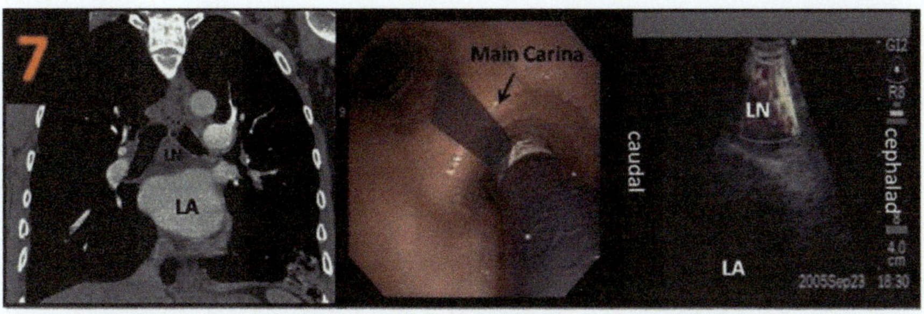

Figure 16. The subcarinal station shown on CT scan (left panel) can easily be visualized with both EUS (right panel) but of course also with EBUS. During EUS, the subcarinal station identifies as a round, hypoechogenic sharply edged structure located in between the esophagus and the pulmonary artery. The upper rim of this artery corresponds in general with the main carina and is helpful during EUS. The main carina is visualized by means of endoscopy during EBUS. The inferior border is the roof of the lower lobe bronchus on the left and the bottom of the bronchus intermedius on the right. There are no unique ultrasound features that correspond to this definition although endoscopy during EBUS is helpful [21]. Courtesy of Septimiu Murgu, MD and Henri Colt,MD; Bronchoscopy International www.bronchoscopy.org

Stations 8 and 9 are the paraoesophageal and pulmonary ligament nodes, respectively, and are situated inferior to the inferior margins of station 7 lymph nodes. The superior border of these lymph nodes is as such defined by the inferior margin of the subcarinal area. Station 8 nodes are located along the left atrium (Figures 17, 18), whereas station 9 nodes are lying within the pulmonary ligament (Figure 19). Although the latter is a structure that cannot be seen with endoscopic ultrasound, station 9 nodes are located just cranial to the diaphragm, which is readily identifiable with EUS-FNA. Stations 8 and 9 lymph nodes can be thus approached by means of EUS-FNA. Occasionally, station 8 nodes can be found by EBUS-TBNA. However, and as suggested above, one has to take into account the inferior stretch of the subcarinal nodes making this station in addition to station 9 becomes invisible for EBUS-TBNA. When performing EUS-FNA, one cannot confuse a lesion or lymph node with the esophagus. When performing EBUSTBNA, the esophagus can be seen as a multilayered structure with a hyperechogenic line in the middle corresponding with air not to be misinterpreted as a lymph node. The discrimination between the left- and right-sided nodes is the midline. Although no formal ultrasound characteristics for the midline are available, the relative position of the endoscope to the descending aorta can help.

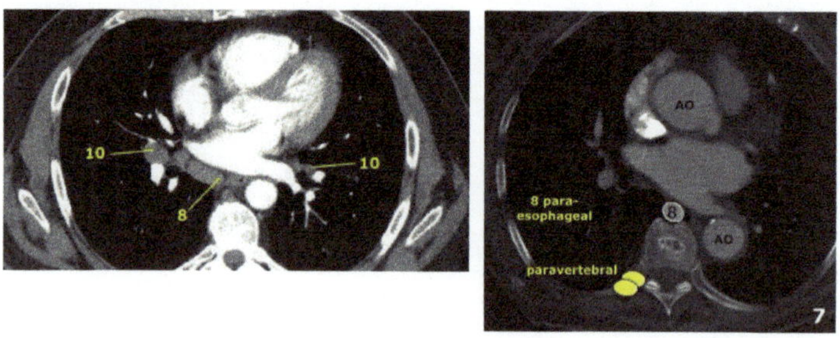

Figure 17. Station 8 Paraesophageal nodes: these nodes are below the carinal nodes and extend caudally to the diaphragm. On the left an image below the carina. To the right of the esophagus a station 8 node [111].

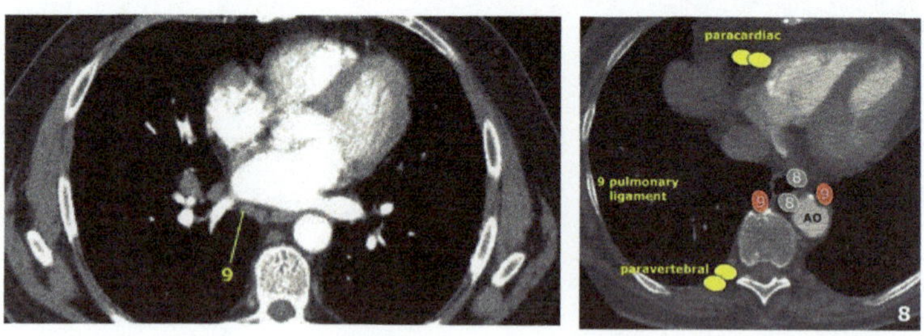

Figure 18. Station 9. Pulmonary ligament nodes: pulmonary ligament nodes are lying within the pulmonary ligament, including those in the posterior wall and lower part of the inferior pulmonary vein. The pulmonary ligament is the inferior extension of the mediastinal pleural reflections that surround the hila [111].

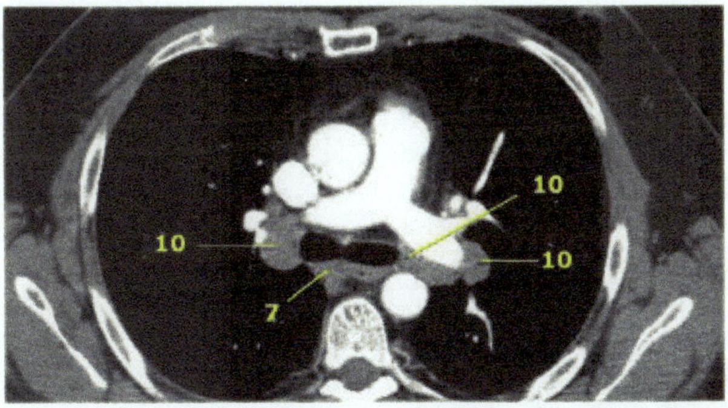

Figure 19. Hilar nodes Hilar nodes are proximal lobar nodes, distal to the mediastinal pleural reflection and nodes adjacent to the intermediate bronchus on the right. Nodes in station 10 - 14 are all N1-nodes, since they are not located in the mediastinum [111].

Station 10 or hilar lymph nodes are situated immediately adjacent to the main stem bronchus but caudal to the inferior border of azygos vein on the right and superior rim pulmonary veins and artery on the left. These nodes can be seen and sampled by EBUS-TBNA (Figures 20, 21). The inferior margin of station 10R is the interlobar region. There is no unique ultrasound feature that defines that border, but because a bronchoscopic view is available during EBUS-TBNA, the secondary carina or the upper lobe split off can serve as surrogate here. EUS-FNA has been thought to be unable to see and sample hilar stations. However, there is no doubt that in certain cases, station 10 nodes located medially from the main stem bronchi can be assessed. Endoscopists should be aware of this because misinterpretation could lead to overstaging [114].

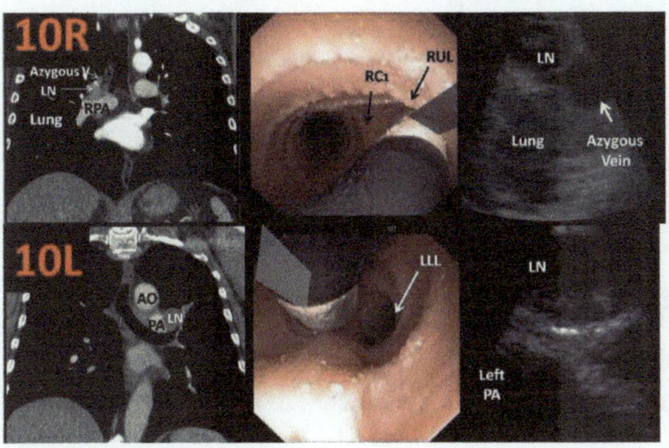

Figure 20. Station 10 lymph nodes: sagittal CT, endobronchial view and corresponding EBUS [106]. Courtesy of Septimiu Murgu, MD and Henri Colt,MD; Bronchoscopy International www.bronchoscopy.org

Once the secondary carina is reached, station 11 lymph nodes (or interlobar nodes) are encountered. From this station on, the nodes can only be approached by EBUS-TBNA and not by EUS-FNA. These nodes are located just underneath the mucosa of the secondary carina on the left. There is a division between 11s and 11i on the right side. The former indicate the nodes between upper lobe and intermediate bronchus, the latter are situated in between middle and lower lobe ultrasound landmarks are not available; however, the synchronous endoscopic view enables the identification of the relevant lobe split offs.

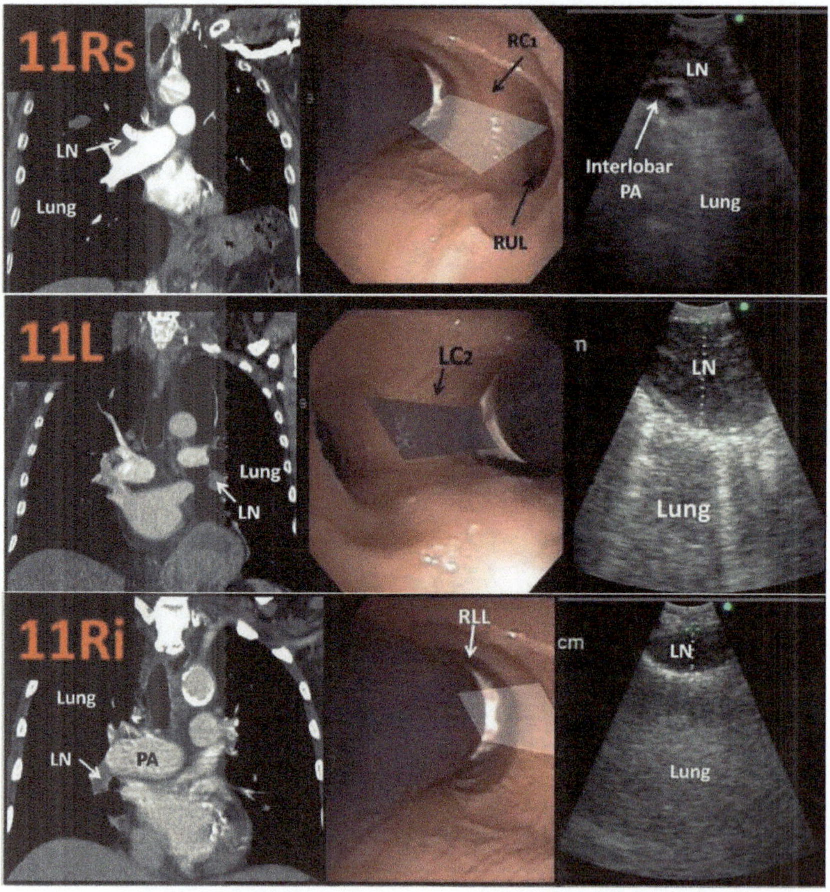

Figure 21. Station 11 lymph nodes (hilar nodes): Sagittal CT, endoscopic view and corresponding EBUS [106]. Courtesy of Septimiu Murgu, MD and Henri Colt,MD; Bronchoscopy International www.bronchoscopy.org

Once the lobar bronchi originate, then **station 12** is reached. Again, there are no unique ultrasound borders, only the endoscopic view can help for guidance. **Stations 13 and 14** are segmental and subsegmental nodes. Frequently, the EBUS-TBNA endoscope is too large to approach the segments and subsegments and their lymph nodes.

In closing, the new IASLC map maintains the lymph node stations of the other maps, but it also groups those that are anatomically proximal in lymph node areas in order to make the lymph node classification easier, especially in patients who will not undergo surgery. In this map, all the lymph node stations are defined by anatomically precise limits that are easy to recognize with imaging techniques and inspection during invasive explorations or thoracotomy. The innovations of this lymph node map are:

- The creation of a supraclavicular lymph node area that includes the supraclavicular, lower cervical (caudal on the lower edge of the cricoid cartilage) and the suprasternal fossa lymph nodes. If these lymph nodes are invaded by a tumor, they are classified as N3, regardless of the side of the tumor.
- The widening of the subcarinal lymph node station. It now includes all the lymph nodes from the tracheal bifurcation until the upper edge of the lower left lobar bronchus and the lower edge of the intermediary bronchus. If they are affected by tumors, these lymph nodes are classified as N2. This new subcarinal station includes lymph nodes that before, at least according to the Japanese map, were hilar (adjacent to the lower sides of the main bronchi), that could be classified as N1 or N3, depending on the side of the tumor. The larger size of this subcarinal station will mean an increase in N2 tumors in detriment of N1 and N3 tumors.
- The incorporation of precise limits for station number 10, the hilar station, which facilitates the prospective collection of data in order to clarify the prognostic role of this station, whose placement on other maps has always been controversial.
- The shift in the midline of the upper mediastinum from the tracheal anatomical midline to the left paratracheal margin exclusively affects the upper and lower right and left paratracheal stations. This modification implies that the affected lymph nodes that are to the left of the anatomical midline, but to the right of the new left paratracheal line, will be N2 for tumors of the right lung, but N3 for those of the left lung.

1.4. Changes to M descriptors [25, 39]

The patients with lung cancer studied for the 7th edition of the TNM Classification of Malignant Tumors presented the following survival rates at 1 and 5 years: T4 any N M0, 53% and 16%; pleural dissemination, 45% and 6%; contralateral pulmonary nodule(s), 46% and 3%, and distant metastasis, 22% and 1%; in this latter case, with significantly lower survival rates than previously cited [39]. With such references, it was decided to subdivide the M component into M1a (presence of pleural dissemination or contralateral pulmonary nodule(s)) and M1b (distant metastasis).

Subclassify the M1 component in (Table 7):

- M1a: Intrathoracic metastasis.
- M1b: Extrathoracic (distant) metastasis.
- Reclassify pleural dissemination (malignant pleural effusions, pleural nodules) and malignant pericardial effusions as a metastasis descriptor: from T4 to M1a.
- Subclassify M1 by additional nodules in the contralateral lung as M1a.
- Subclassify M1 by distant metastases as M1b.
- The MX and pM0 designation has been eliminated from the AJCC/UICC TNM system.

M factor definitions	6th ed descriptor	7th ed descriptor
Metastasis cannot be assessed.	MX	M0
Malignant pericardial effusion.	T4	M1a
Pleural dissemination (malignant pleural effusions, pleural nodules).	T4	M1a
Additional nodules in the contralateral lung (same histology).	M1	M1a
Distant metastasis.	M1	M1b

Table 7. M descriptor changes: comparison between 6th and 7th edition of the TNM Classification of Malignant Tumors [39].

1.4.1. Additional changes

- Introduction of a new accurate definition of visceral pleural invasion (VPI); VPI is a pT2 descriptor (Table 8). To avoid confusion, the abbreviation PL is employed instead of P which is also used for designation of pTNM in distinction from cTNM. The IASLC also recommends the use of elastic stains to distinguish between PL0 and PL1 when hematoxylin and eosin (H&E) sections are not helpful [71].

PL category	Definition	T status	
PL0	Tumor within the subpleural parenchyma or, invading superficially into the pleural connective tissue below the elastic layer.	PL0 is not a T descriptor and the T component should be assigned on other features.	
PL1	Tumor invades beyond the elastic layer.	pT2	Indicates VPI
PL2	Tumor invades to visceral pleural surface.		
PL3	Tumor invades the parietal pleura.	pT3	

Table 8. Classification of visceral pleural invasion (VPI): Proposed modification of Hammar Classification [115]

- Clinical TNM staging now is valid for SCLC, and stratification by stage I to III should be included in clinical trials of early stage disease [116].
- Pathologic TNM staging must be used for all SCLC cases [117]..The International Staging Committee of the IASLC has confirmed that the survival of patients with SCLC worsened as the T and N categories increased [116]. It was also observed that, except in stage IIA, which had only 55 patients for analysis, the 5-year survival worsened as the stage progressed: IA, 38%; IB, 21%; IIA, 38%; IIB, 18%; IIIA, 13%; IIIB, 9%, and IV, 1%. Based on this, the proposal to use the TNM system for staging SCLC was confirmed.
- Carcinoid tumors are now included within the TNM classification [118], a new staging system for neuroendocrine tumors. Lung carcinoids are staged in the same way as carcinomas.

Even though the 6th TNM classification specified that it was not applicable to carcinoid tumors, several studies have used it, finding prognostic differences among the stages. The IASLC has also confirmed that those classified as stage I lived significantly more than those in stage II, and these significantly more than those in stages III–IV; therefore, the new TNM classification of 2009 is recommended to describe the extension of these tumors [118].

Knowing the previous arguments for reorganizing some sections of the T and M components, a sophisticated statistical study was carried out with 17,726 patients whose tumors were better staged [119]. The different survival curves for each stage were obtained, which, without overlapping among them, presented worse levels as the tumor extension increased. This confirms the new stage grouping (Table 9), whose 5-year survivals for each stage were, according to clinical and pathological staging, respectively, the following: IA, 50% and 73%; IB, 43% and 58%; IIA, 36% and 46%; IIB, 25% and 36%; IIIA, 19% and 24%; IIIB, 7% and 9%, and IV, 2% and 13%.

6th ed	7th ed	N0	N1	N2	N3
T/M descriptors					
T1 (=2cm)	T1a	IA	IIA	IIIA	IIIB
T1 (>2 cm =3 cm)	T1b	IA	IIA	IIIA	IIIB
T2 (>3 cm =5 cm)	T2a	IB	IIA(IIB)	IIIA	IIIB
T2 (>5 cm = 7 cm)	T2b	IIA	IIB	IIIA	IIIB
T2 (>7 cm)		IIB(IB)	IIIA(IIB)	IIIA	IIIB
T3 (direct invasion)	T3	IIB	IIIA	IIIA	IIIB
T4 (same lobe nodules)		IIIB(IIIA)	IIIA(IIIB)	IIIA(IIIB)	IIIB
T4 (extension)	T4	IIIA(IIIB)	IIIA(IIIB)	IIIB	IIIB
M1 (ipsilateral nodules)		IIIA(IV)	IIIA(IV)	IIIB(IV)	IIIB(IV)
T4 (pleural or pericardial effusion)	M1a	IV(IIIB)	IV(IIIB)	IV(IIIB)	IV(IIIB)
M1 (contralateral nodules)		IV	IV	IV	IV
M1 (distant)	M1b	IV	IV	IV	IV

Table 9. Stage Grouping Comparisons: Sixth Edition Versus Seventh Edition Descriptors, T and M Categories, and Stage Groupings.

Cells in bold indicate a change in the stage from the sixth edition. Adjacent stage in parentheses represents staging from the sixth edition. T = primary tumor; N0 = no regional lymph node metastasis; N1 = metastasis in ipsilateral peribronchial and/or ipsilateral hilar lymph nodes and intrapulmonary nodes, including involvement by direct extension; N2 = metastasis in ipsilateral mediastinal and/or subcarinal lymph node(s); N3 = metastasis in contralateral mediastinal, contralateral hilar, ipsilateral or contralateral scalene, or supraclavicular lymph node(s); M = distant metastasis [65].

Stage groupings were modified due to changes to the TNM descriptors (Table 5).

1. TNM grouping categories that were down-staged:
    a. T2 smaller tumors, now T2a (>3 cm =5 cm), N1M0 are down-staged from IIB to IIA.
    b. T4 tumors due to additional nodules in primary lobe, now T3, are down-staged from IIIB to IIB (N0) or to IIIA (N1-2).
    c. M1 cases due to additional nodules in other ipsilateral lobe(s), now T4, are down-staged from IV to IIIB (N2-3) or to IIIA (N0-1).
    d. T4 tumors due to other factors, N0-1 are down-staged from IIIB to IIIA.
2. TNM grouping categories that were up-staged:
    a. T2 larger tumors, now T2b (>5 cm =7 cm), N0M0 are up-staged from IB to IIA.
    b. T2 tumors >7 cm, now T3, are up-staged: T3N0M0 from IB to IIB and T3N1M0 from IIB to IIIA.
    c. Tumors with pleural nodules or malignant pleural (or pericardial) effusion were reclassified from T4 to M1a, therefore are up-staged from stage IIIB to IV [120].

The main limitations are derived from the retrospective character of some databases that were not designed to study the TNM classification and lack precise anatomical details about the tumor extension, the number and lymph node stations affected or the differences between the different forms of M1 disease. For this reason, the IASLC itself has initiated a prospective project aimed at once again updating the TNM classification in 2016, validating all the T, N and M descriptors, especially those who have not been until now. Thus, a large international database is being constituted that, correcting the geographical omissions and disproportions in the therapeutic modalities, includes patients with non-small-cell tumors, small-cell tumors and their neuroendocrine subtypes.

In conclusion, the IASLC staging classification is unquestionably a major advance. The size of the database, the broad international spectrum, the careful and detailed analysis, as well as the internal and external validation, are tremendous achievements and relatively unique among types of cancer [121].

So, the main advantages of the new classification would be:

- The size of the database, the largest ever collected for any cancer type.
- For the first time, data was collected from different countries.

- The timeframe of 10 years allowed for 5 years follow-up.
- Cases included all treatment modalities.
- Pathologic and clinical staging where considered in survival analysis.
- The statistical analysis included meticulous internal and external validation.
- Changes to the TNM descriptors and stage groups were derived strictly from the outcome measure of overall survival.

The new TNM system is less intuitive and more complex than the 6th edition, and will be more difficult to learn. The oncology community needs to overcome the higher learning curve in order to offer patients the most appropriate treatment choices based on more accurate prognostic information [120].

2. Electromagnetic navigation bronchoscopy

It is known that diagnostic yield of flexible bronchoscopy is limited by its inability to guide biopsy instruments directly to the lesion. As it was expected, diagnosis success rate is dependent on the size and location of the lesion. The diagnostic yield of flexible bronchoscopy is expected to be between 20 and 84%. However, current nonsurgical techniques available to diagnose small peripheral lung lesions (SPLL) are limited either by low accuracy [122–125] or by potential complications [126–129].

For lesions less than 2 cm in diameter, the diagnostic yield of flexible bronchoscopy is 14% for peripheral lesions in the outer third of the chest and as high as 31% if in the proximal two-thirds [130]. The diagnostic yield of flexible bronchoscopy for mediastinal lymph nodes using transbronchial needle aspiration (TBNA) is reported to be between 15 and 83% [131]. Also, diagnostic yield of TBNA in staging of bronchogenic carcinoma is reported to be between 50 and 60% [132].

Within the past several years, electromagnetic navigation guided bronchoscopy (EGB) has proven very effective at assessing pulmonary nodules accurately with very low complication rates. EGB consists of four elements:

1. Computer software that utilizes thin-slice CT to create a three-dimensional rendering of the lung and tracheobronchial tree, which can then be used for virtual bronchoscopy.
2. A sensor probe that fits through the small working/suction channel of a bronchoscope with a steering mechanism. Because the sensor probe is recognizable within the electromagnetic field, it can be navigated through the small airways of the lung toward peripheral lesions not reachable by conventional bronchoscopy (Figure 22).
3. An electromagnetic field encompassing the patient's thorax, so that the real anatomy can be merged with the computer generated (virtual) anatomy by use of standard "registration points" (e.g., carina, takeoff of the right upper lobe bronchus, bifurcation between the left upper and lower lobes).

4. A hollow, extended working channel (EWC) that can be secured in a small peripheral airway and used to pass diagnostic instruments such as brushes, aspirating needles and biopsy forceps [133].

The ideal patient for EGB should be one with peripheral pulmonary lesion (solid or fatty solid nodule located beyond the visible range of flexible bronchoscopy) detected by chest radiography and CT or presenting with suspicion of cancer by CT morphology or positive positron emission tomography (PET) scan, as well as with a nondiagnostic conventional bronchoscopy in most of these cases; he should have absence of other metastatic lesions accessible for biopsy, a negative TTNA or contraindication for TTNA (severe pulmonary impairment, bleeding diathesis, lesions not accessible by TTNA as judged by a radiologist panel) and contraindication for straightforward curative surgery; in case of associated mediastinal lymph nodes should have a negative transbronchial needle aspiration (TBNA) or difficult to reach with TBNA lymph nodes.

Those patients who should not undergo EGB are those with contraindication to short-acting anesthetic agents, bleeding diathesis, presence of concomitant endobronchial lesion, presence of a pacemaker/defibrillator or a diagnosis by other means (sputum cytology, microbiology) that offers a reliable and easy to control course of treatment.

Navigation aim is to closely approach the target lesion (distance between sensor tip and lesion centre ≤15 mm) and take as many biopsies as possible for each lesion. At every three attempts is advised that the forceps should be withdrawn and the position of the sensor probe in relation to the target lesion checked.

Makris D et al. also recommends that all patients should undertake a CT scan prior to EGB with the following technical criteria: slice thickness 2–3.5 mm, interval between slices (with overlap of 1 mm) 1-2.5 mm, image size 512x512 pixels and dicom format [134].

As for anesthesia, Gildea TR et al. considers that all procedures (flexible bronchoscopy, bronchial washings, bronchoalveolar lavage and the actual EGB) can be safely performed using conscious sedation with intravenous 2 mg boluses of both midazolam and morphine with topical lidocaine [135].

In an emblematic study from Gildea TR et al. in 2006, the role of electromagnetic navigation bronchoscopy using super-Dimension/Bronchus System as a novel method to increase diagnostic yield of peripheral and mediastinal lung lesions was investigated. The superDimension/bronchus system is an image-guided localization system, which is designed to guide bronchoscopic tools to predetermined points within the bronchial tree. The device uses three separate technologies that are combined to enable navigation of dedicated tools within the lung in real time.

The first component is the planning software, which converts digital imaging and communications in medicine standards (DICOM) images from a computed tomography (CT) scan into multiplanar images with three-dimensional reconstruction and virtual bronchoscopy of the airways.

The second component is a steerable probe that contains a position sensor attached to an eight-way steerable instrument that has the ability to navigate turns in the endobronchial tree [135].

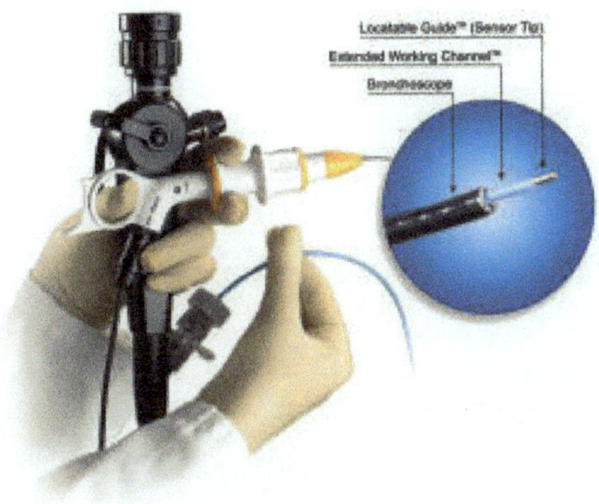

Figure 22. The steerable probe (SP) with bronchoscope [18].

The third component is an electromagnetic (EM) board, which is a field generator connected to a computer containing the planning data. The exact position of the steerable probe when placed within the EM field is depicted on the system monitor.

Registration is the process by which the computer links the five to six virtual fiducial markers to the actual position in the patient. Upon registration completion, the average fiducial target registration error (AFTRE) score was given in millimetres (mm). The AFTRE is the radius of expected difference of the location of the tip of the steerable probe in the actual patient compared with where it is expected to be in the virtual patient [135].

After registration, navigation is performed with simultaneous advancement of the steerable probe toward the target and directing steerable probe to the lesion. The closest distance between the steerable probe tip and the lesion centre is recorded. When navigation is completed, the steerable probe is removed, leaving the extendable working channel through which brushings and TBBXs or TBNA were performed [135].

In this study, biopsies were performed using a C-arm fluoroscopy unit. All instruments were visualized under fluoroscopy only after navigation was completed to confirm proper function and position of the bronchoscopic tools relative to the lesion and the pleura. Brush biopsies involved two to three passes, and four pieces of tissue were obtained by TBBX. TBNA usually was done with 2 to 4 passes of a combination of 19-G and 22-G needles depending on physician choice [130, 135-139].

Eberhardt et al. [18] reported in 2007 92 peripheral lung lesions biopsies from 89 consecutive subjects. The diagnostic yield of EGB was 67%, which was independent of lesion size. Total procedure time ranged from 16.3 to 45.0 min (mean [± SD] procedure time, 26.9 ± 6.5 min). The mean navigation error was 9 ± 6 mm(range, 1 to 31 mm). They reported two incidences of pneumothorax for which no intervention was required. When analyzed by lobar distribution, there was a trend toward a higher ENB yield in diagnosing lesions in the right middle lobe (88%). They concluded that EGB can be used as an independent bronchoscopic technique without the need for fluoroscopy when compared with other available studies. There was no increased risk of pneumothorax (2 of 89 patients; 2%). The upper lobes tend to have sharper angles in the bronchial tree that may be challenging to navigate even with a steerable sensor probe. The EWC ends close to the tip of the sensor probe and makes it less flexible. This reduces the range of deflection and, consequently, the ability to navigate. It can also make the probe flip into a different position when negotiating some tight angles in the bronchi. Navigation in the lower lobes is more affected by diaphragmatic movement during breathing and could result in larger errors than recorded. This is because the planning data are based on CT scan images acquired in a single breathhold [140, 141].

Eberhardt et al. also showed that the improved yield of EGB compared to conventional transbronchial lung biopsy in small lesions (diameter ≤ 2 cm) can be attributed to the improved precision in navigation. This study has shown the yield, safety, and timesaving with use of the EGB system without the need for fluoroscopy. This system eliminates radiation exposure and could reduce procedure costs. The diagnostic utility of the use of EGB in the biopsy of peripheral lung lesions appears to be equivalent to other advanced techniques like endobronchial ultrasound [142-144].

Apparently, these techniques have pushed bronchoscopic biopsy yields closer to those achieved by CT scan-guided transthoracic needle biopsy and surgery. Given the relative comfort [145] and safety [146] of flexible bronchoscopy, and the recognized risks of both CT scan-guided [147-149] and surgical biopsies [150], there is growing need to develop and refine these techniques. The expanded role of lung cancer screening, in which the vast majority of lesions is benign, makes this all the more important [151]. Multimodality diagnosis by combining ENB with other bronchoscopic and imaging techniques may further enhance the diagnostic yield [140].

3. Autoflorescence Bronchoscopy (AFB)

Visible light perceived by the human eye comprises the whole wavelength range, between 400–700 nm. Conventional bronchoscopy illuminates mucosal structures of the airwaves with the full wave spectrum; therefore, light gets reflected, backscattered or absorbed by the structures it encounters, thus providing the human eye with an image [152]. Tissues show a natural autoflorescence when excited in the 200-460 nm range; however, only the visible part of this range is used in medical applications [153].

However, the light source attached to the bronchoscope can emit only blue light, as a proportion of the blue spectrum excites the cellular chromophores, such as collagen, elastin or keratin, contained in the layers of the submucosa, especially within the connective tissue comprised in the elastic fiber bundles, or on the exterior surface of the cartilages (perichondrium). When excited by blue-violet light in the 400-450 nm spectrum, the excited chromophores of normal cellular lines found in the mucosa display a green tint. Another aspect of the autoflorescence theory refers to the thickness and cellular morphology of the examined tissue. Tumors and premalignant lesions have an increased mucosal thickness and therefore absorb more of the excitation occurring from fluorescence light, in what is called "the architectural effect" [153, 154]. Tissues that underwent a morphological change due to various pathological conditions, predominantly premalignant dysplasia or metaplasia-like phenomenon, are colored differently as the green fluorescence is affected by either alterations of cellular chemistry, morphology or epithelial thickness [155–157]. A wide range of AFB devices are currently available on the market: the Storz D-light system [158], Pentax SAFE-1000 [159], the Xilix LIFE system [158] or the DAFE system by Richard Wolf [160].

The main advantage of AFB is that progressive dysplasia of the mucosal layers also results in a progressive transition from normal green autoflorescence to a red-brown color, specific to precancerous or malignant lesions. This makes early premalignant lesions far easier to spot during bronchoscopy as compared to regular white-light based techniques. Inflammatory reactions, granulomas, scars, dysplasia/metaplasia and early malignant lesions which are hard to spot due to their submucosal confinement are therefore easily spotted due to their dark red-brown appearance, surrounded by normal green tissue [155–157].

The addition of AFB to conventional endoscopy can significantly increase diagnostic rate of early malignant or premalignant lesion, without the need of tumor sensitizers and therefore with no additional complications to standard bronchoscopy techniques. The detection rate of high-grade dysplasia and carcinoma in-situ (CIS) is increased to 88% after using AFB, up from the median 40% detection rate that conventional white-light bronchoscopy provides [161, 162]. However, as already stated, both premalignant lesions and various inflammatory conditions have similar appearances in AFB. Therefore, the specificity is rather low, with a high rate of false positive investigations [163, 164].

Since diffuse reflectance spectroscopy measures directly the changes in the path of white light through tissue scattering and absorption levels, some have theorized that combining autofluorescence with diffuse reflectance probes may enhance the specificity of this method. Preliminary findings have shown that a combination between the two can significantly improve the positive predictive value of AFB without altering the already attained high sensitivity for premalignant and early malignant lesions [165] (Bard MPL et al, 2005). Other attempts to improve specificity by local spectroscopical measurements have shown promising results, making way for one-stop techniques which would combine two types of wavelength measurement and fluorophore weighting [153, 165].

One study investigated the use of AFB in primary lung cancer, after treatment of head and neck cancer, detecting 29% (12/44 patients) of all second primary lung cancers, while detecting early lesions in two patients which would otherwise be missed by conventional imaging methods [166]. Early reports of Lam and his team in asbestos and diesel-exposed individuals showed an 86% sensitivity for moderate to severe dysplasia and CIS in the case of AFB, compared to just 52% for white light bronchoscopy [167]. A multicenter study performed by Lam in 1998 with the LIFE system, on 173 patients (142 biopsy-proven cases of severe dysplasia, CIS or invasive cancer) showed that AFB has a relative sensitivity of 2.71 compared to conventional bronchoscopy, successfully detecting 91 cases in comparison to only 35 with bronchoscopy alone. When considering intraepithelial lesions alone, the relative sensitivity increases to 6.1 for AFB compared to standard bronchoscopy [164].

A correlation between the loss of fluorescence and the grade of dysplasia; therefore, a trained endoscopist can differentiate these gradations to some extent, being even able to identify inflammatory or granulomatous lesions [155]. This would In turn greatly improve the specificity of AFB. A different approach consists in the usage of computer assisted analysis of signals of different wavelengths, represented in a spectrogram which in turn can classify benign from malignant lesions.

4. Narrow-Band Imaging (NBI)

NBI is a novel imaging technique capable of improving the visualization of superficial structures of the respiratory mucosa [168, 169]. NBI is used for an accurate classification of lesions, even though it does not have an established role during routine bronchoscopy [170–172]. High magnification bronchoscopy in combination with NBI can visualize the altered micro-vascularization which is formed in dysplastic or neoplastic lesions [173]. As the tumor progresses, it requires an adequately enlarged blood supply, therefore in most cancers, including those of the lungs and airways, neo angiogenesis is a constant phenomenon through which newly formed vessels are constantly produced in order to supplement local needs. These vessels form irregular aberrant patterns, having unequal diameters, tortuous configurations and uneven segment lengths.

The principle of NBI is simple: three optical filters segment the RGB (red-green-blue) light spectrum in sequence, thus narrowing the bandwidth of the spectral transmittance [174]. This allows for visual marking of capillary structures of the sub-mucosa in deep red color, allowing an easier identification and characterization, as different wavelengths penetrate the tissue at different depths. The filtering system is placed in the optical illumination system and basically contains two narrow wavelength components: NBI-B corresponding to the 400-430 nm range (blue and green visualization) and NBI-G for the 530-550 nm range (red visualization), while a third filter can be installed for an accurate segmentation of the blue-green features, operating in the 430-460 nm range; the optical light-source usually operates in the 400-700 nm wavelength range. All current models include a 2-filter system, which emphasizes capillaries in the superficial mucosal layers by the 400-430 nm light, coloring them in shades of brown, while deeper mucosal or submucosal vessels are displayed in cyan by using the 530-550 nm filter. Modern systems allow for easy switch between the normal WLI and the enhanced NBI operations [168].

Limitations of the technology arise from the fact that not all lung malignancies develop submucosal neo vascularization visible from the airways, therefore potential false-negative NBI findings can be frequent when used in combination with WLB. Its sensitivity may be however increased when used in conjunction with other specific techniques such as AFB; however, its role in the screening process for lung malignancies is yet to be determined. A step further in this direction would be the standardization of imaging findings, based on clinical descriptions and classification of abnormal airway vascularity. High magnification bronchoscopy can improve the specificity of the technique, as it may allow a more clear description of the vascular patterns [168]. Good prospects come from new techniques such as probe-based confocal laser endomicroscopy which can provide an in situ diagnosis of malignancy if used in conjunction with any endoscopic technique.

5. Probe-based Confocal Laser Endomicroscopy (pCLE)

Gastrointestinal applications of pCLE are numerous, the system being successfully tested in real-life conditions [175]. It can be used for identifying premalignant lesions otherwise invisible to classic endoscopic techniques, such as Barrett's esophagus [176], classification of polipous lesions at colonic level [177], gastric metaplasia or early stage lesions at all levels of the digestive tracts [178, 179]. The technique requires injection of fluorescein or another fluorophore, followed by endoscopic imaging of the dye to identify mucosal details such as mucosal and vessel architecture to distinguish among normal, dysplastic, and neoplastic tissue. The use of fluorescein as an in-vivo contrast agent for detecting vascular structures has been deemed safe by several studies [180]. It thus allows for better visualization of vascular structures, serving as an overall tissue contrasting agent as it may leak beyond capillary confinement.

The imaging microprobe is connected to 30,000 fiber-optic threads that enable point-to-point real-time detection at 12 frames/sec. The microprobe's flexibility and size (1.5 mm in diameter) allow for great user maneuverability to scan tissues in situ at angles that would not be possible with any available confocal microscope objective. The mini-probe is inserted through a working channel of any standard bronchoscope and can reach the alveolar duct. A laser generator emits 488 nm blue argon laser light which is transmitted through the optical fibers and excites the elastin scaffold of the acinus. In turn, a real time image of the elastic fibers which sustain the alveoli, as well as the microvessel architecture is revealed. The probe can be translated over a larger tissue sample, and the images later reconstructed in order to extend the field of view covered [181]. A monitor attached to an imaging unit is available for real-time visualization of cellular images, the device being capable of recording full length movies which can be recorded and later on analyzed with dedicated software [182].

This technology is still in its early stages; however, it was deemed safe by regulatory organisms in the United States of America for applications in patient settings. In conjunction with safe contrasting agents such as fluorescein [183] or methilen blue [184], it can be used for the in vivo histologic assessment of the bronchial epithelium at all levels of the airway system [185–187]. Several studies reported good initial results in control groups of healthy smokers or patients with chronic obstructive pulmonary disease for diagnosing various forms of parenchymal lung disease [188, 189]. A pCLE investigation seems to be a quick and safe procedure for patients with various pulmonary conditions, with minimal side-effects related to both the technique and the contrasting fluorescent agents used for imaging. General consensus is that further studies are needed in order to extent the diagnostic capabilities and enhance its sensibility in comparison with standard cytological and histological techniques.

Author details

Mihai Olteanu[1], Costin Teodor Streba[1], Bogdan Oprea[1], Raluca Marinas[1], Mimi Floarea Nitu[1], Emilia Crisan[1,2] and Tudorel Ciurea[1]

1 University of Medicine and Pharmacy of Craiova, Romania

2 "Marius Nasta" Pulmonology Institute, Bucharest, Romania

References

[1] Lopez-Encuentra A, Garcia-Lujan R, Rivas JJ, Rodriguez-Rodriguez J, Torres-Lanza J, Varela- Simo G. Comparison between clinical and pathologic staging in 2,994 cases of lung cancer. Ann Thorac Surg 2005; 79:974–979; discussion, 979.

[2] Mountain CF. Revisions in the international system for staging lung cancer. Chest 1997; 111 (6): 1710-1717.

[3] Lung. In: American Joint Committee on Cancer. AJCC Cancer Staging Manual. 6th ed. New York, NY: Springer, 2002, pp 167-181.

[4] Silvestri GA. A seismic shift in staging. J Thorac Oncol 2007; 2 (8): 682-683.

[5] Goldstraw P Crowley JJ; on behalf of the IASLC International Staging Project. The International Association for the Study of Lung Cancer International Staging Project on Lung Cancer. J Thorac Oncol 2006; 1 (4): 281-286.

[6] Rami Porta R. Nueva clasificación TNM del cáncer de pulmón. Arch Bronconeumol 2009; 45 (4): 159-161.

[7] Sobin LH, Gospodarowicz MK, Wittekind C. eds. TNM Classification of Malignant Tumours, 7th ed., 2010, Wiley-Blackwell.

[8] Rami-Porta R, Crowley JJ, Goldstraw P. The revised TNM staging system for lung cancer. Ann Thorac Cardiovasc Surg 2009; 15 (1): 4-9.

[9] Groome PA, Bolejack V, Crowley JJ, Kennedy C, Krasnik M, Sobin LH, Goldstraw P; IASLC International Staging Committee; Cancer Research and Biostatistics; Observers to the Committee; Participating Institutions. The IASLC Lung Cancer Staging Project: validation of the proposals for revision of the T, N, and M descriptors and consequent stage groupings in the forthcoming (seventh) edition of the TNM classification of malignant tumours. J Thorac Oncol 2007; 2 (8): 694-705.

[10] Krasnik M, Vilmann P, Larsen S, Jacobsen G, Preliminary experience with a new method of endoscopic transbronchial real time ultrasound guided biopsy for diagnosis of mediastinal and hilar lesions Thorax. 2003 December; 58(12): 1083–1086.

[11] Herth F J F, Eberhardt R, Vilmann P, Krasnik M, Ernst A, Real-time endobronchial ultrasound guided transbronchial needle aspiration for sampling mediastinal lymph nodes, Thorax. 2006 September; 61(9): 795–798.

[12] Herth FJF, Krasnik M, Yasufuku K, R Rintoul R, Ernst A, Endobronchial Ultrasound-guided Transbronchial Needle Aspiration, J Bronchol 2006;13:84–91

[13] Wong M, Yasufuku K, Nakajima T, Herth FJ, Sekine Y, Shibuya K, Iizasa T, Hiroshima K, Lam WK, Fujisawa T, Endobronchial ultrasound: new insight for the diagnosis of sarcoidosis, Eur Respir J. 2007 Jun; 29(6):1182-6.

[14] Herth FJF, Ernst A, Eberhardt R, Vilmann P, Dienemann H, Krasnik M, Endobronchial Ultrasound-guided Transbronchial Needle Aspiration of Lymph Nodes in the Radiologically Normal Mediastinum. Eur Respir J 2006; 28: 910-914.

[15] Hwangbo B, Kim SK, Lee HS, Lee HS, Kim MS, Lee JM, Kim HY, Lee GK, Nam BH, Zo JI, Application of endobronchial ultrasound-guided transbronchial needle aspiration following integrated PET/CT in mediastinal staging of potentially operable non-small cell lung cancer. Chest. 2009 May;135(5):1280-7. Epub 2008 Dec 31.

[16] Ernst A, Anantham D, Eberhardt R, Krasnik M, Herth FJ. Diagnosis of mediastinal adenopathy-real-time endobronchial ultrasound guided needle aspiration versus mediastinoscopy. J Thorac Oncol. 2008 Jun;3(6):577-82.

[17] Herth FJ, Yasufuku K, Eberhardt R, Hoffmann H, Krasnik M, Ernst A. Resistance index in mediastinal lymph nodes: a feasibility study. J Thorac Oncol. 2008 Apr;3(4): 348-50.

[18] Herth F, Eberhardt R, Mulay T, Anantham D, Ernst A, Resistance index through EBUS in enlarged mediastinal lymph nodes correlates with malignant involvement, CHEST. October 2007;132(4_MeetingAbstracts):465c-466.

[19] Nakajima T, Yasufuku K, Suzuki M, et al. Assessment of epidermal growth factor receptor mutation by endobronchial ultrasound-guided transbronchial needle aspiration CHEST 2007;132(2):597-602.

[20] Nakajima T, Yasufuku K, Suzuki M, et al. Chemosensitivity-related aberrant methylation profiling of non-small cell lung cancer by endobronchial ultrasound-guided transbronchial needle aspiration CHEST 2007;132(4_MeetingAbstracts):466a-466.

[21] Tournoy KG, Annema JT, Krasnik M, Herth FJ, van Meerbeeck JP Endoscopic and endobronchial ultrasonography according to the proposed lymph node map definition in the seventh edition of the tumor, node, metastasis classification for lung cancer. J Thorac Oncol. 2009 Dec;4(12):1576-84.

[22] Annema JT, van Meerbeeck JP, Rintoul RC, Dooms C, Deschepper E, Dekkers OM, De Leyn P, Braun J, Carroll NR, Praet M, de Ryck F, Vansteenkiste J, Vermassen F, Versteegh MI, Veseliç M, Nicholson AG, Rabe KF, Tournoy KG. Mediastinoscopy vs endosonography for mediastinal nodal staging of lung cancer: a randomized trial. JAMA. 2010 Nov 24;304(20):2245-52.

[23] Hwangbo B, Lee G, Lee H, et al. Transbronchial and transesophageal fine-needle aspiration using an ultrasound bronchoscope in mediastinal staging of potentially operable lung cancer CHEST 2010;138(4):795-802, Herth FF, Krasnik M, Kahn N, Eberhardt R, Ernst A. Combined endoscopic-endobronchial ultrasound-guided fine-needle aspiration of mediastinal lymph nodes through a single bronchoscope in 150 patients with suspected lung cancer CHEST 2010;138(4):790-794.

[24] Herth FJ Nonsurgical staging of the mediastinum: EBUS and EUS. Semin Respir Crit Care Med. 2011 Feb;32(1):62-8. Epub 2011 Apr 15

[25] Edge SB, Byrd DR, Compton CC, Fritz AG, Greene FL, Trotti A. eds. Part I. General information on cancer staging and end-results reporting. 1. Purposes and principles of cancer staging. In: Edge SB, Byrd DR, Compton CC, Fritz AG, Greene FL, Trotti A. eds. AJCC Cancer Staging Manual. 7th ed., 2010, Springer; pp. 3-14.

[26] Herth FJ, Eberhardt R, Vilmann P et al. Real-time endobronchial ultrasound guided transbronchial needle aspiration for sampling mediastinal lymph nodes. Thorax 2006; 61: 795–798.

[27] Ernst A, Eberhardt R, Krasnik M, Herth FJ. Efficacy of endobronchial ultrasoundguided transbronchial needle aspiration of hilar lymph nodes for diagnosing and staging cancer. J Thorac Oncol 2009; 4: 947–950.

[28] Tournoy KG, Rintoul RC, van Meerbeeck JP et al. EBUS-TBNA for the diagnosis of central parenchymal lung lesions not visible at routine bronchoscopy. Lung Cancer 2009; 63: 45–49.

[29] Ernst A, Anantham D, Eberhardt R et al. Diagnosis of mediastinal adenopathy real-time endobronchial ultrasound guided needle aspiration versus mediastinoscopy. J Thorac Oncol 2008; 3: 577–582.

[30] Detterbeck FC, Jantz MA, Wallace MB et al. Invasive mediastinal staging of lung cancer. ACCP evidence based clinical practice guidelines, 2nd edition. Chest 2007; 132: 202S–220S..

[31] Tournoy KG, Govaerts E, Malfait T, Dooms C. Endobronchial ultrasound-guided transbronchial needle biopsy for M1 staging of extrathoracic malignancies. Ann Oncol first published online July 5, 2010 doi:10.1093/annonc/mdq311

[32] American Cancer Society. Cancer facts and figures, 1998. Atlanta, GA: American Cancer Society, 1998.

[33] A. Ernst, F.J.F. Herth (eds.), Endobronchial Ultrasound, DOI 10.1007/978-0-387-09437-3_1, ª Springer ScienceþBusiness Media, LLC 2009

[34] Silvestri GA, Gould MK, Margolis ML, et al. Noninvasive staging in non-small cell lung cancer: ACCP evidenced-based clinical practice guidelines (2nd edition). Chest. 2007; 132: 178–201

[35] Bhutani MS, Hawes RH, Hoffmann BJ. A comparison of the accuracy of echo features during endoscopic ultrasound (EUS) and EUS-guided fine-needle aspiration for diagnosis of malignant lymph node invasion. Gastrointest Endosc. 1997; 31: 550–553.

[36] Okamoto H, Watanabe K, Nagatomo A, et al. Endobronchial ultrasonography for mediastinal and hilar lymph node metastases of lung cancer. Chest. 2002; 121: 1498–1506.

[37] Yasufuku node staging in non-small cell carcinoma. Do we have to accept the compromise? Eur J Cardiothorac Surg. 2001; 20: 652–654.

[38] Rami-Porta R, Ball D, Crowley J, Giroux DJ, Jett J, Travis WD, Tsuboi M, Vallières E, Goldstraw P; International Staging Committee; Cancer Research and Biostatistics; Observers to the Committee; Participating Institutions. The IASLC Lung Cancer Staging Project: proposals for the revision of the T descriptors in the forthcoming (seventh) edition of the TNM classification for lung cancer. J Thorac Oncol 2007; 2 (7): 593-602.

[39] Postmus PE, Brambilla E, Chansky K, Crowley J, Goldstraw P, Patz EF Jr, Yokomise H; International Association for the Study of Lung Cancer International Staging Committee; Cancer Research and Biostatistics; Observers to the Committee; Participating Institutions. The IASLC Lung Cancer Staging Project: proposals for revision of the M descriptors in the forthcoming (seventh) edition of the TNM classification of lung cancer. J Thorac Oncol 2007; 2 (8): 686-693.

[40] Dr. A. De la Guerra. New TNM Classification for Lung Cancer. Part II: A review. Doctors Lounge Website. Available at: http://www.doctorslounge.com/index.php/articles/page/342.

[41] Strand TE, Rostad H, Møller B, Norstein J. Survival after resection for primary lung cancer: a population based study of 3211 resected patients. Thorax 2006; 61 (8): 710-715.

[42] Suzuki K, Nagai K, Yoshida J, Nishimura M, Takahashi K, Yokose T, Nishiwaki Y. Conventional clinicopathologic prognostic factors in surgically resected nonsmall cell lung carcinoma. A comparison of prognostic factors for each pathologic TNM stage based on multivariate analyses. Cancer 1999; 86 (10): 1976-1984.

[43] van Rens MT, de la Rivière AB, Elbers HR, van Den Bosch JM. Prognostic assessment of 2,361 patients who underwent pulmonary resection for non-small cell lung cancer, stage I, II, and IIIA. Chest 2000; 117 (2): 374-379.

[44] Hung JJ, Hsu WH, Hsieh CC, Huang BS, Huang MH, Liu JS, Wu YC. Post-recurrence survival in completely resected stage I non-small cell lung cancer with local recurrence. Thorax 2009; 64 (3): 192-196.

[45] Casali C, Storelli E, Morandi U. The prognostic impact of tumor size in resected stage I non-small cell lung cancer: evidence for a two thresholds tumor diameters classification. Lung Cancer 2006; 54 (2): 185-191.

[46] Mountain CF, Carr DT, Anderson WA. A system for the clinical staging of lung cancer. Am J Roentgenol Radium Ther Nucl Med 1974; 120 (1): 130-138.

[47] Ruffini E, Filosso PL, Bruna MC, Coni F, Cristofori RC, Mossetti C, Solidoro P, Oliaro A. Recommended changes for T and N descriptors proposed by the International Association for the Study of Lung Cancer - Lung Cancer Staging Project: a validation study from a single-centre experience. Eur J Cardiothorac Surg 2009; 36 (6): 1037-1044.

[48] Fukui T, Mori S, Hatooka S, Shinoda M, Mitsudomi T. Prognostic evaluation based on a new TNM staging system proposed by the International Association for the Study of Lung Cancer for resected non-small cell lung cancers. J Thorac Cardiovasc Surg 2008; 136 (5): 1343-1348.

[49] Kassis ES, Vaporciyan AA, Swisher SG, Correa AM, Bekele BN, Erasmus JJ, Hofstetter WL, Komaki R, Mehran RJ, Moran CA, Pisters KM, Rice DC, Walsh GL, Roth JA. Application of the revised lung cancer staging system (IASLC Staging Project) to a cancer center population. J Thorac Cardiovasc Surg 2009; 138 (2): 412-418.

[50] Li Z, Yu Y, Lu J, Luo Q, Wu C, Liao M, Zheng Y, Ai X, Gu L, Lu S. Analysis of the T descriptors and other prognosis factors in pathologic stage I non-small cell lung cancer in China. J Thorac Oncol 2009; 4 (6): 702-709.

[51] Kameyama K, Takahashi M, Ohata K, Igai H, Yamashina A, Matsuoka T, Nakagawa T, Okumura N. Evaluation of the new TNM staging system proposed by the International Association for the Study of Lung Cancer at a single institution. J Thorac Cardiovasc Surg 2009; 137 (5): 1180-1184.

[52] Mountain CF. Revisions in the international system for staging lung cancer. Chest 1997; 111 (6): 1710-1717.

[53] Naruke T, Tsuchiya R, Kondo H, Asamura H. Prognosis and survival after resection for bronchogenic carcinoma based on the 1997 TNM staging classification: the Japanese experience. Ann Thorac Surg 2001; 71(6): 1759-1764.

[54] Warren S, Gates O. Multiple primary malignant tumors: a survey of the literature and a statistical study. Am J Cancer 1932; 16: 1358-1414.

[55] Howe HL (ed). A review of the definition for multiple primary cancers in the United States. Workshop proceedings from December 4-6, 2002, in Princeton, New Jersey. Springfield (IL): North American Association of Central Cancer Registries, May 2003.

[56] Martini N, Melamed MR. Multiple primary lung cancers. J Thorac Cardiovasc Surg 1975; 70 (4): 606-612.

[57] Facility Oncology Registry Data Standards (FORDS): Revised for 2009. Chicago, Illinois: Commission on Cancer, American College of Surgeons; 2002.

[58] Johnson CH, Adamo M (eds.), SEER Program Coding and Staging Manual 2007. National Cancer Institute, NIH Publication number 07-5581, Bethesda, MD 2008 revision. Appendix C - Site-Specific Coding Modules. Part 3 C30.0 -C39.9: pgs 375-526.

[59] Shen KR, Meyers BF, Larner JM, Jones DR; American College of Chest Physicians. Special treatment issues in lung cancer: ACCP evidence-based clinical practice guidelines (2nd edition). Chest 2007; 132 (3 Suppl): 290S-305S.

[60] Deslauriers J, Brisson J, Cartier R, Fournier M, Gagnon D, Piraux M, Beaulieu M. Carcinoma of the lung. Evaluation of satellite nodules as a factor influencing prognosis after resection. J Thorac Cardiovasc Surg 1989; 97 (4): 504-512.

[61] Martini N, Melamed MR. Multiple primary lung cancers. J Thorac Cardiovasc Surg 1975; 70 (4): 606-612.

[62] Shen KR, Meyers BF, Larner JM, Jones DR; American College of Chest Physicians. Special treatment issues in lung cancer: ACCP evidence-based clinical practice guidelines (2nd edition). Chest 2007; 132 (3 Suppl): 290S-305S.

[63] Urschel JD, Urschel DM, Anderson TM, Antkowiak JG, Takita H. Prognostic implications of pulmonary satellite nodules: are the 1997 staging revisions appropriate? Lung Cancer 1998; 21 (2): 83-87.

[64] Rao J, Sayeed RA, Tomaszek S, Fischer S, Keshavjee S, Darling GE. Prognostic factors in resected satellite-nodule T4 non-small cell lung cancer. Ann Thorac Surg 2007; 84 (3): 934-938.

[65] Goldstraw P, Crowley J, Chansky K, Giroux DJ, Groome PA, Rami-Porta R, Postmus PE, Rusch V, Sobin L; International Association for the Study of Lung Cancer International Staging Committee; Participating Institutions. The IASLC Lung Cancer Stag-

ing Project: proposals for the revision of the TNM stage groupings in the forthcoming (seventh) edition of the TNM Classification of malignant tumours. J Thorac Oncol 2007; 2 (8): 706-714.

[66] Molina JR. The case of a good satellite: outcomes of resected ipsilateral same-lobe satellite pulmonary nodules. Chest 2009; 136 (3): 660-662.

[67] Pennathur A, Lindeman B, Ferson P, Ninan M, Quershi I, Gooding WE, Schuchert M, Christie NA, Landreneau RJ, Luketich JD. Surgical resection is justified in non-small cell lung cancer patients with node negative T4 satellite lesions. Ann Thorac Surg 2009; 87 (3): 893-899.

[68] Sobin LH, Wittekind C eds. Lung and pleural tumours. In: Sobin LH, Wittekind C eds. UICC International Union Against Cancer, TNM classification of malignant tumours, 6th ed. New York: Wiley-Liss, 2002; pp. 97-107.Even so, some authors use the term as a synonym for pleural nodules.

[69] Sobin LH, Wittekind C eds. Lung and pleural tumours. In: Sobin LH, Wittekind C eds. UICC International Union Against Cancer, TNM classification of malignant tumours, 6th ed. New York: Wiley-Liss, 2002; pp. 97-107.Even so, some authors use the term as a synonym for pleural nodules.

[70] Hammar SP. Common tumors. In: Dail DH, Hammar SP, eds. Pulmonary pathology, 2nd ed. New York: Springer-Verlag, 1994; pp. 1123–1278.

[71] Travis WD, Brambilla E, Rami-Porta R, Vallières E, Tsuboi M, Rusch V, Goldstraw P; International Staging Committee. Visceral pleural invasion: pathologic criteria and use of elastic stains: proposal for the 7th edition of the TNM classification for lung cancer. J Thorac Oncol 2008; 3 (12): 1384-1390.

[72] Mountain CF. Revisions in the international system for staging lung cancer. Chest 1997; 111 (6): 1710-1717.

[73] Antony VB, Loddenkemper R, Astoul P, Boutin C, Goldstraw P, Hott J, Rodriguez Panadero F, Sahn SA. Management of malignant pleural effusions. Eur Respir J 2001; 18 (2): 402-419.

[74] American Thoracic Society. Management of malignant pleural effusions. Am J Respir Crit Care Med 2000; 162 (5): 1987-2001.

[75] Antunes G, Neville E, Duffy J, Ali N; Pleural Diseases Group, Standards of Care Committee, British Thoracic Society. BTS guidelines for the management of malignant pleural effusions. Thorax 2003; 58 (Suppl 2): ii29-ii38.

[76] Sahn SA. Pleural diseases related to metastatic malignancies. Eur Respir J 1997; 10 (8): 1907-1913.

[77] Heffner JE, Nietert PJ, Barbieri C. Pleural fluid pH as a predictor of survival for patients with malignant pleural effusions. Chest 2000; 117 (1): 79-86.

[78] Osaki T, Sugio K, Hanagiri T, Takenoyama M, Yamashita T, Sugaya M, Yasuda M, Yasumoto K. Survival and prognostic factors of surgically resected T4 non-small cell lung cancer. Ann Thorac Surg 2003; 75 (6): 1745-1751.

[79] Sugiura S, Ando Y, Minami H, Ando M, Sakai S, Shimokata K. Prognostic value of pleural effusion in patients with non-small cell lung cancer. Clin Cancer Res 1997; 3 (1): 47-50.

[80] Mott FE, Sharma N, Ashley P. Malignant pleural effusion in non-small cell lung cancer--time for a stage revision? Chest 2001; 119 (1): 317-318.

[81] Kameyama K, Huang CL, Liu D, Okamoto T, Hayashi E, Yamamoto Y, Yokomise H. Problems related to TNM staging: patients with stage III non-small cell lung cancer. J Thorac Cardiovasc Surg 2002; 124 (3): 503-510.

[82] Sawabata N, Matsumura A, Motohiro A, Osaka Y, Gennga K, Fukai S, Mori T; Japanese National Chest Hospital Study group for Lung Cancer. Malignant minor pleural effusion detected on thoracotomy for patients with non-small cell lung cancer: is tumor resection beneficial for prognosis? Ann Thorac Surg 2002; 73 (2): 412-415.

[83] Osaki T, Sugio K, Hanagiri T, Takenoyama M, Yamashita T, Sugaya M, Yasuda M, Yasumoto K. Survival and prognostic factors of surgically resected T4 non-small cell lung cancer. Ann Thorac Surg 2003; 75 (6): 1745-1751.

[84] Rodriguez Panadero F. Lung cancer and ipsilateral pleural effusion. Ann Oncol 1995; 6 (Suppl 3): S25-S27.

[85] Ohta Y, Tanaka Y, Hara T, Oda M, Watanabe S, Shimizu J, Watanabe Y. Clinicopathological and biological assessment of lung cancers with pleural dissemination. Ann Thorac Surg 2000; 69 (4): 1025-1029.

[86] Sugiura S, Ando Y, Minami H, Ando M, Sakai S, Shimokata K. Prognostic value of pleural effusion in patients with non-small cell lung cancer. Clin Cancer Res 1997; 3 (1): 47-50.

[87] Maruyama R, Yokoyama H, Seto T, Nagashima S, Kashiwabara K, Araki J, Semba H, Ichinose Y. Catheter drainage followed by the instillation of bleomycin to manage malignant pericardial effusion in non-small cell lung cancer: a multi-institutional phase II trial. J Thorac Oncol 2007; 2 (1): 65-68.

[88] Kunitoh H, Tamura T, Shibata T, Imai M, Nishiwaki Y, Nishio M, Yokoyama A, Watanabe K, Noda K, Saijo N; JCOG Lung Cancer Study Group, Tokyo, Japan. A randomised trial of intrapericardial bleomycin for malignant pericardial effusion with lung cancer (JCOG9811). Br J Cancer 2009; 100 (3): 464-469.

[89] Kaira K, Takise A, Kobayashi G, Utsugi M, Horie T, Mori T, Imai H, Inazawa M, Mori M. Management of malignant pericardial effusion with instillation of mitomycin C in non-small cell lung cancer. Jpn J Clin Oncol 2005; 35 (2): 57-60.

[90] Naruke T, Tsuchiya R, Kondo H, Asamura H, Nakayama H. Implications of staging in lung cancer. Chest 1997; 112 (4 Suppl): 242S-248S.

[91] Osaki T, Sugio K, Hanagiri T, Takenoyama M, Yamashita T, Sugaya M, Yasuda M, Yasumoto K. Survival and prognostic factors of surgically resected T4 non-small cell lung cancer. Ann Thorac Surg 2003; 75 (6): 1745-1751.

[92] Alon BN, Anson BL. Pleural effusion in patients with non-small cell carcinoma--stage IV and not T4. Lung Cancer 2007; 57 (1): 123.

[93] Mott FE, Sharma N, Ashley P. Malignant pleural effusion in non-small cell lung cancer-time for a stage revision? Chest 2001; 119 (1): 317-318.

[94] Kameyama K, Huang CL, Liu D, Okamoto T, Hayashi E, Yamamoto Y, Yokomise H. Problems related to TNM staging: patients with stage III non-small cell lung cancer. J Thorac Cardiovasc Surg 2002; 124 (3): 503-510.

[95] Leong SS, Rocha Lima CM, Sherman CA, Green MR. The 1997 International Staging System for non-small cell lung cancer: have all the issues been addressed? Chest 1999; 115 (1): 242-248.

[96] Naruke T, Tsuchiya R, Kondo H, Asamura H, Nakayama H. Implications of staging in lung cancer. Chest 1997; 112 (4 Suppl): 242S-248S.

[97] Rusch VW, Asamura H, Watanabe H, Giroux DJ, Rami-Porta R, Goldstraw P; Members of IASLC Staging Committee. The IASLC lung cancer staging project: a proposal for a new international lymph node map in the forthcoming seventh edition of the TNM classification for lung cancer. J Thorac Oncol 2009; 4 (5): 568-577.

[98] Rusch VW, Crowley J, Giroux DJ, Goldstraw P, Im JG, Tsuboi M, Tsuchiya R, Vansteenkiste J; International Staging Committee; Cancer Research and Biostatistics; Observers to the Committee; Participating Institutions. The IASLC Lung Cancer Staging Project: proposals for the revision of the N descriptors in the forthcoming seventh edition of the TNM classification for lung cancer. J Thorac Oncol 2007; 2 (7): 603-612.

[99] Rusch VW, Asamura H, Watanabe H, Giroux DJ, Rami-Porta R, Goldstraw, on Behalf of the Members of the IASLC Staging Committee. The IASLC lung cancer staging project: a proposal for a new international lymph node map in the forthcoming seventh edition of the TNM classification for lung cancer. J Thorac Oncol 2009;4:568-577.

[100] Rusch VW, Crowley J, Giroux DJ, Goldstraw P, Im JG, Tsuboi M, Tsuchiya R, Vansteenkiste J; International Staging Committee; Cancer Research and Biostatistics; Observers to the Committee; Participating Institutions. The IASLC Lung Cancer Staging Project: proposals for the revision of the N descriptors in the forthcoming seventh edition of the TNM classification for lung cancer. J Thorac Oncol 2007; 2 (7): 603-612.

[101] The International Association for the Study of Lung Cancer (IASLC) lymph node map, including the proposed grouping of lymph node stations into "zones" for the purposes of prognostic analyses. (Reprinted from Rusch VW, on Behalf of the Mem-

bers of the IASLC Staging Committee. The IASLC lung cancer staging project: a proposal for a new international lymph node map in the forthcoming seventh edition of the TNM classification for lung cancer. J Thorac Oncol. 2009;4:568-577.

[102] Lee JG, Lee CY, Bae MK, et al. Validity of International Association for the Study of Lung Cancer proposals for the revision of N descriptors in lung cancer. J Thorac Oncol2008; 3:1421 –1426.

[103] Annema JT, Rabe KF. EUS in non-small cell lung cancer. In RH Hawes, P Fockens (Eds.), Endosonography. Philadelphia: WB Saunders, 2006:61–72.

[104] Kramer H, van Putten JW, Douma WR, Smidt AA, van Dullemen HM, Groen HJ. Technical description of endoscopic ultrasonography with fine-needle aspiration for the staging of lung cancer. Respir Med 2005; 99:179-185.

[105] Navani N, Spiro SG, Janes SM, Mediastinal staging of NSCLC with endoscopic and endobronchial ultrasound, Nat Rev Clin Oncol. 2009 May; 6(5): 278–286. doi: 10.1038/nrclinonc.2009.39

[106] Murgu S, Colt H, University of California, Irvine, The EBUS Bronchoscopist: Exploring the mediastinum with endobronchial ultrasound, Module 1, 2011, available at http://www.bronchoscopy.org/education.

[107] van Overhagen H, Brakel K, Heijenbrok MW, et al. Metastases in supraclavicular lymph nodes in lung cancer: assessment with palpation, US, and CT. Radiology 2004;232:75– 80.

[108] Kumaran M, Benamore RE, Vaidhyanath R, et al. Ultrasound guided cytological aspiration of supraclavicular lymph nodes in patients with suspected lung cancer. Thorax 2005;60:229 –233.

[109] Sihoe AD, Lee TW, Ahuja AT, Yim AP. Should cervical ultrasonography be a routine staging investigation for lung cancer patients with impalpable cervical lymph nodes? Eur J Cardiothorac Surg 2004;25: 486–491.

[110] Prosch H, Strasser G, Sonka C, et al. Cervical ultrasound (US) and US-guided lymph node biopsy as a routine procedure for staging of lung cancer. Ultraschall Med 2007;28:598–603.

[111] Robin Smithuis Radiology department of the Rijnland Hospital in Leiderdorp, the Netherlands, available at http://www.radiologyassistant.nl/en/4646f1278c26f#.

[112] von Bartheld MB, Rabe KF, Annema JT. Transaortic EUS-guided FNA in the diagnosis of lung tumors and lymph nodes. Gastrointest Endosc 2009;69:345–349.

[113] Malay Sharma, Vishal Arya and CS RameshBabu (2011). Techniques of Linear Endobronchial Ultrasound, Ultrasound Imaging - Medical Applications, Igor V. Minin and Oleg V. Minin (Ed.), ISBN: 978-953-307-279-1, InTech, Available from: http://

www.intechopen.com/books/ultrasound-imaging-medical-applications/techniques-of-linear-endobronchial-ultrasound

[114] Dooms C, Vansteenkiste J, Van RD, De LP. Esophageal ultrasoundcontrolled fine needle aspiration for staging of mediastinal lymph nodes in patients with resectable lung cancer: do we always see the reality? J Thorac Oncol 2009;4:1043–1045.

[115] Hammar SP. Common tumors. In: Dail DH, Hammar SP, eds. Pulmonary pathology, 2nd ed. New York: Springer-Verlag, 1994; pp. 1123–1278.

[116] Shepherd FA, Crowley J, Van Houtte P, Postmus PE, Carney D, Chansky K, Shaikh Z, Goldstraw P; International Association for the Study of Lung Cancer International Staging Committee and Participating Institutions. The International Association for the Study of Lung Cancer lung cancer staging project: proposals regarding the clinical staging of small cell lung cancer in the forthcoming (seventh) edition of the tumor, node, metastasis classification for lung cancer. J Thorac Oncol 2007; 2 (12): 1067-1077.

[117] Vallières E, Shepherd FA, Crowley J, Van Houtte P, Postmus PE, Carney D, Chansky K, Shaikh Z, Goldstraw P; International Association for the Study of Lung Cancer International Staging Committee and Participating Institutions. The IASLC Lung Cancer Staging Project: proposals regarding the relevance of TNM in the pathologic staging of small cell lung cancer in the forthcoming (seventh) edition of the TNM classification for lung cancer. J Thorac Oncol 2009; 4 (9): 1049-1059.

[118] Travis WD, Giroux DJ, Chansky K, Crowley J, Asamura H, Brambilla E, Jett J, Kennedy C, Rami-Porta R, Rusch VW, Goldstraw P; International Staging Committee and Participating Institutions. The IASLC Lung Cancer Staging Project: proposals for the inclusion of broncho-pulmonary carcinoid tumors in the forthcoming (seventh) edition of the TNM Classification for Lung Cancer. J Thorac Oncol 2008; 3 (11): 1213-1223.

[119] Goldstraw P., editors. Staging manual in thoracic oncology. Orange Park, FL, USA: Rx Press; 2009.

[120] Dr. A. De la Guerra. New TNM Classification for Lung Cancer - Part I: The changes. Doctors Lounge Website. Available at: http://www.doctorslounge.com/index.php/articles/page/340.

[121] Detterbeck FC, Boffa DJ, Tanoue LT. The new lung cancer staging system. Chest 2009; 136 (1): 260-271.

[122] Torrington KC, Kern JD. The utility of fiberoptic bronchoscopy in the evaluation of the solitary pulmonary nodule. Chest 1993;104:1021–1024.

[123] Fletcher EC, Levin DC. Flexible fiberoptic bronchoscopy and fluoroscopically guided transbronchial biopsy in the management of solitary pulmonary nodules. West J Med 1982;136:477–483.

[124] Shure D, Fedullo PF. Transbronchial needle aspiration of peripheral masses. Am Rev Respir Dis 1983;128:1090–1092.

[125] Geraghty PR, Kee ST, McFarlane G, Razavi MK, Sze DY, Dake MD. CT-guided transthoracic needle aspiration biopsy of pulmonary nodules: needle size and pneumothorax rate. Radiology 2003;229:475–481.

[126] Kazerooni EA, Lim FT, Mikhail A, Martinez FJ. Risk of pneumothorax in CT-guided transthoracic needle aspiration biopsy of the lung. Radiology 1996;198:371–375.

[127] Ohno Y, Hatabu H, Takenaka D, et al. CT-guided transthoracic needle aspiration biopsy of small (, or520 mm) solitary pulmonary nodules. AJR Am J Roentgenol 2003;180:1665–1669.

[128] Kato R, Katada K, Anno H, Suzuki S, Ida Y, Koga S. Radiation dosimetry at CT fluoroscopy: physician's hand dose and development of needle holders. Radiology 1996;201:576–578.

[129] Baaklini W, Reinoso M, Gorin A, et al. Diagnostic yield of fiberoptic bronchoscopy in evaluating solitary pulmonary nodules. Chest 2000;117:1049-1054.

[130] Rajamani S, Mehta AC. Transbronchial needle aspiration of central and peripheral nodules. Monaldi Arch Chest Dis 2001;56:436–445.

[131] Horrow EM, Wajdy A, Blum J, Harkin T, Gasparini S, Addrizzo-Harris DJ, Arroliga AC, Wight G, Mehta A. The utility of transbronchial needle aspiration in the staging of bronchogenic carcinoma. Am J Respir Crit Care Med 2000;161:601–607.

[132] Daryl P. Pearlstein, MD, Society of Thoracic Surgeons in San Diego, Calif., February 2011.

[133] Markis D, Scherpereel A, Leroy S, et al. Electromagnetic navigation diagnostic bronchoscopy for small peripheral lung lesions. Eur Respir J 2007;29:1187-1192.

[134] Gildea TR, Mazzone PJ, Karnak D, Meziane M, Mehta AC. Electromagnetic navigation diagnostic bronchoscopy: a prospective study. Am J Respir Crit Care Med 2006;174:982–989.

[135] Goldberg SN, Raptopoulos V, Boiselle PM, Edinburgh KJ, Ernst A. Mediastinal lymphadenopathy: diagnostic yield of transbronchial mediastinal lymph node biopsy with CT fluoroscopic guidance-initial experience. Radiology 2000;216:764–767.

[136] Schenk DA, Chambers SL, Dardak S, Komadina KH, Pickard JS, Strollo PJ, Lewis RE, Patefield AJ, Henderson JH, Tomski SM. Comparison of Wang 19-gauge and 22-gauge needles in the mediastinal staging of lung cancer. Am Rev Respir Dis 1993;147:1251–1258.

[137] Wang KP, Britt EJ. Needle brush in the diagnosis of lung mass or nodule through flexible bronchoscopy. Chest 1991;100:1148–1150.

[138] Reichenberger F, Weber J, Tamm M, Bolliger CT, Dalquen P, Perruchoud AP, Soler M. The value of transbronchial needle aspiration in the diagnosis of peripheral pulmonary lesions. Chest 1999; 116:704–708.

[139] Eberhardt R, Anantham D, Herth F, Feller-Kopman D, Ernst A, Electromagnetic Navigation Diagnostic Bronchoscopy in Peripheral Lung Lesions, CHEST 2007;131:1800–1805.

[140] Becker HC, Herth F, Ernst A, et al. Bronchoscopic biopsy of peripheral lung lesions under electromagnetic guidance: a pilot study. J Bronchol 2005;12:9–13.

[141] Paone G, Nicastri E, Lucantoni G, et al. Endobronchial ultrasound-driven biopsy in the diagnosis of peripheral lung lesions. Chest 2005;128:3551–3557.

[142] Kikuchi E, Yamazaki K, Sukoh N, et al. Endobronchial ultrasonography with guide-sheath for peripheral pulmonary lesions. Eur Respir J 2004;24:533–537.

[143] Kurimoto N, Miyazawa T, Okimasa S, et al. Endobronchial ultrasonography using a guide sheath increases the ability to diagnose peripheral pulmonary lesions endoscopically. Chest 2004;126:959–965.

[144] Herth FJ, Ernst A, Becker HD. Endobronchial ultrasoundguided transbronchial lung biopsy in solitary pulmonary nodules and peripheral lesions. Eur Respir J 2002;20:972–974.

[145] Herth FJ, Eberhardt R, Becker HD, et al. Endobronchial ultrasound-guided transbronchial lung biopsy in fluoroscopically invisible solitary pulmonary nodules: a prospective trial. Chest 2006;129:147–150.

[146] Lechtzin N, Rubin HR, White P Jr, et al. Patient satisfaction with bronchoscopy. Am J Respir Crit Care Med 2002; 166:1326–1331.

[147] Suratt PM, Smiddy JF, Gruber B. Deaths and complications associated with fiberoptic bronchoscopy. Chest 1976;69:747–751.

[148] Sawabata N, Ohta M, Maeda H. Fine-needle aspiration cytologic technique for lung cancer has a high potential of malignant cell spread through the tract. Chest 2000;118:936–939.

[149] Gupta S, Krishnamurthy S, Broemeling LD, et al. Small (</=2-cm) subpleural pulmonary lesions: short- versus longneedle-path CT-guided biopsy; comparison of diagnostic yields and complications. Radiology 2005;234:631–637.

[150] DeCamp MM Jr, Jaklitsch MT, Mentzer SJ, et al. The safety and versatility of videothoracoscopy: a prospective analysis of 895 consecutive cases. J Am Coll Surg 1995;181:113–120.

[151] International Early Lung Cancer Action Program Investigators, Henschke CI, Yankelevitz DF, et al. Survival of patients with stage I lung cancer detected on CT screening. N Engl J Med 2006;355:1763–1771.

[152] Hirsch FR, Prindiville SA, Miller YE, et al. Fluorescence versus white-light bronchoscopy for detection of preneoplastic lesions: a randomized study. JNatl Cancer Inst 2001;93:1385—91.

[153] Hüttenberger D, Gabrecht T, Wagnières G et al. Autofluorescence detection of tumors in the human lung——Spectroscopical measurements in situ, in an in vivo model and in vitro. Photodiagnosis Photodyn Ther. 2008;5(2):139-47.

[154] Qu J, MacAulay S, Lam S, Palcic B. Laser-induced fluorescence spectroscopy at endoscopy: tissue optics, Monte-Carlo modeling and in vivo measurements. Optical Engineering 1995;34(11):3334—43.

[155] Nakhosteen JA, Khanavkar B. Autofluorescence Bronchoscopy: The Laser Imaging Fluorescence Endoscope. In: Interventional Bronchoscopy. Prog Respir Res. Bolliger CT, Mathur PN (eds). Basel, Karger, 2000, 30:236–242.

[156] Becker HD. Bronchoscopy and computer technology. In: Thoracic Endoscopy: Advances in Interventional Pulmonology. Simoff MJ, Sterman DH, Ernst A (Eds). Massachusetts, USA; Blackwell Publishing, 2006: 88–118.

[157] Morgan R, Ernst A. Advanced diagnostic bronchoscopy. In: Introduction to bronchoscopy. Ernst A (Ed). New York, USA. Cambridge University Press, 2009: 134–141.

[158] Herth FJ, Ernst A, Becker HD. Autofluorescence bronchoscopy—a comparison of two systems (LIFE and D-Light). Respiration 2003;70:395—8.

[159] Homasson JP, Capron F, Angebault M, Nguyen Bich N. Lung autofluorescence. Preliminary study of two systems without laser illumination or photosensitization. Review of Pneumological Clinics 2001;57:202—7.

[160] Goujon D, Zellweger M, Radu A, et al. In vivo autofluorescence imaging of early cancers in the human tracheobronchial tree with a spectrally optimized system. Journal of Biomedical Optics 2003;8:17—25.

[161] Kurie JM, Lee JS, Morice RC, et al. Autofluorescence bronchoscopy in the detection of squamous metaplasia and dysplasia in current and former smokers. J Natl Cancer Inst 1998;90:991—5.

[162] Wagnieres GA, Star WM, Wilson BC. In vivo fluorescence spectroscopy and imaging for oncological applications. Photochem Photobiol 1998;68:603—32.

[163] Lam S, MacAulay C, Hung J, et al. Detection of dysplasia and carcinoma in situ with a lung imaging fluorescence endoscope device. J Thorac Cardiovasc Surg 1993;105:1035–1040.

[164] Lam S, Kennedy T, Unger M, et al. Localization of bronchial intraepithelial neoplastic lesions by fluorescence bronchoscopy. Chest 1998;113:696–702.

[165] Bard MP, Amelink A, Skurichina M, den Bakker M et al. Improving the specificity of fluorescence bronchoscopy for the analysis of neoplastic lesions of the bronchial tree

by combination with optical spectroscopy: preliminary communication. Lung Cancer. 2005;47(1):41-7.

[166] Lee P, de Bree R, Brokx HA, et al. Primary lung cancer after treatment of head and neck cancer without lymph node metastasis: is there a role for autofluorescence bronchoscopy? Lung Cancer. 2008;62(3):309-15.

[167] Lam S, Hung J, Kennedy SM, et al: Detection of dysplasia and carcinoma in situ by ratio fluorometry. Am Rev Respir Dis 1992;146: 1458–1461.

[168] Yamada G, Kitamura Y, Kitada J et al. Increased microcirculation in subepithelial invasion of lung cancer. Intern Med. 2011;50:839-43.

[169] Vincent BD, Fraig M, SilvestriGA. Apilot study of narrow band imaging compared to white light bronchoscopy for evaluation of normal airways, pre-malignant and malignant airways disease. Chest. 2007;131(6):1794–1799.

[170] Kaltenbach T, Sano Y, Friedland S et al. American Gastroenterological Association (AGA) institute technology assessment on image-enhanced endoscopy. Gastroenterology 2008; 134: 327–40.

[171] Tajiri H, Niwa H. Proposal for a consensus terminology in endoscopy: how should different endoscopic imaging techniques be grouped and defined? Endoscopy 2008; 40: 775–8.

[172] Ohtani K, Lee AM, Lam S. Frontiers in bronchoscopic imaging. Respirology. 2012;17(2):261-9.

[173] Shibuya K, Hoshino H, Chiyo M, Iyoda A, Yoshida S, et al. High magnification bronchovideoscopy combined with narrow band imaging could detect capillary loops of angiogenic squamous dysplasia in heavy smokers at high risk for lung cancer. Thorax 2003;58:989-995.

[174] Gono K, Obi T, Yamaguchi M, Ohyama N, et al. Appearance of enhanced tissue features in narrow-band endoscopic imaging. J Biomed Opt. 2004;9(3):568-77.

[175] Liu H, Li YQ, Yu T, Zhao YA, Zhang JP, et al. Confocal endomicroscopy for in vivo detection of microvascular architecture in normal and malignant lesions of upper gastrointestinal tract. J Gastroenterol Hepatol 2008;23:56e61.

[176] Pohl H, Rosch T, Vieth M, Koch M, Becker V, et al. Miniprobe confocal laser microscopy for the detection of invisible neoplasia in patients with Barrett's oesophagus. Gut 2008;57: 1648e53.

[177] Buchner AM, Shahid MW, Heckman MG, Krishna M, Ghabril M, et al. Comparison of probe-based confocal laser endomicroscopy with virtual chromoendoscopy for classification of colon polyps. Gastroenterology 2009;138:834e42.

[178] Hoffman A, Goetz M, Vieth M, et al. Confocal laser endomicroscopy: technical status and current indications. Endoscopy. 2006;38:1275–1283.

[179] Hsiung PL, Hardy J, Friedland S, et al. Detection of colonic dysplasia in vivo using a targeted heptapeptide and confocal microendoscopy. Nat Med. 2008;14:454–458.

[180] Wallace MB, Meining A, Canto MI, Fockens P, Miehlke S, et al. The safety of intravenous fluorescein for confocal laser endomicroscopy in the gastrointestinal tract. Aliment Pharmacol Ther 2010;31:548e52.

[181] Thiberville L, Salaun M, Lachkar S, Dominique S, Moreno-Swirc S, et al. Human in vivo fluorescence microimaging of the alveolar ducts and sacs during bronchoscopy. Eur Respir J 2009;33:974e85.

[182] Newton RC, Kemp SV, Yang GZ et al. Imaging parenchymal lung diseases with confocal endomicroscopy. Respir Med. 2012;106(1):127-37.

[183] Fuchs FS, Zirlik S, Hildner K, Frieser M, Ganslmayer M, et al. Fluorescein-aided confocal laser endomicroscopy of the lung. Respiration 2011;81:32e8.

[184] Thiberville L, Salaun M, Lachkar S, Moreno-Swirc S, Bourg-Heckly G. In-vivo confocal endomicroscopy of peripheral lung nodules using 488nm/660nm induced fluorescence and topical methylene blue. Eur Respir Soc Berlin 2008:263se4s

[185] Thiberville L, Moreno-Swirc S, Vercauteren T, Peltier E, Cave C, et al. In vivo imaging of the bronchial wall microstructure using fibered confocal fluorescence microscopy. Am J Respir Crit Care Med 2007;175:22e31.

[186] Musani AI, Sims M, Sareli C, Russell W, McLaren WJ, et al. A pilot study of the feasibility of confocal endomicroscopy for examination of the human airway. J Bronchology Interv Pulmonology 2010;17:126e30.

[187] Lane PM, Lam S, McWilliams A, Leriche JC, Anderson MW, et al. Confocal fluorescence microendoscopy of bronchial epithelium. J Biomed Opt 2009;14:024008.

[188] Newton RC, Kemp S, Elson DS, Yang G-Z, Thomas CMR, et al. Confocal endomicroscopy in diffuse lung diseases – initial results and future directions. Am J Respir Crit Care Med 2010; 181:A6620.

[189] Newton RC, Kemp S, Yang GZ, Darzi A, Sheppard M, et al. Tracheobronchial amyloidosis and confocal endomicroscopy. Respiration 2011;82:209e11.

Chapter 10

Endoscopy of Larynx and Trachea with Rigid Laryngo-Tracheoscopes Under Superimposed High-Frequency Jet Ventilation (SHFJV)

Alexander Aloy and Matthaeus Grasl

Additional information is available at the end of the chapter

1. Introduction

1.1. History (an overview)

1.1.1. Indirect laryngoscopy

Knowing that almost all laryngeal and tracheal diseases are visible at the surface of the mucous membranes it is of particular interest to visualize these structures.

Endoscopic examinations of the larynx and the trachea are essential in the otorhinolaryngological field and had their beginning over 200 years ago. Before the 1800`s only autopsy specimen could clarify laryngotracheal diseases.

In 1807 the physian Phillip Bozzini (Germany) reported about a speculum called "the light conductor, or a simple apparatus for the illumination of the internal cavities and spaces in the living animal body" [1].

In 1816 Ludwig Mende (Germany), a gynaecologist & obstetrician and forensic doctor examined first the inner part of the larynx at a living human being. He looked at a larynx of a suicidal person, who had cut through the soft tissue of the supraglottic area [2].

In 1827 L. Senn (Switzerland) successfully examined the larynx of a child with a small mirrow, cited in [3].

In 1829 Benjamin Guy Babington (Great Britain) developed a larynx-mirrow "glottoscope" and could illuminate the upper parts of the larynx. The instrument combined an epiglottic retractor with a laryngeal mirror. He presented it in the Hunterian Society of London [4].

In 1854 the Spanish singer, voice teacher and scientist Manuel García, living in London, succeeded in performing the auto-laryngoscopy. He first visualized his own larynx, using a dental mirror and a second hand-held mirror to reflect sunlight. Garcia tranfered the method to patients (Figure 1) and could analyse directly the phonation. He presented his invention to the Royal Society in 1855 [5]. The importance of this technique was unrealised first. But in 1862 he was granted an honour of medical degree followed by many international distinctions.

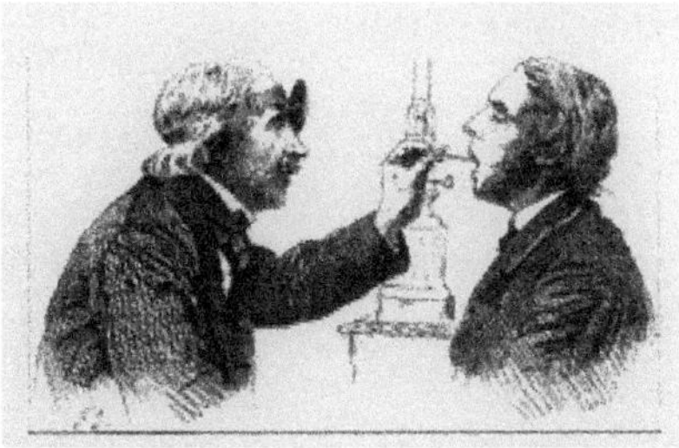

Figure 1. Manuele Garcia`s laryngoscopy.

In 1857 Ludwig Türk, a neurologist and professor of laryngology in Vienna (Austria), unsuccessfully tried Garcia`s mirror under the use of the ophthalmoscope [6] which was invented by Hermann v. Helmholtz (Germany), a physiologist and physicist in 1851[7].

Johann Nepomuk Czermak, professor of physiology at the University of Pest (Hungary) assumed Türk`s mirror, completed this procedure using light-concentration by a concave head mirror (Figure 2), and presented it 1858 the Viennese medical community [8].

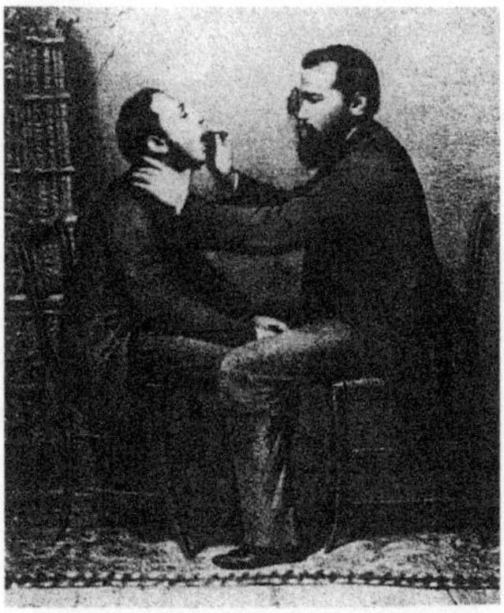

Figure 2. Johann Nepomuk Czermak performing the indirect laryngoscopy using natural lighting.

This method propagated rapidly and is still in use, but with electric light source.

In 1878 Max Joseph Oertel (Germany) describes his invention: the laryngo-stroboscopy via a perforated disc. But the feasibility of this apparatus was not implemented until 1895 when the eletricity has been installed [9].

Important milestones for the investigation and treatment of laryngeal diseases were the beginnings of the anaesthesia 1846 using ether by William Morton (USA) [10] and the introduction of antisepsis by Joseph Lister (Scotland) who performed first 1867 surgery under antiseptic conditions [11]. A fundamental progress was the introduction of the cocain as an anaesthetic and analgetic agent in 1884 by the laryngologist Edmund Jelinek (Austria) [12].

1.1.2. Direct laryngoscopy

The direct inspection of the larynx is essential in cases of endotracheal intubation and can be performed by spatulate instruments like the straight Miller-spaculate (Robert A. Miller 1941, USA), especiallly for children [13] or the slightly arcuated Macintosh-spatulate (Robert R. Macintosh, 1943, Great Britain) [14].

But this is not the topic of this historical overview.

The real interest consists in tube-shaped instruments with lighting for direct inspection of the larynx, which is only practicable under anaesthesia or deep sedation.

The first laryngologist who directly vizualized the larynx using a tongue depressor and a mirror for illumination was Albert von Tobold (Germany) in 1864. He removed with this method laryngeal papilloma [15].

In 1895 the laryngologist Alfred Kirstein (Germany) first described direct inspection of the vocal cords. He had modified an oesophagoscope for this purpose and called this device an autoscope (electroscope) [16].

In 1897 Gustav Killian a laryngologist (Germany) removed at first with success via a rigid bronchoscope a bronchial foreign body. It was a piece of bone in the right main bronchus [17]. This practical invention was affiliated in professional circles with enthusiasm because the dramatical death rate of 50 percent in case of tracheobronchial foreign bodies could be minimized continuously. This technique persisted for almost 70 years as the standard diagnosis and therapeutic procedure for bronchopulmonar diseases.

In 1910 Gustav Killian constructed a special laryngoscope, not a tube but a spatula, with a mouth gag (hypopharynx was clear visible) that could be fixed to a supporting construction by a hook, the „suspension-laryngoscopy" (Figure 3). The inspection of the larynx was easier by the hanging position of the head and laryngotracheal surgery could be done with both hands [18].

Wilhelm Brünings 1910 [19] and Arthur Hartmann 1911 [20] (both Germany) improved Kirsteins electroscope with proximal electric lighting at the handgrip.

Paul H. Holinger 1947 (USA) created a laryngoscope using an U-shaped handgrip and had a better view to the anterior commissure [21].

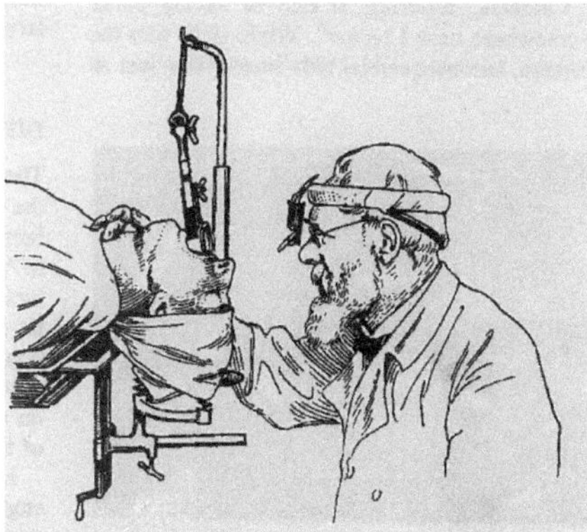

Figure 3. Gustav Killian performing a supension laryngoscopy. The patient`s head is suspended by attaching the laryngoscope to the "gallows".

1961 Oskar Kleinsasser (Germany) published [22] his development of a new instrument for magnified endolaryngeal observation and photography. He used a chest holder. A combination of a wide-angle telescope and a telephoto lens guaranteed excellent depth of field for still and motion fotography.

In 1970 Geza J. Jako (USA) refered about his development of a laryngosope, a modified Holinger-Yankauer tube with an ellipsoidal proximal and a round distal aperture. It is made of stainless stell with the inside surface matt to decrease glare. On each side of the instrument there is a built-in tube for the insertion of fiberoptic light pipes. The laryngoscope with a special holder is suspended on an instrument table over the patient`s chest and was developed for laser surgery in the larynx [23].

1970 M. Stuart Strong (USA) coupled the carbon dioxide laser to the surgical microscope. The laser provides precise cutting and also haemostasis of small vessels and is manipulated with a joystick and a foot-pedal [24].

In 1979 Hilko Weerda et al. (Germany) designed an expandable laryngoscope which derived from the Kleinsasser-tube and the Killian-Lynch-suspension laryngoscope consisting of an upper and lower blade. Their distance and angle of twist are variable [25].

The rigid laryngotracheal endoscopy made a qualitative leap with the introduction of the Hopkins-fibreglass-optics with their unachievable splendour and precision with endoscopic resolutions which allow a hundredfold magnification when used additionally. Prof. Harald H Hopkins (Great Britain) developed it the 1960 th with Karl Storz Ltd. Company with limited liability (Germanny) [26].

1.1.3. Jet ventilation

First attempts to sustain the pulmonary gas exchange without periodical alterations of gas volumes were done by Franz Volhard in an animal experiment with dogs in 1908 [27]. He performed an "artificial respiration" by leading in oxygen with a very low flow via a trans-laryngeal tracheal tube which did not fill out the diameter of the trachea.

This method indeed enabled sufficient oxygenation but hypercapnia occurred rapidly.

In 1909 Samuel J. Meltzer et al. (USA) enhanced Volhard`s method by applicating the oxygen with high velocity and named it "diffusion respiration". With this high insufflation flow partially elimination of carbon dioxide was practicable.

Clinical application was implemented at first in 1954 by Lothar Barth (Germany) and was used for bronchoscopies and for bridging short apnoea phases over a period of lung resections [29]. Because of insufficient elimination of carbon dioxide it could be applied only 15 -20 minutes. Therefore a broad distribution did not take place.

In 1967 R. Douglas Sanders developed a method enabling a continuously ventilation during bronchoscopy [30]. Two cannulas are placed into the endoscope and 15 to 20 breathing gas portions are applicated periodically during the inspiration phase. Because of the injector effects the primarily very small-sized tidal volumes receive an enhancement. The Venturi effect additionally entrains air through the open proximal end of the endoscope and both result in a sufficient pressure and flow at the end of the endoscope for inflating the lungs. Subsequently gas exchange occurs compareable to conventional breaths (Figure 4). This method simplified general anaesthesia for bronchoscopy and is still in use in surgery of the thorax, published by E. Gebert et al. [31] and Shaotsu Thomas Lee [32].

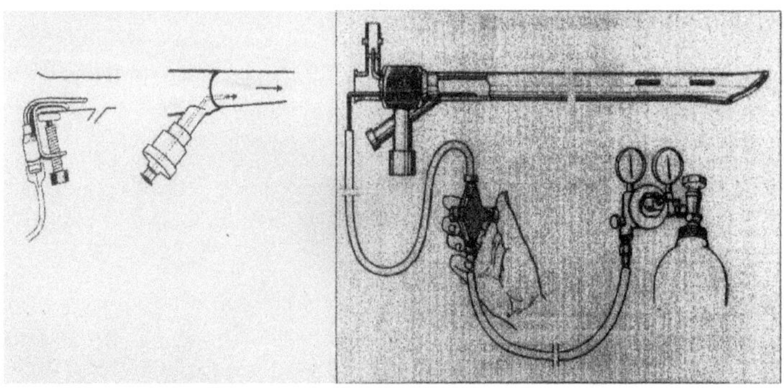

Figure 4. The injector apparatus of R. Douglas Sanders.

In 1971 Jane L. Bradley et al. (Great Britain) described improvements of Sanders` pulmonary ventilation for bronchoscopy. She fixed the proximal injector needle at the bronchoscope and the distal needle became an integral part of the bronchoscope, oxygen feeding was assured and interruption of the oxygen flow was regulated electronically [33].

In 1972 Paul Peter Lunkenheimer et al. succeeded a further advancement by oscillating the gas mixture, which was insufflated into the airways. A membrane vibration generator placed at the proximal end of the bronchoscope enabled it. Such oscillations of the breathing gas with frequences from 1200 to 6000 per minute led in a satisfactory manner to a gas exchange with widely minimisation of intrathoracic pressure fluctuations [34]. An additional integrated carbon dioxide absorber increased elimination of carbon doxide [35].

In 1980 Demond J. Bohn et al. published at first a successfully ventilation with this technique in an animal experiment [36]. With a piston pump sinuoidal vibrations with a frequency from 900 to 1500 per minute were tranfered to the breathing gas, elimination of the carbon dioxide is carried out by a cross-flow of fresh mixture. At this way of high frequency oxygenation a superposition of spontaneous breathing is not feasible.

In 1977 and 1980 Ulf H. Sjöstrand (Sweden) published about his invention of high-frequency positive pressure ventilation. He modified a conventional lung ventilator by the application of special valve configuration and could reduce the compressible gas volume. Tidal volumes from 200 to 300 ml with a frequency of 60 to 80 per minute were applicable [37, 38].

Miroslav M. Klain et al. (USA) developed 1976 the high-frequency ventilation. A high pressure jet is conditioned into small-sized single gas quantities by an assessable valve and then applicated via a catheter with a low inner diameter. The breathing gas quantities leave the catheter as a clocked high frequency jet. This jet activates a suction mechanism (entrainment) and the tidal volume is augmented. In a frequency range of 100 to 200 per minute a sufficient gas exchange can be perpetuated in a completely open system towards the atmosphere [39-41].

This high frequency jet ventilation is the initial point of all following developments.

In particular Alexander Aloy and colleagues are engaged practically and scientifically since 1990 over more than twenty years in this field of ventilation [42].

His and contemporarely applicatioins and publications are presented in the next following parts of this chapter.

2. Microlaryngoscopy and endolaryngeal microsurgery

Direct laryngoscopy via the transoral route allows the immediate entry to the inner laryngeal and tracheal structures and has now an extreme importance for the special field of laryngological diagnoses and surgical treatments in the otorhinolaryngologic discipline.

A laryngoscope holder is adhered to the chest selfholding by a mount as a supension similar to a gallow.

The binoccular vision and bi-manual manipualtion via the forward spaced microscopy facilitates detailed diagnoses and treatment at the vocal cords and circumjacent areas [43-45].

2.1. Indications

Microlaryngocopy is particulary helpful in the need of diagnosis and treatment of the vocal chords or surrounding areas, which are first seen by indirect laryngoscopy. The microlaryngoscopy for staging and excision biopsy of tumours is part of a panendoscopy of the upper aerodigestive tract. Absolute indications are the strong suspicion of precancerous or cancerous epithelial diseaes as well as constringent processes. But also benign lesions like polyps, cysts and oedemas have to be operated soon, because it is often found that the opposite vocal chord reacts with a dent, oedema or epithelial thickening. These secondary alterations prolongate healing. Inflammatory epithelial reactions are to be treated with inhalations before in few hard going cases operation is done. Rigid laryngoscopy is a domain for the elimination of foreign bodies in larynx and trachea as well as the surgical treatment of laryngeal or glottic webs. Laryngotracheal injuries and the placement respectively the removal of laryngotracheal endoprosthesis, medialization of vocal chords after palsy of an inferior laryngeal nerve by relining and surgical widening of the glottis are further areas of application of laryngotracheoscopy.

2.2. Contraindications

Special endangering of patients life by anaesthesia when medical conditions such as apoplectic stroke, heart infarction, aneurysm, severe cardiadic arrhythmias, aggravated pulmonary, liver and renal diseases are contraindication for general anaesthesia and consecutively for microlaryngoscopy. Unfrequent contraindications are severe malformations of the jaws, cervical spine diseases like Morbus Bechterew and local spasticity [43].

2.3. Description of the instruments

The design of the instrumental equipment represents the association of the representational problems and their solution. The present instrumentation indicates the requirement on average in the German-speaking language room and is to be adapted individually for particular purposes:

2.3.1. Laryngoscope

The mostly used laryngoscope tube at our institution, the Deaprtment of Ototrhinolaryngolgy of the Medical Universitiy, is that of Kleinsasser with a length of of 80 to 200 mm and a distal diameter of 8 -16 mm (Figure 5). The medium-sized closed coverage type for adults is used predominantly in the endolarynx. An overlong small-bore universal applicable laryngoscope is used in children and adults with difficult adjustabel areas of the endolarynx - especially the anterior commissure, the interary and subglottic region. The proximal end of the tube is differently shaped in dependency to the size for adults and children. The side of the tubes turned to the teeth is flat for spreading the pressure to the teeth as uniform as possible. At both sides of the proximal end mounting parts are placed to fix the cold light rod eighter at the left or right side [43].

The spatulated laryngosope of Weerda et al. [46] has an upper and lower blade which is inserted in a closed position and once inside the larynx the distance and angle of twist of the blades is variable. This instrument has adapters for suction and jet stream ventilation and is suitable in particular for the root of the tongue, the vallecula, supraglottis and hypopharynx.

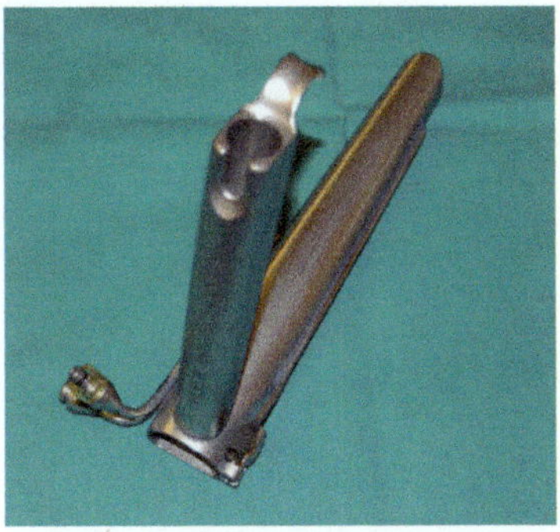

Figure 5. The Kleinsasser laryngoscope already adapted for jet ventilation (see also part 3 of this chapter).

When laser is used the tubes and spatulas are adapted according to the needs. The inner surface coating should be non-reflecting, opal or black. On the lateral outside cannulas for suction of smoke are mounted.

2.3.2. Laryngoscope holder

The laryngoscope holder is eighter placed on patient`s chest with a broad rubber ring or it is put on a robust instrument table [43, 47] respectively a holding bow [48] just over his chest to avoid pressure on the anaesthetized chest and to minimize movement of the instrument.

2.3.3. Example for a configuration of a microscope combining modern vizualisation technologies with a user friendly platform

1. Light source:
   - 2 x 300 W xenon,
   - automatic iris control for adjusting the illumunation to the field of view,
   - individual light treshhold setting,
   - focus light link: working distance controlled light intensity,
   - display of remaining lamp life time.
2. Microscope:
   - free to move at a tripod or as a ceiling mounted,
   - motorized focus,
   - working distance 200-500 mm,
   - motorized zoom 1:6 zoom ratio,
   - 10 x magnetic widefield eyepieces with integrated eyecups,

- autofocus with 2 visible laser dots - automatic mode with magnetic brakes,
- binocular observer ocular,
- multifunctional programmable handgrips,
- magnetic clutches for all system axes,
- central user interface,
- XY robotic movement in 3 axes (variable speed),
- system setup: autobalance,
- navigation interface,
- interface for micromanipulator,
- intraoperative fluorescence,
- laseradapter.

3. Video, fotography, Television for decumentation and teaching:
   - HD video touchscreen on extended arm,
   - integrated video still image capturing on HDD and USB-media,
   - integrated HD video camera,
   - integrated SD or HD video recording and editing,
   - adapatation of consumer (SLR) photo/video camera,
   - video-in for external SD video sources,
   - patients data transfer from/to PACS.

2.3.4 Instruments

Instruments are small at the tip, thin, long (25 cm) and flexible.

All instruments should be manipulated freehanded, which is easily trainable and backing of the arms becomes dispensable. The set of microsurgical instruments should be kept in a basic amount. It includes double-spoon forceps, scissors: straight, laterally and upwards arcuated, acutenaculum, sickle and peeling knifes, suction tubes and coagulation probes.

Instruments for laser microlaryngological surgery are of nonreflecting surface. Protectors are neccessary for the subglottic area when tubeless ventilation is applicated. Additional when the vocal chords are treated the false cords and also the contralateral intact side is to be moved sidewards.

2.4. Beginning and protection activities

The often "poor risk" patients need preoperatively a careful investigation and treatment to make them capable for anaesthesia. Dental record is essential before insertion of the laryngoscope. When indicated patients have to go for remediation preoperatively. Dental impression trays equally spread the pressure of the laryngoscope at the teeth of the upper jaw and can bridge a dental gap.

Patients lie in dorsal position on the operating table and the correct posture of the head is the dorsal flection in flat bedding. Using adequate laryngoscope types it enables even in patients with a thick and short neck to adjust the larynx. If there are anamnestic indications concerning pathologies at the cervicale spin an orthopaedic specialist has to decide if the head position during laryngoscopy will be tolerated well.

In case of laser application all persons in the operating room have to wear special glasses. When CO_2 laser is in use eyeglass lenses are sufficient. Patients face and eyes are to be protected by a humid green woven fabric. The doors to the operating room where laser is used must be signalized.

2.5. Anaesthesia and ventilation during micro laryngotracheoscopy (basic considerations)

Please see the next part of this chapter.

2.6. Insertion of the laryngoscope

First of all a teeth protector for the lower and upper jaw is placed in position. The insertion of the laryngoscope should be performed not until the patient is full relaxed and in sufficient depth of narcosis. The laryngoscope should be as large as possible enabling best lighting and overview of the larynx. In cases of preexisting laryngotracheal intubation the ventilation tube is moved by two fingers to the left side and the laryngoscope is inserted from the right side under the illumination of a cold light which is piped inside of the tube to the distal end. The tongue should not be pinched between the teeth and the laryngoscope at the same time. The epiglottis is loaded up by the laryngoscope. If the laryngeal skeleton is to be pressed from outside to inward in cases of the need to expose the anterior commissure the laryngoscope should be inserted only into the area of the false cords. In cases of a small, weak or U-shaped epiglottis it can happen that the epiglottis is enrolled and the suprahyoidal part is folded and compressed when the laryngoscope is inserted. Consecutively inspection of the anterior commissure is hindered and a postoperative oedema can occur. Solving of this problem is to clamp the epiglottis when inserting the laryngoscope. The laryngoscope is positioned few millimeters above the anterior commissure. The dorsal lying ventilation tube can be used as a guidance till the exposition of the false and vocal chords.

Next is to underpin the laryngoscope at the mobile laryngoscopy-table and to move it slowly upwards. When a distending laryngoscope is inserted at maximum aperture laterally between the spatulas parts of the tongue can be pinched and it protrudes into the lumen of the laryngoscope. This can be prevented by covering the closed distending-laryngoscope with a finger of a medical glove which is forming a lateral wall when the laryngoscope is opened [49].

2.7. Inspection of the larynx and the circumjacent areas

At the begin of the introduction of the laryngocope the structures are inspected by looking with the naked eyes using the lighting inside the laryngoscope: base of the tongue, valleculae, epiglottis: lingual and laryngeal surface area and free margin, aryepiglottic fold, pharyngoepiglottic fold, the processus vocalis and tubercula cuneiformia respectively corniculata, the arytaenoid cartilage, the sinus piriformis bilateral, the posterior hypopharyngeal wall and postcricoid area. After fixation of the laryngoscope under the use of the microscope the false and vocal chord, the sinus Morgagni, the anterior and posterior commissure as well as the subglottic space and the upper parts of the trachea are to be seen under a magnification of up to 40.

2.8. Microlaryngoscopic diagnoses and surgical therapies

(*most frequent clinical symptom is hoarseness*)

2.8.1. Tumours

Diagnosis and therapy of precancerous lesions and carcinomas of the larynx, especially the vocal chords are still a central domain of laryngoscopy. Any unclear or suspicious epithelial alteration is to be exstirpated and examined by histology. As followup exam after radiotherapy microlaryngoscopy is qualified in particular.

2.8.1.1. Precancerous lesions

Chronic hyperplastic laryngitis is an epithelial thickening of laryngeal mucous membrane affecting both vocal chords with a spread over their complete length. In this dermatoid epithelium often *leukoplakia* lies as milky area, slightly opacity of the surface or as verrucous, thick, white coating. A second group of cornification of the epithelium is the circumscript *keratosis* which is located nearly only at one vocal chord. The surface can be plain, tubercular, verrucous or papillary with all transitions. Histological differentiation of the keratosisis is for all benign types is grade I, when few atypic cells are seen grade II and when a carcinoma in situ is diagnosed grade III. A carcinoma in situ becomes in a high rate an apparent carcinoma and is to be treated as such a malignant tumour. The human papilloma virus induced *solitary hyperceratotic "adult"papilloma* has a high rate of recurrence after surgery and is to be distinguished from the *"juvenile" papilloma* which also occurs in adults but never turns to a malignization. Precancerous lesions are always movable over the muscle of the vocal chord without problems.

2.8.1.2. Squamous scell carcinomas

Carcimomas in situ and apparent carcinomas primarily originate bilateral from an enlarged area and are named wallpaper carcimomas respectively superficial spreading carcinomas. Additionally, not infrequently, multiple focuses of seperated carcinomas confluence later. Difficult relocatability, solid or swallen areas and superficial exulceration are important signs of deeper invasion. A relatively rare shape of growth is excessive polypus/exophytic like. Because of tumour infiltration the blood supply suffers and necroses occur. To identify the superficial spread of the tumours it is additonally necessary to investigate the infraglottic area as well as the ventriculus Morgangni and the false chord via a 30 ° and 70° rigid fiberoptics.

A huge advantage of endolaryngeal microsurgery is the possibility to get biopsies from all locations without contusion. In cases of palliative tumour size reduction ("debulking") laryngeal tumour masses can easily be reduced to avoid a tracheotomy. Small-sized tumours can be removed in one piece as an "excision biopsy".

Clear guidelines applied for endoscopic resections of carcinomas include the selective und reluctant production of the indication by a laryngologist experienced in microlaryngologic diagnosis and surgery. Resection is only permitted when the complete tumour circumference over his borders is easily visible with the microscope. Otherwise an external approach is to be chosen allowing simultaneously reconstruction of the glottis. The careful histological investigation is a condition precedent in cases of microlaryngeal resection. When resection was not in healthy tissue an immediate revision surgery is necessary [43].

Laser surgery in the larynx demands special safety precautions, instruments, anaesthesiological procedures, experiences of the mircosurgeon and knowlegde of histopathological appraisal. Because bleeding is the most common complication of laser surgery of tumours of the upper aerodigestve tract every clinic performing this surgery should have a clear concept of managing it. When these conditions are respected even enlarged function receiving and organ saving operations in the larynx and hypopharynx with good oncological results are quite practicable [49].

2.8.2. Benign lesions

Polyps are only seen at the vocal chords predominantly at one side inserting at the anterior two third at the slope of the vocal chord. They have a diameter on average of 5 mm, bigger one`s are floating in the glottic area. Petiolated pendolous polyps sustain longer, broad based polyps are juvenile and have a thin transparent epithelium (Figure 6). Polyps never degenerate into a carcinoma. If a polyp persists a longer period at the contralaeral side contact reaction in shape of excavation, epithelial thickening or oedematous swelling occurs. This is not to be treated when the polyp is resected.

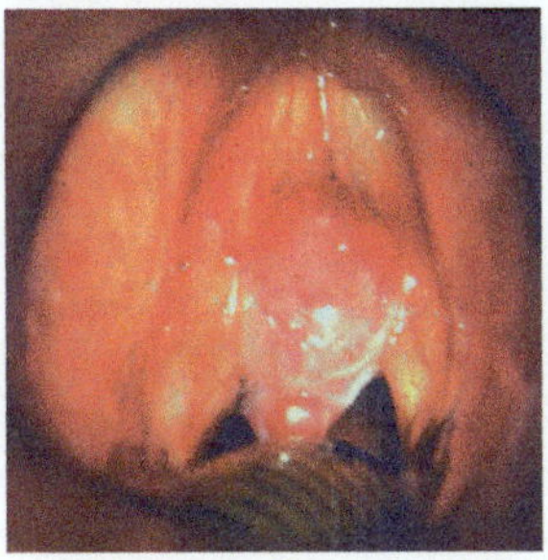

Figure 6. Large vocal chord polyp in the anterior part of the glottis.

Vocal chords nodules are seen exclusively in women with powerful voice formation. They present as a symmetric swelling of the epithelium of the vocal chords in typical localisation at the border between the first and second third. In up to 50 % the diagnosis of nodules by indirect laryngoscopy is wrong – microlaryngoscopy shows cysts or polyps. Morphodiffentiation compared to polyps is difficult but in any case they are no fibroepithelioma. Microlaryngeal resection and postoperative phonatric training is indicated.

In hyperactive children vocal nodes impress as soft spindling swelling in the middle of both vocal chords. Operative resection is not necessary because by no longer than the puberty they involute spontaneously. Phoniatric therapy is useful. Laryngeal papillomas are to be excluded.

The *varix chordis* is found in patients with vocal overstressing at the surface or margin in the middle or posterior part of one vocal chord. Under microscpy one or various capillaries lead to a bloodblaster. Laser coagulation followed by vocal training is a promising therapy.

Laryngeal cysts are frequent and located typically at three areas:

1. *vocal chord cysts* are with about 50 % the most frequent and in most cases as one chamber at the subglottic slope of the anterior third of a vocal chord with a diameter of about 5 mm. Their inner lining is squamous epithelium. The content matter is a muddy aqueous-milky detritus. Under microscopy the subepithelial content glimmers yellowish. They are removed gentle under protection of the muscle layer.

2. *vestibular fold cysts* are found nearly exclusively in elderly patients. The first mode, originating from the minor salivary glands, presents with one chamber and is pedunculated at the roof of the ventriculus laryngis (Morgagni) with a prolapse into the glottis. They are neither a real prolapse nor an inner laryngocele and can be mutated oncocytoid, which is a benign age-related metaplastic dyschylic transformation. They can be removed easily by cutting through the peduncle. The second mode is characterized by multiple chambers, often bilateral, inside the vestibular fold and metaplastic transformed epithelium. The excision is hindered by the deep location and the botryoid extension, which promotes relapses.

3. *epiglottic cysts* are located always at the same position, deep in the vallecula epiglottica slightly paramedian at the lingual surface of the epiglottis. In ten percent they occur multiple, only the bigger one cause dysphagia and have to be operated. This can be complicated by prominent venes. The inner layer of the wall of the cysts is squamous epithelium enclosing a milky pale yellow fluid. The complete sac of the cyst is to be removed.

The *Reinke-oedema* or *polypoid chorditis* is a frequent disease mostly in heavy smokers. The extention ranges from marginal spindle shaped swelling to bulky floating bulges with stridor. In most cases both vocal chords are involved, but asymmetrically. With longer persistence of the Reinke-oedema the epithelium keratinizes. Patients develop a compensatory phonation by the vestibular folds which are to be reversed by postoperative voice therapy. Surgery begins with plain and clean cutted margins at the tip of the processus vocalis of the arytaenoid cartilage where the oedema is pronounced. The anteroir commissure is not involved and an epithelial debridment there should be prevented to avoid synechias. The subepthelial mucous is to be sucked carefully.

Chronical hyperplastic laryngitis is predominantly seen in 90 percent in heavy smoking men. Additional working place associated noxious agents as heat, dust and noice-induced overuse of the voice are said to be at least co-factors. Microlaryngoscopic findings are typical. The thickening of the epithelium begins always at the anterior third of the vocal chords and spreads to the whole vocal chords and inner larynx. In advanced cases of expanse leucoplakia and a pathological secretion of a yellow viscous mucous adheres. Sometimes the disease progresses per acute exacerbation. Signs of this procedure are slit shaped ulcers at the free margin of the vocal chords and crimson bulges of oedema at the border from squamous to cylindrical epithelium. Carcinoma can follow. Resection of nearly all hyperplastic area via microlayngoscope is the symptomatic therapy of choice. It lasts about 4 to 8 weeks till re-epithelisation of a vocal chord is finished. In this period a stingent ban on smoking is to order.

Contact granuloma and *contact pachydermia* are two pathogenetic identical but independent diseases caused by vocal abuse and strike of the processus vocales against each other with following formation of granulation tissue. This can be connected with dysphagia, odynophagia, scratching, sensation of foreign body and haemoptysis. Sometimes granulomas are rejected spontaneously. In other cases the granuloma persists over months and years which are forming bilateral cranial and caudal from the processus vocalis lip-like bulges (in America the Jackson`s "contact ulcer", which is not realy an ulcer - there is no loss of substance) and dash against each other during phonation. All transitions to the typical dish-shaped epitheliazed contact pachyderms are seen. Despite careful microsurgical resection and postoperatvive voice training local recurrences frequently arise.

Intubation granulomata are caused by too large sized larynotracheal tubes which excoriate the processus vocales almost one-sided (Figure 7). Depending on their growth they get a pendualted form and can be rejected and expectorated spantaneously. Recurrences after resection are seen not infrequently, additionally applicaion of cortison should minimize them.

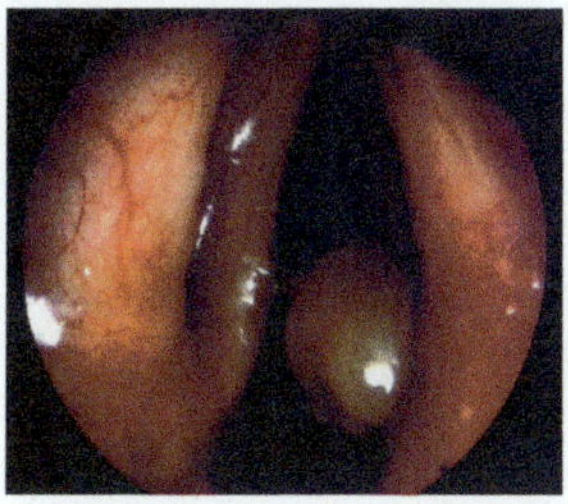

Figure 7. Intubation granuloma in the posterior third of the right vocal chord.

"Juvenile" papillomata are to be revoved repeatedly because of their tendency of frequent recurrences: optionally by cold instruments, laser, ultrasound, cryocautery or electrocoagulation. Additional mitomycin is applied. It is of importance to work organ preserving. The

essential advantage nowadays is that the surgical percedure is performed endolaryngeal and therefore the affected children do not need a tracheostomy.

Haemangioma of the larynx are congenital and become symptomatical several months postpartal with the general growth. They are treated by laser resection and additional long-term application of cortisone and recently by propranolol alone.

The incidence of laryngeal *mycosis* is increasing caused by more patients with immunosuppressive therapy and AIDS. In Europe candida albicans and aspergillosis as endomycosis are of clinical relevance. The affection of the larynx is predominantly secondary, the mucous membrane is discrete swollen and reddened, typical off-white coatings are seen only exceptionally and it looks like a chronic laryngitis. The basic concept of the diagnosis is still the microbiological demonstration of the pathogenic agent. Systemic antimycotic drugs are given.

Laryngeal *synechia* can be differentiated by location into anterior vocal chords ones, posterior interarytaenoid ones and false chord ones. Anterior synechia can be congenital and are very rare and then aquired more frequent as complication after microlaryngeal surgery. Resection of the narrowing and movement blocking scar tissue is difficile and recurrences many times arise. Cortison and mitomycin is applied additionally. Subglottic annulare stenosis *"pinhole aperture synechia"* are sequels of artificial ventilation and are resectable with out the need of inserting a dilitator. *"Cricoidal stenosis"* caused by diminution of the cricoidal cartilage are funnel-shaped and not to be treated endolaryngeal but resected by an external approach.

Unilateral pareses of the *inferior laryngeal nerv* are treated by a phoniatric training, improvement of voice in defintive unilateral pareses demands an injection of the vocal chord for example with Teflon®. In cases of *acute bilateral paresis* of the *inferior layryngeal nerve* a tracheotmy is only to be avoided when a larynologist performs immediately a posterior chordectomy including a resection of the processus vocalis or partial arytaenoidectomy or a (temporary) laterofixation of the vocal chord or applicates Botulinum toxin [50].

2.9. Disadvantages

General anaesthesia is essential for microscopic laryngoscopy because of the required length of time and the inconveniences to the patient if not applied. Risks of general anaesthesia can be deminished by a close prepoerative examination of all vital functions. It is in the responsibility of the laryngologist to estimate the practicability of tracheal intubation after the induction of anaesthesia. Patients with compromized airways in a severe degree have to be tracheotomized in local anaesthesia before microscopic laryngoscopy is performed. A set of instruments for a coniotomy is to be provided. In some cases the anterior larynx cannot be adjusted without the risk of damage of the upper teeth. Exposure can be achieved by using smaller laryngoscopes and additionally by impressing the larynx.

2.10. Complications

It is not an unusal finding that cardiadic arrhythmias occur during direct laryngoscopy but they clear all spontaneously. Continuous anaesthetical monitoring discovers them and medication can stop them if necessary.

Obtruction of the airway by compression or kinking of the flexible intratracheal ventilation tube is a serious problem and the prevention requires constant attention from both, the anaesthesiologist and the endoscopist.

Post-extubation laryngospasm is a severe complication and are to be kept to a minimum if anaesthetic experts anticipate and prevent them.

Although the incidence of dental fracture is very low the chipping of enamel by friction is seen more especially when the laryngoscope is in contact with unprotected teeth.

If the operative manipulation leads to a dramatic narrowing of the airway by oedema an elective tracheotomy is to be performed. Minor oedemas in the larynx are treated by intravenious applied cortisone. Cortisone is additionally given to prevent postoperatively the formation of endo-laryngotracheal citatrices and following synechiae and webs.

Tearing, contusion and haematoma of the lips, tongue or pharyngeal wall can be avoided by gentle introduction of the laryngoscope.

In few cases an overexpansion causes a palsy of the hypopharyngeal or glossopharyngeal or lingual nerve. Although very seldom taste disturbances are refered.

Bleedings after biopsies are staunched by swabing with adrenalin resepctively by well-directed monopolar cauterization. Bleeding is the main complication after laser surgery.

2.11. Postoperative procedures

Untill recover of one`s voice is recured a rest is indicated with avoidance of susurration, coughing and harrumph. Coughing depressing and secretolythic agents are helpful in this phase. A normal theme of speech is considered as possible after healing of the alteration and laryngological investigation. Phoniatric exercises are a useful help for voice rehabilitation especially in cases of functional causation and after removal of a Reinke-oedema or a chronic laryngitis or resection of a vocal chord or an arytaenoidectomy. Antibiotics are prescribed only when enlarged surgical operations like partial endoscopic tumorresection or arytaenoidectomies were performed. Humid inhalations are to be recommended in any case.

3. Low-frequency and high-frequency jet ventilation: Technical basics and special considerations for clinical application

The supraglottic jet ventilation is a technique whereby the ventilation gas is emitted by a jet injector above the glottic level via an endoscope. The superimposed high-frequency jet ventilation, used by us [51], represents a supraglottical jet ventilation and needs an endoscope, a jet laryngoscope, with two integrated jet nozzles for ventilation. Ng [52] localizes the jet nozzles for the supraglottic jet ventilation at the distal end of the endoscope nearby the tip of the endoscope and thus immediately in front of the glottis. On the contrary we put the jet nozzles more proximal far away from the tip of the endoscope. Initially this ventilation technique was applicated preferential in laryngeal interventions without reduction in cross section of the glottic level. Further clinical experience pointed out that this technique is also implementable in cases of severe stenosis in front of the tip of the endoscope.

3.1. Construction of the jet laryngoscope

The jet laryngoscope used by us and first described by Aloy et al. 1990 [53] is originally a larynx endoscopy tube [54] which was modified by incorporation of fix jet nozzles (Figure 8).

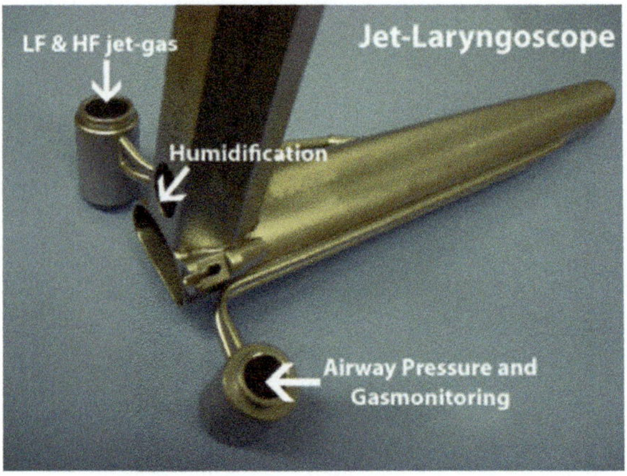

Figure 8. Jet laryngoscope according to KLEINSASSER for SHFJV® according to ALOY (Carl Reiner Jet Laryngoscope, Carl Reiner Ltd. Company with limited liability, Viennna, Austria) with a connexion for the low-frequency (LF) and high-frequency (HF) jet gas at the left proximal side. Opposite at the right side there is the connexion of the monitoring. At the basis of the grip of the laryngoscope lies the aperture for the feeding of the moistened and warmed-up ventilation gas.

The findings of flow dynamic measurements at the lung simulator served for the basic conception of the construction of this jet laryngoscope. Experiences with nozzles suspended in standard laryngoscopes achieved success. To attain a sufficient tidal volume, under the utilization of the Venturi Effect, the size of the jet nozzle as well as its localisation and adjustment play a major role. This was demonstrated in corresponding investigations. The gas jet, entering the laryngoscope, must not be directed to the opposite wall but should be targeted to the caudal direction at the virtual central point of the distal end of the tube finding the continuation median in the trachea. The optimal angle of incidence is 18 degrees. As aperture of the nozzles which influences the effectivity of the jet beam 1.8 mm was chosen. At the right side of the laryngoscope there is a conduction fixed ending at the tip of the laryngoscope used for the measurement of the ventilation pressure and oxygen concentration (Figure 9).

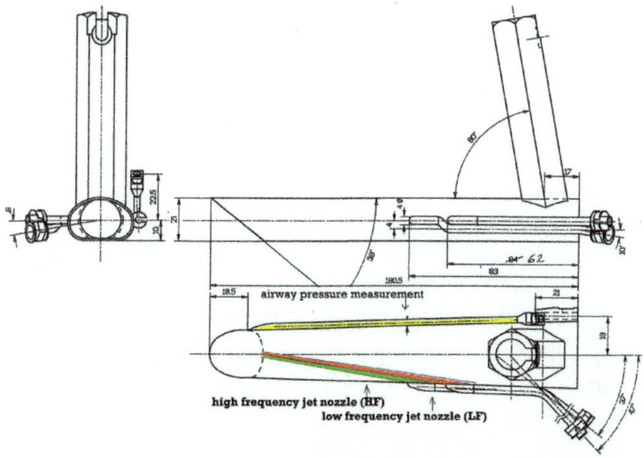

Figure 9. Schematical drawing of the gas flow in the jet laryngoscope (two jet nozzles) and of the pressure measurement and oxygen concentration (FIO_2) at the tip of the endoscope (yellow nozzle).

3.2. Ventilation technique

The simultaneous application of a jet stream with low- (normo- upto lowfrequent) frequency (12-20 impulses per minute; 0.2 - 0.3 Hz) and a further jet stream with high-frequency is performed via a jet nozzle. The low-frequent jet produces a high, superior pressure plateau representing the inspiration phase with a sufficient tidal volume (Figure 10). This is followed by breathing space of expiration.

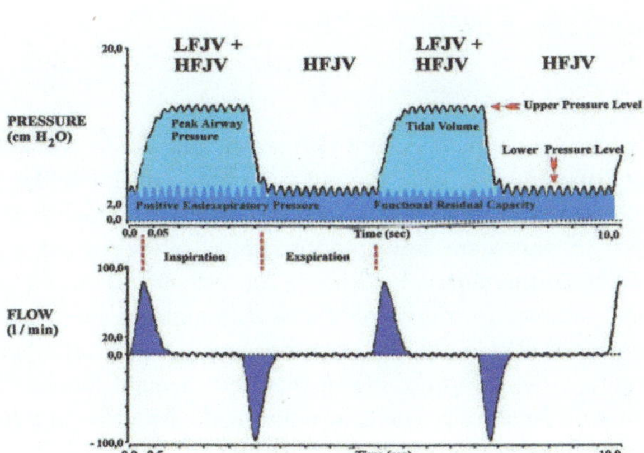

Figure 10. Relationship of pressure and flow during simultaneous low-frequency and high-frequency jet ventilation.

On the other hand via a second nozzle during the low-frequent inspiration and the subsequent expiration a continous high-frequent gas application is conducted and is additionally superimposed to the low-frequent jet ventilation causing a minimal enhancement of the inspiratory pressure plateau. In the expiration sphase of the low-frequent jet ventilation there exists only the high-frequent jet. The high-frequent jet portion (frequency from 20 to1500 impulses per minute; 0.3 to 25 Hz) produces a lower pressure plateau corresponding to an end-espiratory pressure plateau, corresponding to an end-expiratory pressure (PEEP).

3.3. Pressure profile in the lung

Ventilation via a complete open system with two different pressure plateaus is generated.

The periods of inspration and exspiration of the normo-frequent as well as the high-frequent jet gases are to be adjusted variable. It is a *time- and pressure controlled ventilation* at two pressure plateaus with decelerating flow.

3.4. Adjustment of the respirator

Variable parameter of the low-frequency jet ventilation:

Working pressure of the gas leaving the jet nozzle: 0.03-0.04 bar/kg body weight.

Frequency: 12-20 impulses/min (adults), 20-30 impulses/min (children).

Inspiration/Exspiration ratio: primary 1:2 or 1:1.

Variable parameter of the high-frequency jet ventilation:

Working pressure of the gas leaving the jet nozzle: 0.02 bar/kg body weight.

Frequency variable: 100-1500 impulses/min.

Inspiration/Exspiration ratio: primary 1:2 or 1:1.

3.5. Respirator

The development of the jet ventilation with two jet streams made it mandatory to design a specific respirator (Figure 11). An electronic respirator enabling the low- and high-frequent gas application was developed. Simultaneously the pinside of the endoscope measured ventilation pressures are digital and graphically represented, just as the adjusted and measured FIO_2. Furthermore a laser mode is practicable reducing automatically the FIO_2. The ventilation parameters are recorded and an integrated pressure limitation reacts to a too high pressure and also to a pressure drop. Therefore a barotrauma can be avoided with greatest certainty. After the input of patients body weight the ventilation is started with a default setting of the device. The connection with the jet laryngoscope is made by two not confusable jet hose couplings. Moreover the respirator includes different usable ventilation modes for the application of bronchoscopy and infraglottic one-lumen catheter techniques.

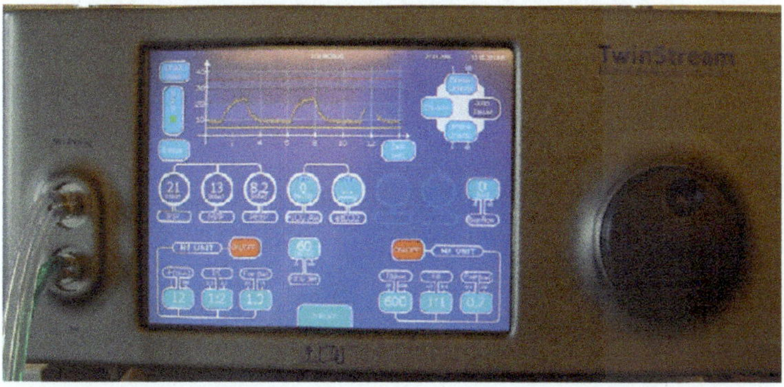

Figure 11. Jet respirator for the combined high-frequent and low-frequent jet ventilation (Twin Stream ™ multimode respirator, Carl Reiner Ltd. Company with limited liability, Vienna, Austria). The continuous airway pressure is displayed in the left upper corner. The top right part shows the adjustable pressure limitation. In the middle left the digital airway pressure and in the center of the display the inspiratory oxygen concentration is displayed. On the lower left side the low-frequency jet unit can be seen and on the right there is the high-frequency jet unit.

3.6. Physical effects during ventilation

3.6.1. Gas velocity

The applicated ventilation gas (oxygen/air mixture) is a fluid with 1 to 1.5 bar of pressure of at the nozzle. At the tip of the laryngoscope a decompression of a 100 fold occurs so that there are registrated pressures of 20 mbar. The flow velocity can achieve at the discharge of the nozzle up to 300 m/sec, but at the tip of tube it is also distinctly shortened and represents less than 100 m/sec [55].

3.6.2. Characteristics of the gas flow – Computational fluid dynamics

The computational fluid dynamics performed by us shows that during application of superimposed high-frequency jet ventilation via the jet laryngoscope an *asymmetric bi-directional gas flow* occurs in the jet laryngoscope (Figure 12).

3.6.3. Free-jet

The gas stream emitted from the particular jet nozzle is a free jet inducing an entrainment of surrounding air at the rim caused by an occurring discontinuity [56]. This entrainment is also the reason why the oxygen concentration adjusted from the respirator is diminished at the tip of the endoscope. The beams respectively the stream becomes progressively broader and his velocity decelerates (Figure 13).

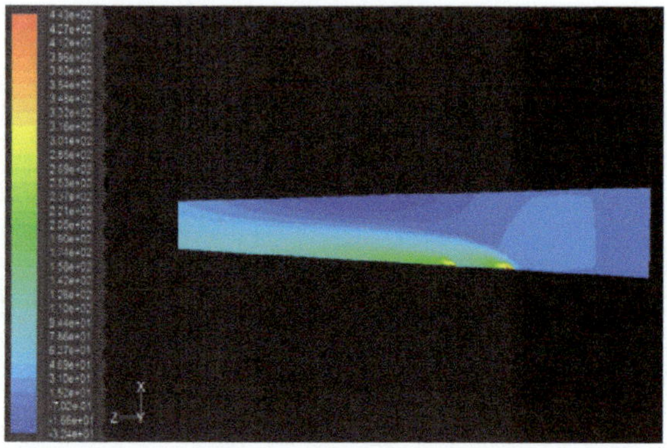

Figure 12. Charactristics of the gas flow in the jet endoscope: flow of the gas leaving the nozzles with high velocity (yellow) towards left side to the virtual tip of the endoscope. Additionally a fluid flow exists towards left side with decreasing velocity (light blue) directed to the tip of the endoscope. At the opposite side of the endoscope there is a flow (dark blue) toward right side outwards.

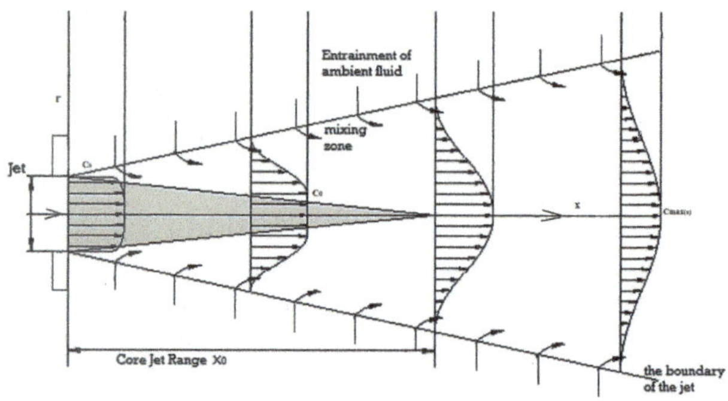

Figure 13. Schema of the characteristics of the free jet as it ejects from the nozzle. A typical deformation of the profile of the beams respectively the stream and an entrainment of the (rim) boundary zone is demonstrated.

3.6.4. Characteristics of pressure in the jet laryngoscope

The described position of the nozzles causes a typical behaviour of the pressure, as shown in Figure 14. In front of the nozzles a negative pressure occurs, which comes to its maximum immediately after the aperture of the jet nozzles.

Due to the nozzles ending in the first section of the jet laryngoscope the Venturi–effect takes place far away from the surgical area, suction and spraying of blood is prevented.

Only after the nozzles the pressure in the laryngoscope increases.

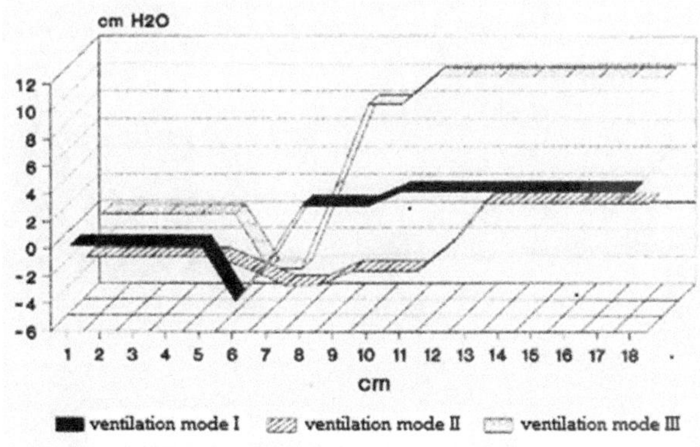

Figure 14. Characteristics of the pressure in the jet laryngoscope under the application of three different ventilation modes. On the outside (left) of the endoscope a moderate negative pressure originates when gas is emitted at jet nozzles. In the area of the nozzles the pressure becomes strongly negative. Then a positive pressure originates in the direction of the tip of the endoscope (right).

3.6.5. The Joule Thomson effect

Real gases cool when expanding without performing work (against an external pressure) [57, 58]. The increase of the volume enlarges the median distance of the gas molecules. Work is to be applied against the intermolecular attracting forces. The potential energy of the system grows at the cost of the kinetic energy of the gas molecules and therefore the temperature drops. Due to this effect during prolonged mechanical ventilation, heating and humidification of the respiratory gas is needed to avoid damage to the mucous membrane in the trachea.

3.7. Influence on physical effects

3.7.1. Moistening and warming of the respiratory gas

Further development of the jet laryngoscopes allows now the continuous moistening and warming of the respiratory gas. The gas is supplied via a so-called bias-flow to a moistening device and is moistened and warmed inside (Figure 15).

3.7.2. Entrainment of the gas

Due to the installation of an aperture in the grip of the endoscope oxygen enters the laryngoscope replacing the entrainment of surrounding air. Therefore the oxygen concentration remains the same as it leaves the jet nozzles. Thereby at first the entrainment of the air in the laryngoscope is reduced and as second the ventilation gas is moistened and as third it is warmed-up. Although physical effects cannot be eliminated completely, they can be diminished in their intensity nevertheless.

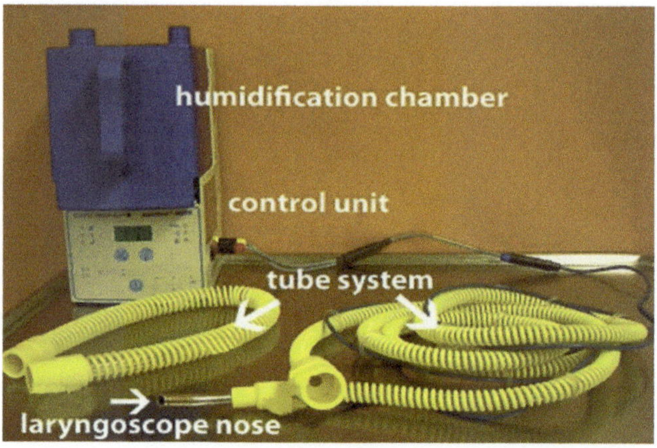

Figure 15. Device for moistening and warming-up of the respiration gas. The central unit (white) incorporates the electronical control unit. The humidifying chamber (blue) for single or multiple use is fixed at the central unit. The tubing system (yellow) is splitted in a short tube which transports the ventilation gas coming from the respirator to the humidifying chamber, and in a long tube which transports the now moistioned and warmed-up gas from the humidifier chamber to the jet laryngoscope. The distal part of the long tube is metallic and is connected to the jet laryngoscope.

Recent developments and clinical experiences with superimposed high-frequency jet ventilation demonstrate that a broad spectrum of clinical application is practicable [59].

This method is suitable for laryngotracheal diseases in adults and also excellent in infants and children [60, 61]. Additional, special indications for jet ventilation are supraglottic, glottic, subglottic and tracheal stenoses. Further applications are the ventilation during bronchoscopy, the percutaneous dilatation tracheostomy (PDT) [62] and the placement of airway stents and the treatment of acute respiratory distress syndrome (ARDS).

4. Tubeless laryngotracheal surgery via jet ventilation

Endolaryngeal and -trachel surgery always burdens from the situation in the operation area which is to share with the anaesthesiologists. An endotracheal tube narrows the view for endoscopic examination and surgery in the larynx and in particular in the trachea. Stenotic areas cause respiratory insufficiency and often can not be passed by a tube however small they may be. A safe ventilation technique, the superimposed high-frequency jet ventilation (SHFJV), which allows the laryngotracheal surgeon optimal conditions for diagnosis and surgical procedures was invented by Aloy 1990 [63].This tubeless method, described in detail before, became rapidly the anaesthetic method of choice for laryngotracheal operations at our Department of Otolaryngology in Viennna [64, 65] (Figure 16). The following report stresses out in general our experiences when laryngotracheal surgery is performed under SHFJV.

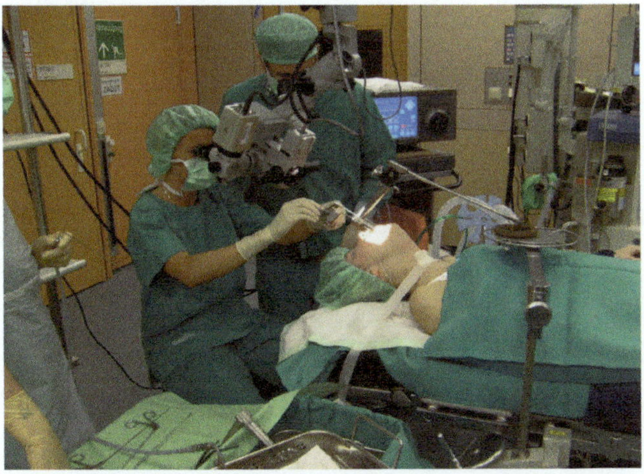

Figure 16. Microlaryngoscopy under superimposed high-frequency jet ventilation (SHFJV)

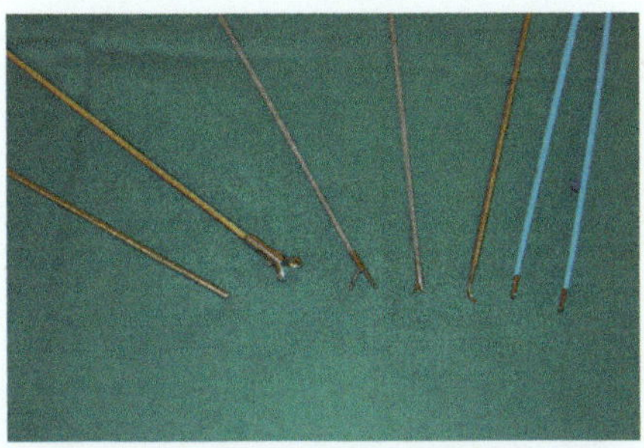

Figure 17. Long micro instruments for the operative procedure in the larynx and in the trachea.

At our department of otorhinolaryngology in Vienna, Austria 2123 micro laryngeal/tracheal surgical interventions were made under SHFJV from 1990 up to December 2011 using micro instruments demonstrated in Figure 17. Diagnoses and number of patients is demonstrated in the following Table 1.

If it becomes necessary that the vocal chords are in a complete standstill in fine phonosurgical interventions it is easy and hazard-free to interrupt the jet ventilation for a few seconds.

We never saw complications associated with jet ventilation which include inadequate oxygenation and ventilation, severe dehydration of the mucosa, gastric distension, regurgitation, and even gastric rupture. Pneumomediastinum or pneumothorax have been reported, and occurs mostly when applying jet ventilation with an obstructed airway [66].

Diagnoses	Total (n=2123)	Percent (100%)
Laryngeal carcinoma	403	19.0
Vocal chord leucoplakia	272	12.8
Laryngeal papillomatosis	122	5.7
Chronic laryngitis	116	5.5
Vocal chord polyp	259	12.2
Reinke`s oedema	221	10.4
Laryngeal/tracheal stenosis	172	8.1
Bilateral vocal chord paralysis	45	2.1
Unilateral vocal chord paralysis	72	3.4
Vocal chord nodule	57	2.7
Vocal chord granuloma	71	3.3
Vocal chord cyst	93	4.4
Vocal chords synechia	53	2.5
Supraglottic cyst	83	3.9
Phonosurgery	32	1.5
Others	52	2.5

Table 1. Diagnoses of patients undergoing micro laryngeal/tracheal surgery with superimposed high-frequency jet ventilation (SHFJV).

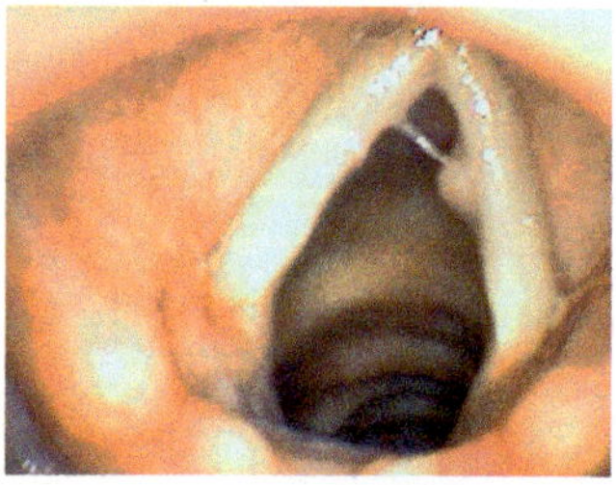

Figure 18. Cyst at the free margin of the right vocal chord anterior half with free access to the operation area.

The continuous pressure control of the SHFJV- device could ward a barotrauma in our application in any case.

4.1. Contraindications of SHFJV in laryngotracheal surgery

The jet ventilation has proven to be most suited for patients with normal, unobstructed airways and normal lung and chest wall compliance (Figure 18). Reduced chest wall compliance such as in obesity (body mass index >35) may lead to unmeant gastric insufflation and distension causing worsening of the respiratory compliance. A significant overbite especially in combination with retrognathia makes laryngotracheal placement of the ventilation laryngoscope impracticable and the incidence of accidental gastric hyperinflation is high.

Expected massive bleeding is an absolute contraindication. However slight bleeding does not reach the trachea and deeper airways because of the high-frequent gas flow with PEEP-effect pressures the blood to the laryngeal respectively tracheal wall and with the expiration it is tranported externally.

5. CO_2 laser micro laryngotracheal surgery during supraglottic jet ventilation

Three characteristics are the basics of the high energy density of laser:

1. monochromaticity: in a high degree with very limited range of wavelengths,
2. coherence: in the laser beam the electromagnetic fields of all photons oscillate synchronously in identical phase, and
3. collimated beam: laser light remains in a narrow spectrum.

With laser light, tissue penetration is mostly a function of wavelight. Long-wavelight laser light such as that from CO_2 laser (operation at 10,600 nm) is completey absorbed by water in the first few layers of cells. The thermal effect is therefore largely limited to the point of entry into the target tissue. This results in explosive vaporisation of the surface tissue of the target with surprisingly little damage to underlying cells. When coupled to an operating microscope the laser vaporizes the lesions with precision, causing minimal bleeding and oedema: an obvious advantage, especially in small pediatric airways.

Technique of CO_2 laser microsurgery	Advantages of CO_2 laser microsurgery
Wavelength: ~10.000 nm; infrared - invisible	Contactless operating
Pilotlaser: red (aiming beam), coaxial	Precise dosing and control
Micromanipulator for application	Reduced bleeding
Focus diameter: 0.3-0.7 mm	Reduced risk of infection
at a distance of 40 cm	Less postoperative pain
Microscopic magnification: 4 to 40-fold	

Table 2. Technique of CO_2 laser microsurgery and advantages of laser surgery.

The pulsed dye laser (PDL) has a shorter wavelength and spares the epithelium, but specifically hits the microvascular supply of the lesion. This has an advantage in the anterior laryngeal commissure because not denuting the epithelium is beneficial, it should limit the occurrence of webs. In certain situations, a laser based resection technique is surgical method of choice for:

1. sessile lesions,
2. lesions in scared areas and

3. lesions near or in the laryngeal ventricle.

Anaesthesia for laryngotracheal interventions can be performed with or without endotracheal tubes [67]. As the most servere complication laser induced combustion is considered. Within 635 laser applications under SHFJV at the Department of Otorhinolaryngology of the Medical University of Vienna we had to see in one case an endlaryngeal fire caused by ignition of an erroneous dry swab which was inserted in the subglottic space for laser prevention of the trachea wall. The fire could be extinguished rapidly. After orotracheal intubation a tracheostomy was performed for the entrence of ventilation. The patient could be discharged from the intensive care unit within 10 days and from hospital after closure of the tracheostomy after 21 days without further essentially respiration problem deriving from this accident, especially there was no stenotic laryngotracheal process [68]. It is clearly to state, that this ignition was not in a causal connection with the SHFJV. The major complication, airway fire, is avoided by SHFJV itself: there is no flammable material in the airway. Other ventilation devices like plastic tubes do not withstand laser strikes and will ignite the longer the laser exposure lasts. Metallic foil-wrapped plastic tubes may injure pharyngeal and laryngotracheal tissues by sharp edges, loose their elasticity and tend to kink. The protective effect is lost if the foil is detached and airway obstruction may occur when parts of the foil is aspirated. The reflexion from the surface bears the risk of damage of surrounding tissues. For a considerable time laser safe endotracheal-tubes are put up for sale. The disadvantage of these tubes is the size of its diameter. Because of the required material safety these tubes have a large outer diameter and a small inner diameter. In case of a larger stenosis it is not possible to use these endotracheal tubes. But just in cases of stenoses jet ventilation has a major advantage. No tube - no fire when the applied oxygen concentration is low ($< 40\%$). The jet ventilation is done with a mixture of oxygen/air. Nitrous oxide should not be used.

The high gas flow dilutes and eliminates the smoke and therefore additional suction for smoke is redundant. Laser laryngotracheal surgery was perfomed with a CO_2 laser (Hercules 5040; Haereus, Germany or Sharplan 1050; Vörösmarty, Israel).

Special indications for CO_2 laser application in combination with SHFJV in laryngeal diseases are the early glottic cancer [69, 70], the papillomatosis and the stenoses. Indispensable precaution is the internal approval for general anaesthea, the adjustability of the inner laryngealtracheal structures with special attention to the anterior commissure and the expectation of low bleeding. The laser surgical procedures under SHFJV lasted from 15 up to 120 minutes, on the average of 42 minutes.

5.1. Circumscribed carcinoma

The preoperative information of the patients include the postoperative bleeding which depends on the extent of the resection. A revision under endotracheal intubation and general anaesthesia and sometimes a tracheotmy will be necessary. The patient has to know that until the definitve histological findings are evident in case of incomplete resection a re-operation will be necessary. Healing of the wound is delayed with functional consequences like hoarseness and transient aphonia. Synechiae and stenoses rarely occure. After histological confirmation of the initial diagnosis the surgery by CO_2 laser with the soft super pulsed mode a nearly char-free cutting via vaporisation is performed.

Dissecting the soft tissue of the tumour is has proven to perform with the micro manipulator fine serrated hither and thihter movements. With this method laser`s physical properties for cutting and coagulation are utilized most effective [71]. Like the study group of our department could show excellent oncological results can be expected in T1a-glottic cancer in comparison to radiotherapy and conventional surgery [72].

Postoperative stridor is mostly due to a swelling of the local mucous membrane and is easy to be treated by cortisone.

5.2. Laryngo/tracheal stenosis

Congenital and aquired stenoses in all regions of the larynx are a prefered indication for CO_2 laser surgery (Figures 19, 20, 21). Tubeless ventilation allows the surgeon to operate in an already narrow area.

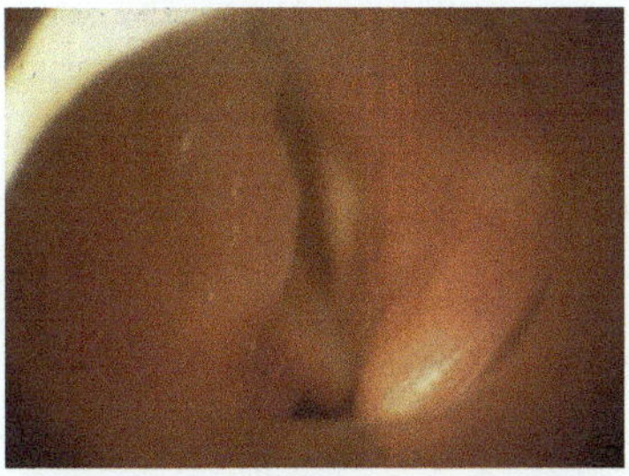

Figure 19. View through the ventilation laryngoscope in position. Tumour caused massive stenosis. In the area of the posterior commissure a residual lumen exists, enabling patient`s spontaneous but stridulous breathing.

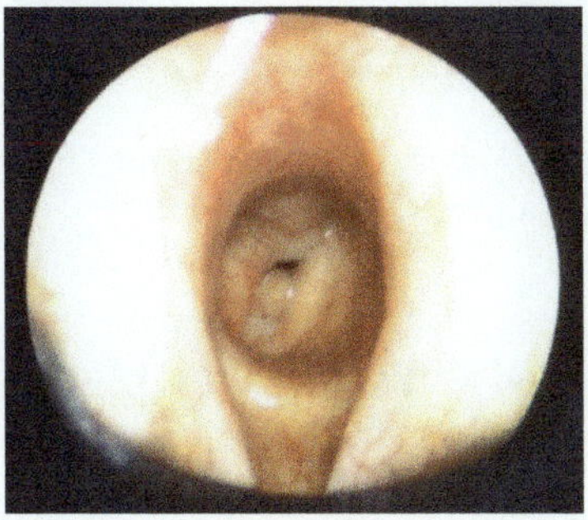

Figure 20. High grade subglottic stenosis with a substantially reduced lumen.

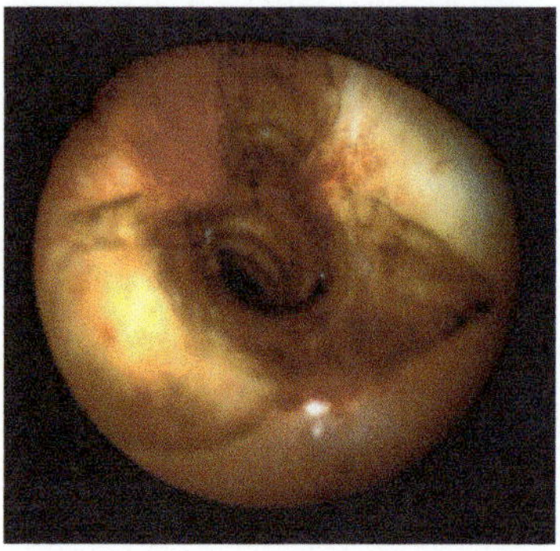

Figure 21. Star-shaped opening of a glottic/subglottic stenosis with CO_2 laser under SHFJV.

5.3. Laryngeal papillomatosis (see also part 6)

Accordingly to their biological behavior with multiple recurrences in juvenile papllomatosis repeated interventions are necessary (Figure 22). The CO_2 laser in combination with SHFJV [73] offers the opportunity of a safe procedure with preserving the funtional important vocal chords.

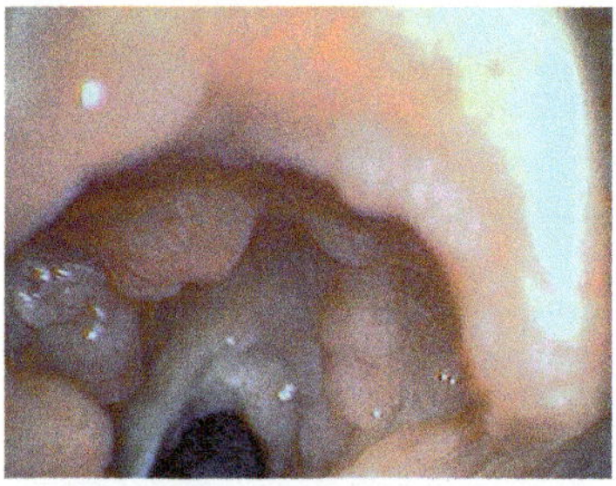

Figure 22. Glottic and supraglottic recurrence of a juvenile papillomas.

(We thank Prof. W. Bigenzahn from the Department for Phoniatry and Logopaedia of the Medical University of Vienna for providing this figure).

6. Tubeless laryngotracheal surgery in infants and children via jet ventilation

Laryngotracheal surgery in infants and children is handicaped by the narrow anatomical area of operations and often additionally by the pathological substrate itself. A special cooperation between the surgeon and the anaesthesist is indispensable. Ventilation via an endotracheal tube with a cuff is most safe to operate. But even this endotracheal tube blocks on the one hand the unobstructed view of the operating field and on the other hand the necessary space for surgical activity and additionally mutates the anatomical structures. In cases of pronounced stenoses in the laryngotracheal area an endotracheal intubation cannot be applied. An alternative procedure is the tracheotomy, especially for infants and children and the postoperative care an enormous burden.

A rigid bronchoscope used for ventilation restricts the visibility of the working space and it may occur that it cannot pass a stenosis. Laryngotracheal surgery in the apnea technique is still in use but is associated with the heightened risk of hypoxemia and hypercapnia.

An improvement of ventilation of the patient during laryngotracheal surgery was established by single-frequency jet ventilation techniques applied either per percutaneous insertion of a needle into the trachea or endotracheal tubes or catheters, or application of a jet nozzle into the endocopy tube [74, 75]. All these techniques have the disadvantage of the risk of hypoxaemia and hypercapnia especially in patients underlying pulmonary and cardiadic aggravated risks and operations with a long continuance. Needles placed transtracheal bear the elevated risk of barotrauma because the gas supply takes place below the stenosis [76].

6.1. Ventilation

As an alternative ventilation technique the jet ventilation presents themselves with 3 modalities:

1. *transtracheal jet ventilation* (Figure 23): for endoscopic laryngeal surgery, also with laser, excellent visibility for the surgeon, even in glottic or supraglottic stenoses with minor complications up to 20 % [77-79]. Very important is the bedding of the child with maximum extension of the head. This allows fixing the mobile trachea between middle finger and thumb. The cricoid membrane is narrow and at best to be felt by a fingernail. The punction with ventilation catheter is to be directed in a caudal direction.

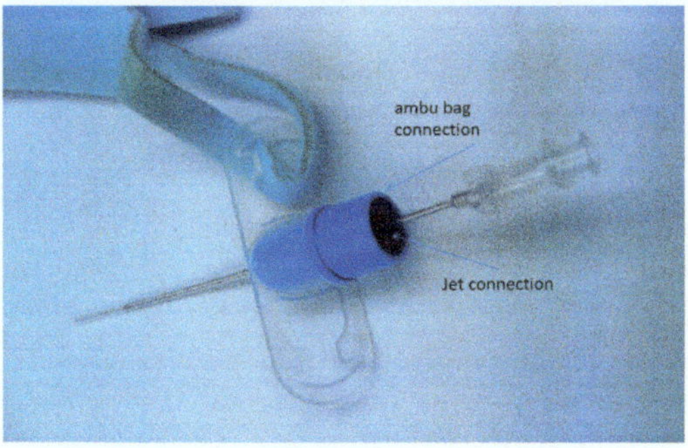

Figure 23. Percutaneous transtracheal jet ventilation catheter (VBM®-Medizintechnik, Germany) for children with steel punction needle.

2. *infraglottic, transoral jet ventilation:* transoral or nasotracheal positioning of a catheter through the glottis deep enough into the trachea. Available if the glottis is not narrowed.

Not available for children because the diameter of the catheter is often more than 5 mm.

3. *supraglottic jet ventilation:* as an alternative method the authors, Grasl et al. 1997 [80], have presented their experiences in the first use of tubeless superimposed high- and low-frequency jet ventilation (SHFJV) with a jet laryngoscope in laryngotracheal surgery in infants and children 28 infants and children. This intervention was spread successively [81]. Because of the absence of an additional jet catheter optimal working conditions with best visibility in primarily narrow areas are created. Nowadays jet laryngoscopes with also two intergrated jet nozzles for children are available in different sizes. The transfer of the jet gas takes place at the proximal section of the laryngoscope and not nearby the glottis. The endoscopes are equipped with an integrated ventilation pressure measurement positioned at the tip. At the grip of the endoscope (Figure 24) there is an aperture for the connection of the moistening and warming of the ventilation gas. On the left side there of upper section of the laryngoscope there are two jet nozzles, on the right side are located a nozzle for the ventilation pressure measurement and a nozzle for the true FIO2 recording. Additional monitorings are the pulsoxymetry, the electrocardiogram and the noninvasive measurement of the blood pressure. We consider because of our complication free experiences the invasive arterial monitoring as needless.

The supraglottic jet ventilation offers the surgeon the opportunity to use the CO_2 laser [82].

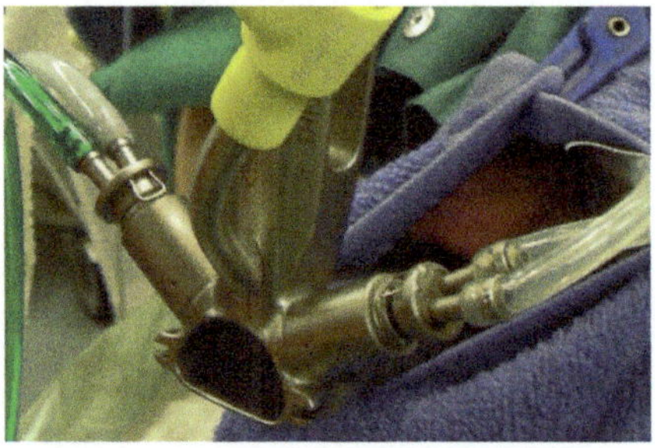

Figure 24. The proximal section of the ventilation laryngoscope for children with all connexions.

6.2. Anaesthesia

Ventilation is carried out by an air/oxygen mixture. If the CO_2 laser is used the inspiratory oxygen concentration is reduced to 40 %. In corresponding dose rate propofol is applied as hynoticum, fentanil or remifentanil as analgesia and rocuronium as short effective relaxant.

Anaesthesia starts with manual ventilation by a conventional respirator. When relaxation takes effect the jet laryngoscope is placed and jet ventilation starts. After the end of the surgical intervention the jet laryngoscope is removed and mask ventilation follows till the patient is awake.

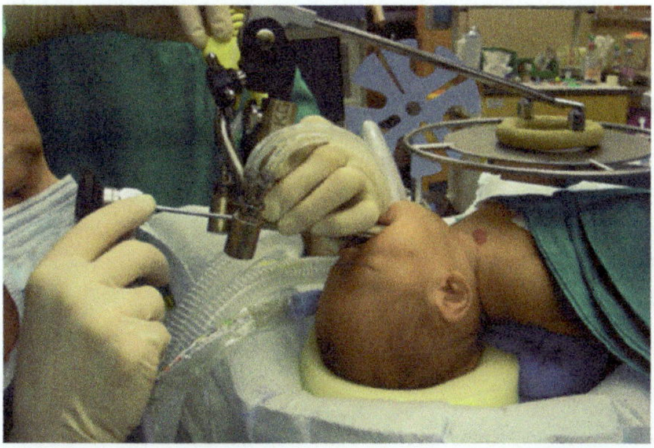

Figure 25. Procedure of an endoscopic surgical intervention under a continuous superimposed high-frequency jet ventilation.

The physiology of the infantile lung offers several specifics. The compliance and also the resistence of the lung make age-related fluctuations. The compliance is significantly lower and the resistance higher than in adults. Due to the resulting time constant a higher ventilation frequence exists. With increasing age an approximation to the values up to that of adults occurs. Subsequently the following considerations for the adjustment of the respirator are: higher frequency of ventilation, ventilation pressure low but not too low, the start calibration of the respirator with body weight specification, orientation at the displayed and measured values of ventilation pressure. As in adults the supraglottic jet ventilation is performed at two different pressure plateaus. With the superior pressure plateau CO_2 is eliminated, the inferior pressure plateau produces the positive end-expiratory pressure (PEEP).

Contraindications for the jet ventilation are: impracticality to bring the jet laryngoscope in the right position, bleeeding in larynx and trachea and the absence of patient`s sobriety.

The superimposed jet ventilation offers the anaesthesist and the surgeon optimal working conditions (Figure 25). Anaesthesia has as advantage the continuous mechanical ventilation with integrated limitation of pressure. The surgean has optimal conditions of visibility with no displacement of anatomical structures by a catheter or endotracheal tube. A further advantage is the safe application of laser surgery.

The youngest patient was two week old. Therefore no age-related limitation exist for the superimposed high-frequency jetventilation.

Up to now at the Department of Otorhinolaryngology of the Medical Universitiy of Vienna 230 infants and children with an age below 14 years were ventilated sufficiently by a therefore extra designed rigid endoscopy tube derived from the Kleinsasser tube [79] during laryngo-tracheal surgery. Diagnoses were: papillomatosis, subglottic stenoses, laryngeal inspection, web, foreign body, vocal chord cyst, vocal chords granuloma and miscellaneous. Movement of foreign bodies becomes much more easy and elegant during the tubeless ventilation: a Fogarty-Catheters© guided behind the foreign body helps to bring him more proximal where he can be gripped and extracted with a forceps [83]. With this SHFJV technique laryngeal stenoses and cardiopulmonal insufficiences do not present special risks. Laryngotracheal surgery under SHFJV can be applied in any child except special general contraindications.

As in adults before effective jet ventilation can start, the laryngoscope tube, adjusted to size of the childlike larynx, is inserted and evaluated for suitability for jet ventilation. Immediately afterward the suspension system is installed and the jet injector needles are attached to the laryngoscope. The steadily ventilation can begin. Up to this point of time the manipulation happens in an anaesthetized but apnoeic patient.

The procedure of the jet ventilation took from 5 up to 130 minutes, on average about 35 minutes. The ventilation assured in any case a sufficient oxygenation and CO_2 elimination.

Only in a few cases during introduction or recovery of the anaesthesia an endotracheal tube had to replace the ventilation tube temporarily caused by adverse anatomical characteristics. A serve laryngospasm never resulted from SHFJV. To eliminate the danger of pneumothorax in the application of SHFJV it is to state that it is an open system with an air supply always above the existing stenoses. Additionally an intergrated monitoring of pressure in the laryngoscope is positioned. The surgical procedure could be performed in any case.

Contraindication for SHFJV in infants und children are in principle the same as in grownups.

The technique of SHFJV has helped us to handle the naturally difficult surgery of the larynx and trachea in infants and children and simplified it considerably.

A very special laryngeal disease in children is the recurrent respiratory papillomatosis (RRP) [84-86].

Only a minority of Human papilloma virus (HPV) carrying mothers will become symptomatic. The route of transmission to the infant in not yet completely understood.

There is no cure for RRP at present and no therapy modality that might eradicate the virus from the respiratory mucosa. Local recurrences are therefore frequently seen.

Vaccination against HPV 6 and 11 across the board should decrease the incidence of children in future.

RRP requires a protracted and repeatedly therapy over years.

The surgical therapy with a removal of the papillomas as much as possible und preservation of normal structures is the procedure of (Figure 26). Scaring from overagressive resections effects dysphonia and airway comprise. Incomplete resections are accepted under these aspects especially in the anterior commissure. It is not practicable to eradicate all virus particles even when clinically all evident papillomas had been removed.

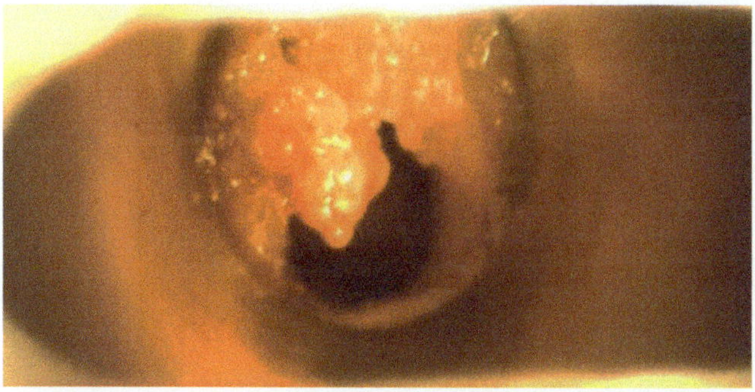

Figure 26. Laryngeal papillomatosis. View through the jet laryngoscope.

We have experiences about 122 surgical interventions under SHFJV in children with RRP.

Near all of them received papilloma ablation by CO_2 laser.

In addition the adjuvant medical therapy plays an increasing role: a-Interferon, and various antiviral agents, of which the most commonly used is the intralesional sidovir.

We cannot confirm, based on our experiences, the theoretical risk in clinical practice that the applicated jet is forcing papilloma fragments deeper into the airways. Our preliminary results provide no indication that the risk of spread of papillomas by jet ventilation into the trachea has increased. A spread of papillomas by an endotracheal tube cannot be entirely excluded.

7. Supraglottic jet ventilation in laryngotracheal stenoses

High degree stenoses in the larynx and trachea represent an acute alarming situation for the affected patients. In a slow increasing stenotic process the narrowing of the laryngeal or tracheal lumen up to 80 % is clinically well tolerated by the patients [87-89]. A further increase of the stenoses, for example caused by a local swelling, is associated with life-threatening dyspnoea and hypoxia. In these cases a tracheotomy is necessary to maintain gas exchange. If an endotracheal intubation is impossible due to the massive narrowing of the laryngotracheal area and ventilation via mask provides sufficient oxygenation tracheotomy is performed under local anaesthesia. An extreme dyspnoea requires oxygenation via a percutaneous transtracheal puncture or surgical cricothyrotomy.

7.1. Applications of the jet ventilation in obstructive supraglottic respectively glottic or infraglottic narrowing of the airways

According to the local spread of pathologies the following anatomical localisations of obstructions exist: *i) supraglottic, ii) glottic, iii) subglottic* and *iv) tracheal.*

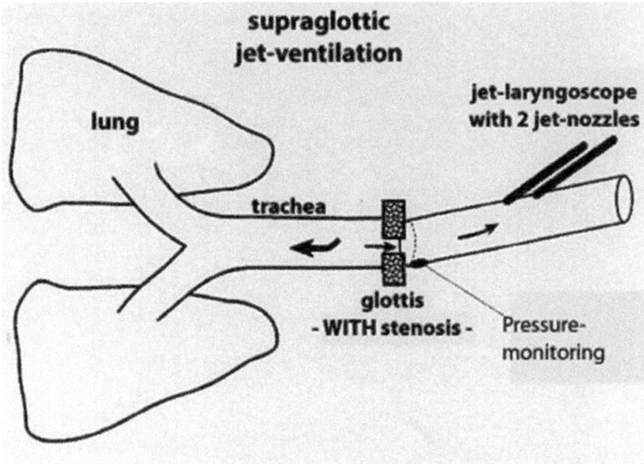

Figure 27. Schematical drawing of the supraglottic jet ventilation with a stenosis in front of the tip of the laryngoscope.

If the glottis is not obstructed any form of jet ventilation can be applied. The narrower the glottic space becomes because of a pathological process the more attention is to be applied to the chosen jet ventilation.

In principle three options are available for jet ventilation with stenosis: *i)* the *transcricoidal punction* – not usable in cases of long-stretched stenoses where the trachea is not to be localized, *ii)* the *transoral infraglottic jet catheter* – not to be inserted through high-grade stenoses and *iii)* the *jet laryngoscope* – a supraglottic jet ventilation with jet gas emission above the glottic area (Figure 27). The first and second techniques are in terms of the location of the jet nozzles infraglottic jet ventilations.

Initially the application of the supraglottic jet ventilation was applied cautious in obstructive pathologies but at an early stage the advantages in severe airway obstructions emphasized [90, 91]. It became apparent that the increasing ventilation pressure, measured at the tip of the laryngoscope, behind an obstruction can not be higher than in front of it.

Therefore this technique is best suited for all kinds of to be expected difficult airway. However absolute requirement is to place the jet laryngoscope ahead the expected obstruction.

If a stenosis is produced at the lung simulator in the level of the fictitious glottis immediately ahead of the laryngoscope the following characteristics with regard to the tidal volumes are observed (Figure 28).

Increasing of the working pressure of the device for both types of ventilation, the low- and high-frequent jet, produces a sufficient respiratory tidal volume (**blue columns**).

With decrease of the compliance (0.05 l/mbar, **red columns**) the tidal volume without stenosis is already low and decreases dramatically with increase of a stenosis, at the identical original setting of the jet ventilator.

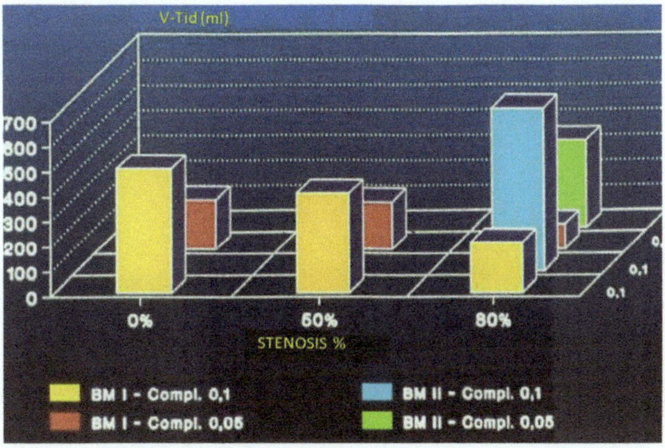

Figure 28. Diagram of the respiratory tidal volume (ml) to be achieved by a supraglottic jet ventilation via a jet laryngoscope in a default setting on the lung simulator: with a narrowing of the cross section for ventilation, at first without stenosis (0 %, left), then with a 50 % stenosis (centre) and at last with a 80 % stenosis (right) all **yellow columns**. The lung compliance was adjusted at 0.1 liter per millibar (l/mbar).

The increase of the working pressures of the ventilators succeeds in achievement of sufficient tidal volumes even in 80 % stenosis (**green column**).

7.2. Computational fluid dynamic

In a jet laryngoscope a flow simulation with ANSYS fluent® was carried out. First, the creation of a three-dimensional image of the jet laryngoscope with the preprocessor Gambit was performed. This was followed by the definition of boundary conditions and input parameters in the solver and the iterative calculation in fluent.

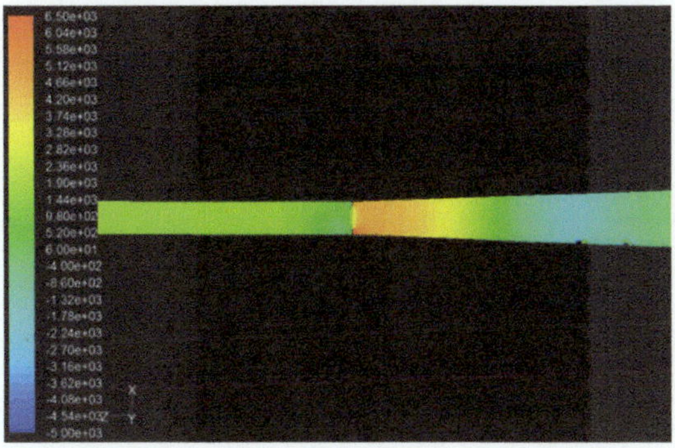

Figure 29. Distribution of pressure in the jet laryngoscope in case of a stenosis. Note the impact pressure in front of the stenosis (Figures 29, 30). The pressure behind the stenosis is lower than the pressure before the stenosis.

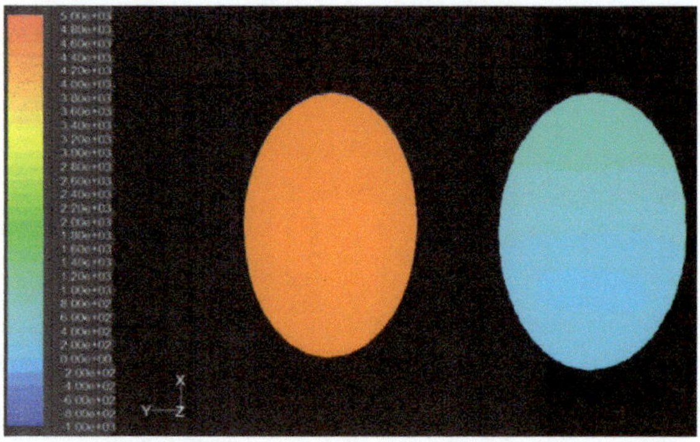

Figure 30. Characteristics of pressure in front and behind the stenosis in the jet laryngoscope. Note the pressure before the stenosis (left) and behind the stenosis (right).

These experimental results show that the pressure behind a stenosis is not higher than the pressure in front of the stenosis.

This simulation of the gas flow at a stenosis at the tip of the endoscope shows in the case of a reduction of the cross-section immediately in front of the tip of the endoscope the occurrence of an impact pressure. This pressure increases continuously at the shock front up to the stagnation point, but the velocity decreases. However the pressure behind the stenosis is lower than ahead the stenosis.

The supraglottic jet ventilation via the jet laryngoscope guarantees even in high grade stenoses (grade II-III according to RT Cotton [92] a sufficient ventilation. The development of a barotrauma can be excluded like experimental results demonstrated. Only in stenosis grade IV when in no way a lumen exists the SHFJV via a jet laryngoscope cannot be applied.

An essential advantage of this technique is that the surgeon has in these difficult situations an absolutely free approach to the larynx and trachea. Because of the absence of inflammable material laser is safe to applicate. The high gas flow avoids the smoke induced obstruction of vision.

Parameter	Setting
Inspiration time	Long-time
Expiration time	Short-time
Driving pressure	High
Ventilation frequency	High

Table 3. Setting of the respirator in stenosis and supraglottic jet ventilation.

Experimental results demonstrate if supraglottic jet ventilation is applicated the ventilation pressure behind a stenosis cannot be higher than in front of a stenosis. The pressure measurement at the tip of the endoscope allows the detection of elevated airway pressures. At the ventilator a pressure limitation can be adjusted and the ventilation stops when the pressure limit is reached. Clinical results with the absence of any complications caused by ventilation confirm this. The supraglottic jet ventilation can be applied in severe high-grade stenoses [93] (Figures 31, 32, 33). All these results are only valid for the type of supraglottic jet ventilation where the jet nozzles are positioned in the proximal section of the jet laryngoscope and not at the tip of the endoscope. Only in the case of grade IV stenosis after Cotton, in which no lumen in the area of the larynx is more available, the SHFJV on the jet laryngoscope cannot be applied.

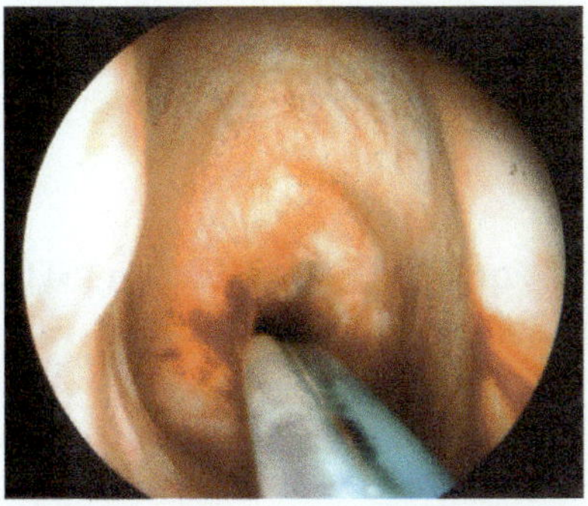

Figure 31. A severe subglottic stenosis: a jet-catheter (Hunsaker Mon®-Jet-Ventilation Tube, Medtronic Xomed® Inc. Jacksonville USA) is placed through this stenosis. Although the visibility conditions are good, the working conditions are difficult for the surgeon caused by the catheter.

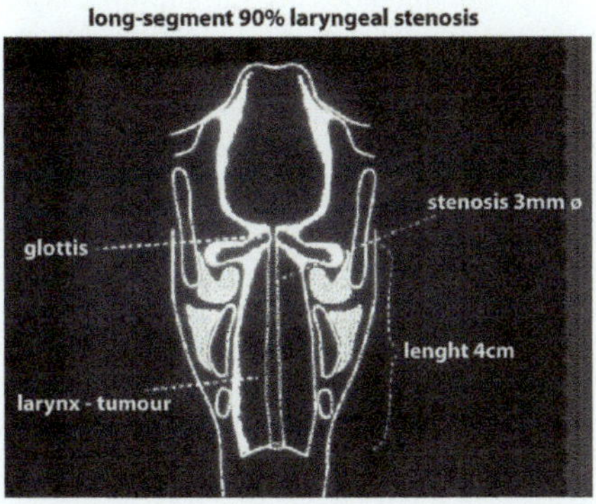

Figure 32. Schematic drawing of a long-segment 90% laryngeal stenosis. The diameter of the stenosis was 3 mm. In this clinical case, it was realizable to achieve a sufficiently ventilation. A transoral jet ventilation with a catheter would not have been possible. The diameter of a jet catheter is more than 3 mm. In the case of transtracheal jet ventilation, it would not have been possible to find the trachea in a simple way.

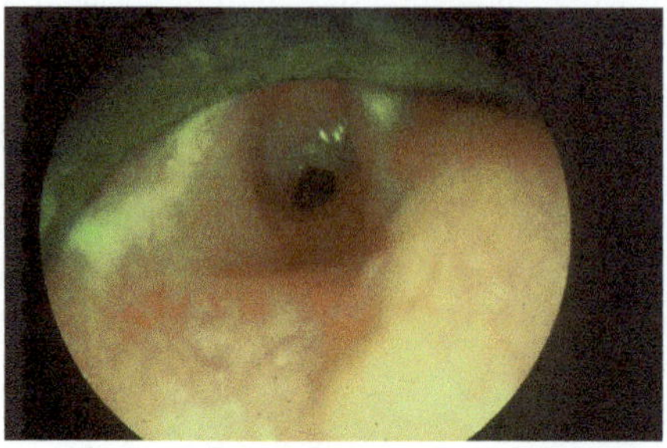

Figure 33. Extended subglottic stenosis. The use of a jet catheter through the glottis would make the outflow of the jet gas impossible.

8. Superimposed high-frequency jet ventilation (SHFJV) for tracheobronchial stent insertion

Central airway obstruction is caused by lung cancer, esophageal carcinoma, thyroid carcinoma, malignant lymphoma, and rather rare carcinoma of the larynx, trachea and hypopharynx. If the airway constriction is not yet in the focus external-beam radiation therapy, endoluminal brachytherapy and photodynamic therapy can be applied.

If curative treatment fails and progessive extended tumour growth infiltrates and advances intraluminal or external compression the effective lumen of the airway becomes dramatically narrow.

Palliative surgical tumour reduction methods are intraluminal laser ablation, electrocautery or mechanical removal. This is followed by implantation of tracheal or bronchial stents for to improve ventilation.

Indications for insertion of tracheobronchial stents are severe stridor and dyspnea in patients with tracheobronchomalacia and extraluminal compression, intraluminal tumour growth and tracheoesophageal fistulas. Airway stents have proved as best practical environmental option to renew and to perpetuate airways in such patients with a serious central airway obstruction.

[94-97]. Endotracheal intervention can be performed under local anaesthesia by fiberoptical bronchoscopy or under general anaesthesia using rigid bronchoscopy or supension laryngoscopy [98]. From the consideraton of anaesthesia a conventional ventilation or jet ventilation can be performed [99, 100].

Suspension laryngoscopy and jet ventilation offers an ideal setting with directly visual control for the precise placement of tracheal and bifurcational airway stents [101].

Low-frequency jet ventilation provides adequate ventilation as well as a non obstructed field during fibre optic bronchoscopy and stent insertion [102].

Airway stent placement requires a combination of surgical techniques and skills with safety and perpetuated ventilation during manipulation. The procedure is to be planned carefully, a constant communication between the surgeon and anaesthesiologist is an indispensable condition.

Stents are made from either metallic expandable prostheses or flexible silicone, with each type having their special indications according to the requirements and are placed either temporary or permanent.

Temporary	Permanent
Decay of a post-stenotic pneumonia	Benig: long-segment stenosis
Improvement of the overall condition Stabilization of a tracheobronchomalcia	complicated injuries
Pretherapeutic until radio/chemotherapy is effective.	functional inoperative patients
	Malign: anatomical and functional inoperative patients
	(lenghts of stenosis, tumour spread,
	overall condition).

Table 4. Indication for temporary and permanent tracheobronchial stents.

8.1. Technique of stent implantation

Usually the stent implantation is carried out under general anaesthesia in most cases via a bronchoscope under conventional ventilation or via a tracheoscope with the opportunity for jet ventilation or with growing extent via a jet laryngoscope [101]. Even in severe tracheal stenosis the jet ventilation is recommended [102, 103]. First at all inspection and then measurement of the stenosis is performed. If necessary a surgical debulking for the enlargement of the tracheal lumen is made.

8.2. Anaesthetic management

During execution of these steps and the placement of the stent a continuous ventilation of the patient is applied, preferential with jet ventilation [104] without phases of apnoea.

Often we really succeed to create a straight axis between the trachea and the jet laryngoscope and under certain circumstances the view extends to the carina.

The advantage of jet ventilation especially via the jet laryngoscope is the continuous automatically ventilation and the operation area with no limitation of visibility. Ventilation is arranged by an air/oxygen mixture applicated via the bronchoscope or the jet laryngoscope.

Through the jet laryngoscope or the rigid bronchoscope a simultaneous low- and high-frequency jet ventilation is applicated.

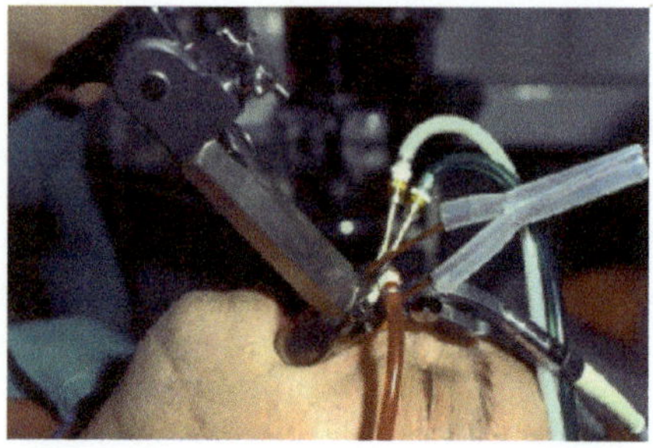

Figure 34. Application of a Y-stent under guidance of two catheters (right and left main bronchus) under superimposed high-frequency jet ventilation.

Anaesthesia is performed as totally intravenous, as hypnoticum propofol continuous, as short-acting relaxant serves rocuronium as a bolus and as short-acting analgesic remifentanil. This kind of anaesthesia has well proven in adults and children [105].

If the stent is to be positioned as a distal Y stent or a tube, it is essential to check that both limbs are patient. The ventilation laryngoscope allows a lot of space for manipulation. Folding and or creasing of a limb of a T or Y tube can disable ventilation with the need of emergent removal of the stent. Additionally, when jet ventilation is used, a totally stent blockage can cause high airway pressures with the risk of a tension pneumothorax. After the placement of a stent, the laryngoscope is removed and the patient may awaken with mask ventilation.

At this moment all equipment and personnel should stay at call in the operating room until the patient is completely awake and ready for transport.

If a stent reaches into the upper trachea, standard intubation in following anaesthesia should be avoided, because this second endotracheal tube may adhere to the stent and remove it during extubation.

8.3. Types of stents

Selfexpanding stents

Wallstent: small-meshed grating, self expanding, for extraluminal caused stenosis.

Gianturco-Z-stent: broad-meshed grating, for example for tracheobronchial malacia.

Silicone stents

For application various sizes and types can be adapted to the particular located situation (Figures 34, 35, 36). Their application is descibed in numerous publications [106, 107]. That includes also the Montgomery -T-tubes [108], the Dumona-Artemis-Stent and also the Orlowski-stent [109] and also the Polyflex® stent is to be allocated to the silicone stents. In the silicone grating polyester fibres are integrated. The application of all these stents can be done under continuous jet ventilation.

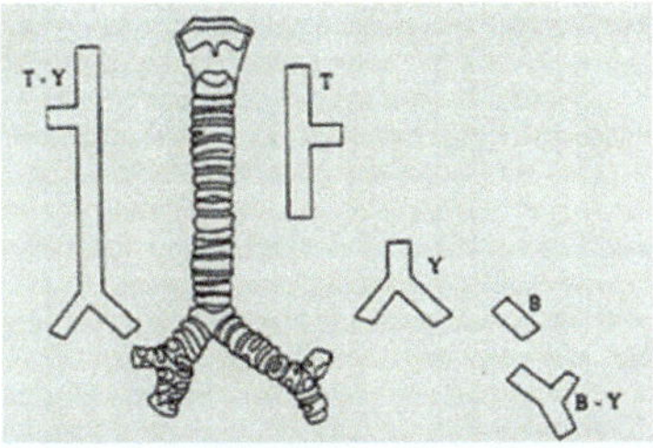

Figure 35. Various forms of silicone stents to be inserted according the respective local anatomical situation. From W. Klepetko et al. Endoluminal Stenting of the Tracheobronchial System. Acta Chirurgica Austriaca 1991;23(3)124-129 [11] with friendly permission of Springer Verlag, Vienna-New York.

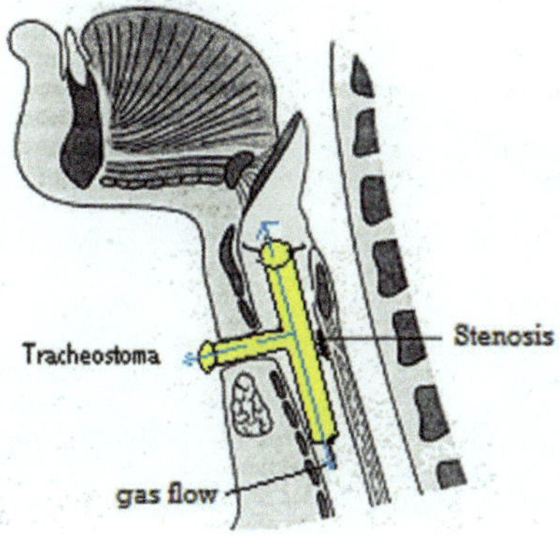

Figure 36. A typical T-tube according Montgomery in correct position.

The T-tube according Montgomery serves to bridge tracheal stenoses in the presence of a tracheotomy.

Polyflex®-Stent

The application of a Polyflex® stent is made with a special application system (Fa. Rüsch®). The stent is produced from silicone with a polyester meshwork and is X-ray shadow giving. The Polyflex® stent includes a stent loader with an insertion tube (Figures 37, 38). Suitable stent dimensions are: diameter: 8-22 mm; length: 2-8 cm.

The most frequently and dangerous complications of anaesthesia (SHFJV) and surgery for patients with airway pathology and stent insertion are listed in Table 5. Bleeding can occur from the underlying pathology or manipulation of the laryngoscope or when tissue is ablated (e.g. by laser). If bleeding originates from friable tissue a significant compromise of ventilation results. Then rapid suction is as necessary as the control of bleeding which reqires a variety of interventions, including epinephrine solution, tamponade with a bronchoscope or balloon-

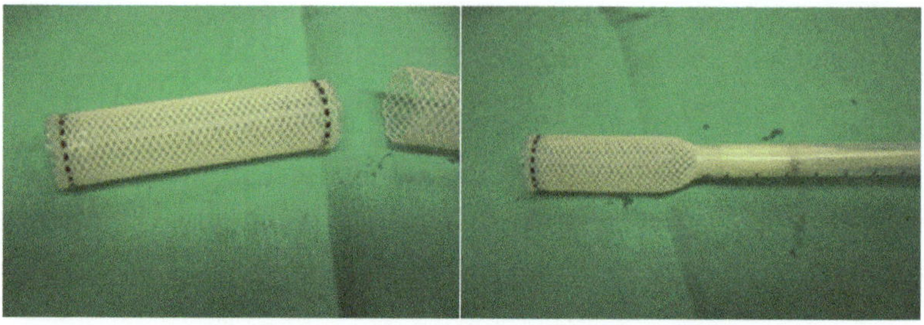

Figure 37. Polyflex®-stent in regular size (left) and after potential expansion with the stent-loader (right). The stent loader can be placed through each jet laryngoscope.

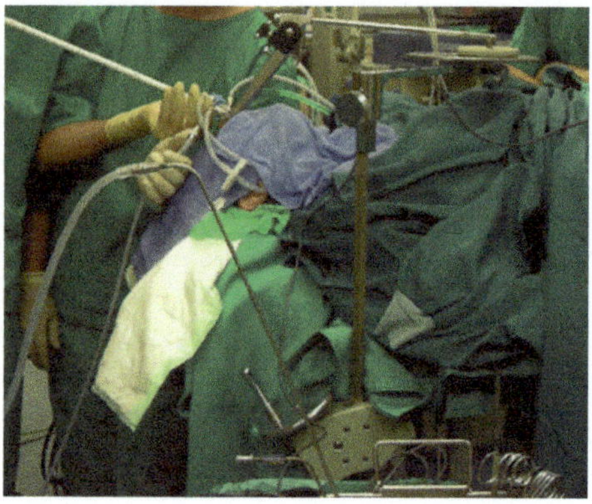

Figure 38. Application of a Polyflex® stent with a stent loader under superimposed jet ventilation. The patient is ventilated continuously by the jet laryngoscope. The stent loader can be adapted and placed into the trachea passing the jet laryngoscope.

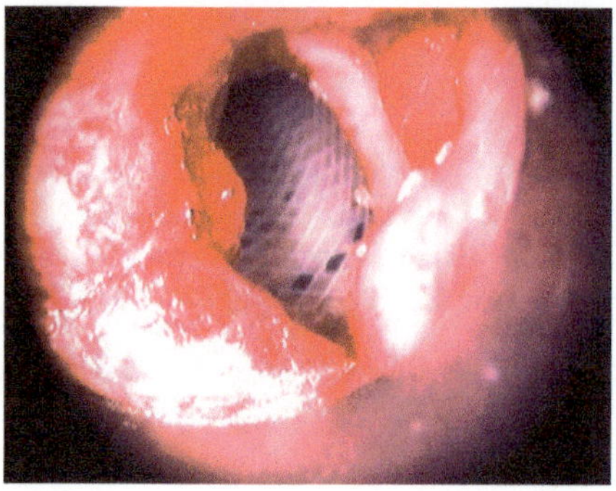

Figure 39. Tracheal stent (Polyflex®-stent) in the trachea.

tipped catheter. Pieces of necrotic or fragmentary tissue as well as clots from bleeding can block the distal airway. SHFJF is not be to be interrupted when they are removed. Airway perforation can be caused by the manipulation at the walls of the trachea or bronchii when the stent is inserted, a subcutaneous emphysema results. An injury of the inner larynx, especially the vocal chords, happens prevalently when difficulties of insertion of the laryngosope tube occur and is rarely severe.

A barotauma occurs suddenly when a mass causes a ball-valve effect or in a distal airway the route of air exit is blocked by a mass and the air pushed behind causes a tension pneumothorax. Typical signs are absence of chest excursion, sudden tachycardia and hypotension. A rapid decompression to prevent a cardiavascular collapse is essential.

The occurrence of inadequate oxygenation and ventilation are always to be observed and this is best to be done by strictly attention to a loud pulsoxymeter which allows quickly an adequate reaction and correction.

Complications of tracheobronchial stent insertion	
Acute complications	**Long-term complications**
Bleeding	Displacement of the stent
Occlusion	Granulation tissue
Perforation	Mucosa impaction of the stent
Vocal chord injury	Oesophagotracheal fistula
Subcutaneous emphysema	
Pneumothorax	
Hypoxaemia	
Hypercapnia	

Table 5. Complications of tracheobronchial stent insertion.

The application of the described stents like silicone stents, wall stents and Polyflex® stents via the jet laryngoscope enables the surgeon due to the excellent field conditions a fast and safe intervention (Figure 39). The anaesthesiologist takes care of an unproblematic ventilation. A ventilation caused barotrauma under supraglottic jet ventilation did not occur in any case at our department. Inside the jet laryngoscope a continuous ventilation pressure measurement with pressure limitation under connection to the respirator is conducted.

9. High-frequency ventilation techniques in adult respiratory distress syndrom (ARDS)

The high frequency ventilation is characterized as a type of artificial respiration where low tidal volume is applicated with a hyper-physiological frequency. Different types of high-frequency jet ventilations were developed and used in the last 30 years [110]. From the numerous potential applicable types of high-frequency ventilations like High-Frequency-Pulsation (HFP), Forced Diffusion Ventilation (FDV) [111, 112] and High Frequency Jet Ventilator (HFJV) only the High Frequency Positive Pressure Ventilation (HFPP), the High Frequency Jet Ventilation (HFJ), the High Frequency Oscillation (HFO) and combined high-frequency ventilation techniques became widely accepted and are used in clinical field (Table 7).

9.1. Theoretical advantages of the high-frequency ventilation

From the aspect of a lung protective ventilation with the option to reduce the end-inspiratory lung volume the risk of ventilation-induced damage of lungs [113] when conventional ventilation is performed should be reduced by the high- frequency ventilation.

However higher end-exspiratory lung volumes can be applied [114]. Simultaneously these tidal volumes are transferred with only marginally pressure variations at a higher frequency and thus the average airway pressure is to be kept at a higher level as it is in conventional ventilation. The high average airway pressure seems to optimize the end-exspiratory lung volume and is protective against the periodic collapse and therefore also avoiding an atalectatic trauma. The perfect mode of application of high-frequency ventilation should permit lung recruitment manoeuvre and thereby shifting the lung under optimizing of the compliance and oxygenation to the exspiratory arm of the pressure/volume relationship. The opened lung is ventilated then with small-sized tidal volumes and slight fluctuation of pressure. This results also in a diminished alveolar distension and a reduced collapse of alveolar tissue. In an experimental laboratory animal study the high-frequency oscillation shows in comparison to a lung protective conventional ventilation an attenuation of activation of alveolar macrophages and neutrophils in lung injury [115].

Clinical indications for high frequency ventilation
Bronchopulmonary fistula
All types of pulmonary reduction of ventilation with no improvement under conventional ventilation therapy
Atalectasis
Pneumonia
Acute lung insuffiency (ALI)
Adult respiratory distress syndrome (ARDS)
Inhalation injury

Table 6. Clinical indications for high-frequency ventilation in adult distress syndrom (ARDS).

9.2. High-frequency oscillatory ventilation (HFO)

Lunkenheimer and co-workers observed already 1994 [116] that normocapnea can be achieved when small gas volumes rates are applicated into the airway of animals with a ventilation frequency of more than 40 Hertz. Using a piston pump sinus-like variations of pressure are

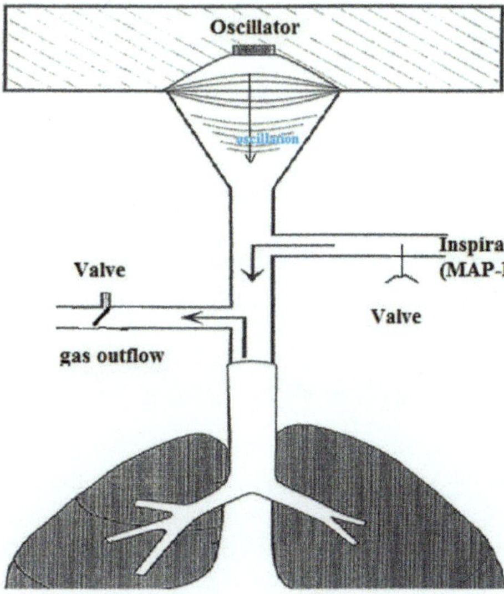

Figure 40. A piston pump puts an oscillation membrane in vibration.

produced and directed to into the lungs (Figure 40). An auxiliary flow of gas (bias-flow) crosses the oscillating gas flow to provide fresh gases. This was followed by the application and further developments of the high frequency oscillation with numerous clinical applications. Although the high frequency oscillation has established in paediatrics it could not be implemented in adults with ARDS because of limited elimination of CO_2. With the improvement of the technical devices this problem of CO_2 elimination could be resolved.

High-frequency oscillation differs from high-frequency jet ventilation by the fact that in addition to the inspiration the expiration is also active, the tidal volume is less.

The frequencies could be higher, however, they are today similar to the jet ventilation usually under 10 Hz. Recently the interest in the high-frequency oscillation has risen again especially for the acute respiratory distress syndrome. The high-frequency pressure oscillations allow the use of a high mean airway pressure to achieve a recruitment of atalectalic lung tissue. At the same time the high mean airway pressure prevents a collapse of lung tissue and high peak airway pressure during inspiration can be avoided.

Different mechanisms of gas transport have been described, like: direct alveolar ventilation in the lung units situated near the airway opening, bulk convective mixing in the conducting convective transport of gases as a result of the asymmetry between inspiratory and expiratory velocity profiles, longitudinal dispersion caused by the interaction between axial velocities and radial transports due to turbulent eddies, molecular diffusion near the alveolo-capillary membrane [117].

9.3. Parameters to be adjusted on the apparatus for high frequency oscillatory ventilation (Figure 41)

Oscillations frequency

3-15 f = Hz

Inspiratory time (I:E) of the pulsation (a single breath cyclus) in %:

33-50%

Mean airway pressure (MAP - Paw = PEEP – post end-expiratory pressure):

3-55 cm H2O

Oscillation pressure –amplitude –delta P:

up to 10 cm H2O

Bias flow:

0-60L/min

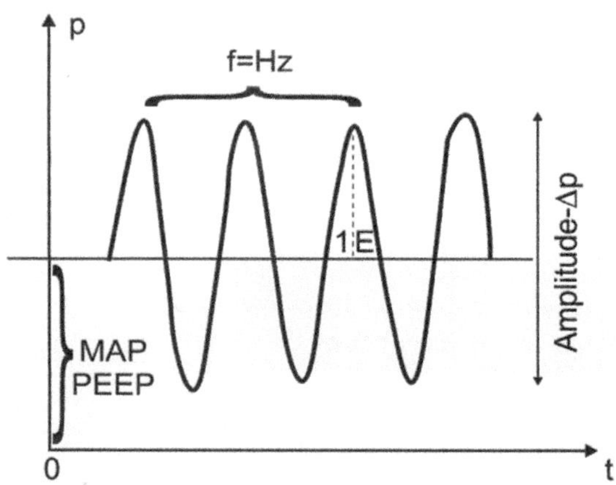

Figure 41. Parameters to be adjusted on the apparatus for high-frequency oscillatory ventilation.

9.4. Combined high-frequency ventilation (CHFJV)

At the first time in 1983 El-Baz et al. introduced the Combined High Frequency Ventilation Technique [118]. Two types of high-frequency ventilation (HFPPV and HFO) were combined.

At a basic frequency of 60 breaths per minute high-frequent gas pulses up to 3000 were superimposed. Further developments combined different types of high frequency ventilation.

The application of an additive, mostly conventional breath with an enlarged tidal volume enables the enhancement of CO_2 elimination. A disadvantage is the usually need of combination of two devices.

Author	Frequency (LF/HF)	Mode (Combination)
El Baz et al. [118]	60/3000	HFPPV HFO
Yeston et al. [119]	2/250	IMV HFO
Keszler et al. [120]	5-7/200	IMV HFJV
Boynton et al. [121]	5-10/1200	IMV HFO
Barzilay et al. [122]	1-5/130-170	IMV HFPPV
Borg et al. [123]	15-20/900-1200	PCV HFO
Jousela et al. [124]	15/360	CMV HFV

Table 7. Authors and their use of combinations of predominately conventional types of ventilation with different high-frequency ventilation techniques. HFPPP… High-Frequency Positive Pressure Ventilation; HFO… High-Frequency Oscillation; IMV… (Intermittend mandatory Ventilation); HFJV… High- Frequency Jet Ventilation; PCV… (Pressure Controlled Ventilation); CMV… (Controlled Mechanical Ventilation); HFV… (High-Frequency Ventilation).

9.5. High-frequency percussive ventilation

Can be considered as a special type of the combined high-frequency ventilation. The high-frequency jet pulse produced by the respirator are superimposed by a apparently conventional pressure controlled higher pressure plateau. A pulsatile jet ventilation with two different high pressure plateaus is generated by only one respirator (Figure 42).

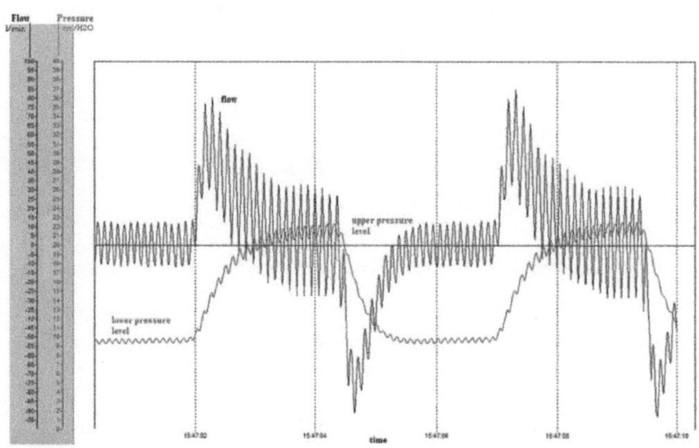

Figure 42. Characteristics of pressure and flow during ventilation with the VDR-4 ventilator. Peak airway pressure: 21 cm/H2O; PEEP: 9 cm/H2O; low-frequency: 12 cycles/min; high-frequency 500 cycles/min; inspiration:exspiration ratio = 1:2.

Phasitron® (Percussionaire® Corporation, Sandpoint, Idaho, USA)

The gas delivered by the respirator is first transmitted to the so-called Phasitron® (Figure 43) where its augmentation of volume, humidification and warming takes place.

The mobile Venturi-body in the Phasitron® is moved forward in the inspiratory phase. This causes a closure of the expiratory aperture and now warmed-up and moisturized air is sucked in by the jet effect.

This prepared column of air lying in front of the Phasitron® is now applied to the lung according to the jet frequency.

a)

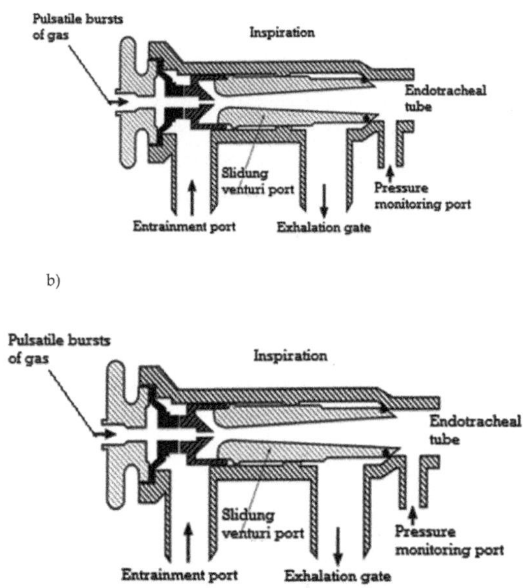

Figure 43. Phasitron®: movement of the Venturi-body during a) inspiration an b) exspiration. During the inspiration moistened and warmed air is drawn in by the entrainment port. During the exspiration the entrainment port is closed.

9.6. Clinical experiences with high-frequency ventilation

9.6.1. High-frequency oscillatory ventilation

The high-frequency oscillatory ventilation is recently moved in the centre of interest especially for application at the acute lung failure [125]. However bronchopulmonal fistulas are indications for this method [126] and from the theoretical point of view for all purposes of lung protection. Without controversy high-frequency oscillatory ventilation is applied in paediatric intensive care since a longer period and has become a routine method.

The best references for their indicated application at ARDS results from two prospective studies [127, 128] and a retrospective clinical trial with application of high-frequency oscillation in combination with a recruitment manoeuvre [129], all showing significantly increase of oxygenation in comparison to conventional ventilation.

9.6.2. Combined high-frequency jet ventilation (CHFJV)

The use of the conventional part of ventilation with low ventilation frequencies with conventional PEEP but higher volume tides guarantees a sufficient CO_2 elimination.

A high-frequent ventilation mode superimposes the conventional mode. Predominantly the oxygenation is enhanced by the high-frequent pulsatile fraction of ventilation.

9.6.3. High-frequency percussive ventilation

In literature concerning the implementation of the high-frequency percussive ventilation in patients with acute lung failure was reduced over a long period to paediatric and adult. More descriptions exist about successful application in patients with ARDS, after inhalation trauma and taumata [130]. In paediatric patient polpulation with an inhalation trauma a lower rate of infection and mortality could be observed. Surprisingly a greater extent of departments apply the high-frequency percussive ventilation in clinical use even though they do not publizise their results.

9.6.4. High-frequency jet ventilation

The high-frequency jet ventilation has become widely accepted in operative interventions in the larynx and trachea. Optimal working conditions with best view for the surgeons are achieved under the application of thin jet catheter and the absence of an endotracheal tube.

Application of high-frequency ventilation in intensive care units in premature patients with respiratory distress syndrome and interstitial pulmonary emphysema is a safe procedure and dimishes peak pressures. In relation to the outcome and mortality from the high-frequenecy jet ventilation did not derive a benefit in comparison to conventional ventilation.

The exclusive application of high-frequency jet ventilation in adults did not prevail. Usually is is applicated as combined high-frequency jet ventilation in cases when the conventional ventilation fails. The literature refers only about case reports or not randomized trials with few cases. However it demonstrates that these ventilation techniques are in use, although expensive, safe in application with a high potential to increase the oxygenation.

9.6.5. Superimposed high-frequency jet-ventilation (SHFJV)

SHFJV is a special type of combined high-frequency ventilation. A respirator produces a low-frequent jet ventilation with a higher pressure level. Simultaneously a superposition with a high-frequent jet ventilation takes place which ensures for itself alone a lower plateau of pressure analogous a positive end-expiraratory pressure (PEEP). Only one respirator generates these two plateaus of pressure. This ventilation technique is primarily used in the operative area of otorinolaryngology, but this Ventilation can be applied also due to ventilation technique of the respirator in the intensive care unit. So we could show in a clinical study [131] that this ventilation technique can lead to a quicker recruitment of the lungs in patients with a respiratory insuffiency. However, further studies are necessary to make more precise and definitive statements.

9.6.6. Potential effects of high-frequent ventilation techniques

First clinical results show that under high-frequency ventilation potentially a fast recruitment of dependent areas of the lung occurs without a simultaneous massive overexpansion of non-dependent areas of the lungs. It is conceivable that the under high-frequency ventilation observed enhanced gas exchange is not so much to be explained by mechanism of increasing diffusion but by pulsatile mechanism leading to a fast recruitment of lung tissue.

Acknowledgements

The authors thank Mr. Heinrich Reiner from the Carl Reiner Corp. in Vienna, Austria, for his understandingful and dynamic help in implementation and propagation of our jet ventilation program at the Medical University of Vienna. Mr. Reiner supported not only the clinical and practical issues but also the scientific ones.

Author details

Alexander Aloy[1*] and Matthaeus Grasl[2]

*Address all correspondence to: alexander@aloy.co.at, matthaeus.grasl@meduniwien.ac.at

1 Department of Anaesthesia and General Intensive Care Medicine, Vienna, Austria

2 Department of Otorhinolaryngology, Head & Neck Surgery, Vienna, Austria

This chapter deals with the history of laryngoscopy and the fruitful scientific and clinical collaboration of anaesthesiologists and laryngologists in development and application of jet ventilation for surgical laryngotracheal interventions via a rigid laryngoscope.

References

[1] Bozzini, Ph. Der Lichtleiter oder die Beschreibung einer einfachen Vorrichtung innerer Höhlen und Zwischenräume des lebenden animalischen Körpers. Weimar: Verlag des Industrie Compoir; (1807).

[2] Mende, L. Von der Bewegung der Stimmritze beym Athemholen; eine neue Entdeckung; mit beygefügten Bemerkungen über den Nutzen und die Verrichtung des Kehldeckels. Greifswald; (1916).

[3] Mackenzie, M. The Use of the Laryngoscope in Diseases of the Throat. Philadelphia: Lindsay and Blaciston; (1865).

[4] Babington, B. Report of the Huntarian Society. The London Medical Gazette. (1829); 3:565.

[5] Garcia, M. Observations on the Human Voice. Proceedings of the Royal Society of London, (1855);7:397-410.

[6] Türk, L. Kehlkopfspiegel und die Methode seines Gebrauchs. Z Ges Ärzte zu Wien. (1858);26:401-409.

[7] Helmholtz von H. Beschreibung eines Augenspiegls zur Untersuchung der Netzhaut im lebenden Auge; Berlin.. Translation in Arch Ophthalmol. (1951);46:565-583.

[8] Czermak JN. Über den Kehlkopfspiegel. Wiener Med Wschr. (1858);8:196-198.

[9] Oertel MJ. Das Laryngo-stroboskop und die laryngostroboskopische Untersuchung. Arch Laryngorhinologie. (1985);3:1-16.

[10] Morton W. Remarks on the Proper Mode of Admininstering Sulfuric Ether by Inhalation. Dutton and Wentworth; (1847).

[11] Lister J. On the Antiseptic Principle of Surgery. The British Medical Journal (1867); 351:245-260.

[12] Jelinek E. Das Cocain als Anästhetikum für den Phaynx und den Larynx. Wiener Med Wschr. (1934);34:1334-1337 and 1364-1367.

[13] Miller RA. A new laryngoscope. Anaesthesiology. (1941);7:205-206.

[14] Macintosh RR. New Inventions. A new laryngoscope. Lancet. (1943);241:205.

[15] Tobold A. Lehrbuch der Laryngoskopie. Berlin; August Hirschwald Verlag, (1869).

[16] Kirstein, A. Autoskopie des Larynx und der Trachea (Laryngoscopia directa, Euthyskopie, Besichtigung ohne Spiegel). Archiv für Laryngologie und Rhinologie. (1895); 3:156-164.

[17] Kollofrath O. Entfernung eines Knochenstücks aus dem rechten Bronchus auf natürlichem Wege und unter Anwendung der directen Laryngoskopie. Münch Med Wschr. (1897);38: 1038-1039.

[18] Killian G. Die Schwebelaryngoscopie. Archiv für Laryngologie und Rhinologie. (1912);26:277-317.

[19] Brünings W. Direct Laryngoscopy: Criteria determinating the appliccability of autoscopy. Direct laryngoscopy, brochoscopy and esophagoscopy. London: Bailliere, Tindall, Cox; (1912);93-95.

[20] Hartmann A. Zur Behandlung der Larynxtuberkulose. In: Hoffmann R (Hrsg) Verh d Vereins dt Laryngologen 1908-1912. Würzburg: Kabitsch; (1913).

[21] Holinger P. A new anterior commissure laryngoscope. Ann Otol Rhinol Laryngol. (1947);56:437-440.

[22] Kleinsasser O. Larynx-Microscope for Early Diagnosis and Differential-Diagnosis for Carcinoma of the Larynx, Pharynx and Oral Cavity. Z Laryng Rhinol. (1961); 40:276-279.

[23] Jako GJ. Laryngoscope for microscopic observation, surgery and photography. The development of an instrument. Arch Otolaryngol (1970);91:196-199.

[24] Strong MS. Microscopic laryngoscopy. A review and appraisal. Laryngoscope. (1970);80:1540-1552.

[25] Weerda H, Pedersen P, Meuret G, Wehmer H, Braune H. A new laryngoscope for endolaryngeal microsurgery. A contribution to inject respiration. Arch Otolaryngol. (1979);225:103-106.

[26] Hopkins, HH. The Application of Frequency Response Techniques in Optics. Proceedings of the Physical Society. (1962);79(5): 889-896.

[27] Volhard F. Über die künstliche Beatmung durch Ventilation der Trachea und eine einfache Vorrichtung zur rhytmischen künstlichen Atmung. Münch Med Wschr. (1908);55:209-211.

[28] Meltzer SJ, Auer J. Continuous respiration without respiration movements. J Exp Med. (1909);11:622-625.

[29] Barth L. Thearpeutic use of diffusion breathing in bronchoscopy. Anaesthesist. (1954);3(5) 227-229.

[30] Sanders RD. Two ventilatory attachments for bronchocopes. Del Med J. (1967); 39:170-176.

[31] Gebert E, Deilman M, Pedersen P. Inject-ventilation in brochoscopy. Anaesthesist. (1979);28(8) 378-389.

[32] Lee S. A ventilating laryngoscope for inhalation anaestesia and augmented ventilation during laryngoscopic procedures. Br. J Anaesth. (1972);44(8) 874-878.

[33] Bradley JL, Moyes RN, Parke FW. Modifications of Sanders` techique of ventilation during bronchoscopy. Thorax. (1971);26(1) 112-114.

[34] Lunkenheimer PP, Raffenbeul W, Keller H, Frank I, Dickhut HH, Fuhrmann C. Application of transtracheal pressure oscillations as modification of "diffusion respiration". Br Anaesth. (1972);44(6) 627-633 .

[35] Lunkenheimer PP, Frank I, Ising H, Keller H, Dickhut HH, Fuhrmann C. Intrapulmonal gas exchange during simulated apnea due to transtracheal periodic intrathoracic pressure changes. Anaesthesist (1973);22(5):232-238.

[36] Bohn DJ, Mijasaka K, Marchak BE, Thomson WK, Froese AB, Bryan AC. Ventilation by high-frequency oscillation. J Appl Physiol (1980);48(4) 710-716.

[37] Sjöstrand U. Review of the physiological rationale for and development of high-frequency positive pressure ventilation. Acta Anaesth Scand [Suppl.] (1977);64:7-27.

[38] Sjöstrand U. High-frequency positive pressure ventilation (HFPPV): a review. Crit Care Med (1980);8(6) 345-364.

[39] Smith RB, Lindholm CE, Klain M. Jet ventilation for fiberoptic bronchoscopy under general anaesthesia. Acta Anaesthesiol Scand. (1976);20(2) 111-116.

[40] Babinski M, Smith RB, Klain M. High-frequency jet ventilation for laryngoscopy. Anesthesiology. (1980);52(2) 178-180.

[41] Klain M, Kezler H. High-frequency jet ventilation. Surg Clin North Am. (1985);65(4) 917-930.

[42] Aloy A, Schachner M, Spiss CK, Cancura W. Tube-free translaryngeal superposed jet ventialtion. Anaesthesist. (1990);39(19) 493-498.

[43] Kleinsaser O. Microlaryngoscopy and endolaryngeal microsurgery. Philadelphia: WB Saunders & Co; (1968).

[44] Jako GJ. Laryngoscope for microscopic obeservation, surgery and photography. Arch Otol. (1970);91(2) 196-199.

[45] Strong MS. Microscopic laryngoscopy. A review and appraisal. Laryngoscope. (1970);80(10) 1540-1552.

[46] Weerda H, Pedersen P, Meuret G, Wehmer H, Braune H. A new laryngoscope for endolaryngeal microsurgery. A contribution to inject respiration. Arch Otolaryngol. (1979);225:103-106.

[47] Ono J, Saito S. Endoscopic microsurgery of the larynx. Ann Otol Rhinol Laryngol. (1971);80(4) 479-86.

[48] Thomas GK. Suspension apparatus for laryngeal microsurgery. Arch Otolaryngol. (1971);94(3) 258-259.

[49] Steiner W, Ambrosch P. Endoscopic Laser surgery of the upper aerodigestiv tract. With special emphasis on cancer surgery. Stuttgart/New York: Thieme; (1997).

[50] Cohen SR, Thompson JW. Use of botulinum toxin to lateralize true vocal cords: a biochemical method to relieve bilateral abductor vocal cord paralysis. Ann Otol Rhinol Laryngol. (1987);96(4) 534-541.

[51] Aloy A, Schachner M, Cancura W. Tubeless translaryngeal superimposed jet-ventilation. Eur Arch Otorhinolaryngol. (1991);248(8) 475-478.

[52] Ng A, Russell WC, Harvey N, Thompson JP. Comparing methods of administering high frequency jet ventilation in a model of laryngotracheal srenosis. Anesth Analg. (2002);95(3): 764-769.

[53] Aloy A, Schachner M, Spiss CK, Cancura W. Tube-free translaryngeal superimposed jet ventilation. Anaesthesist. (1990);39(10) 493-498.

[54] Kleinsasser Operations Laryngoskop; Zepf. Medical Instruments; Germany Tuttlingen

[55] Aloy A, Schragl E, Neth H, Donner A, Kluwick A. Flow pattern of respiratory gases in superimposed high-frequncy jet ventilation (SHFJV) with the jet laryngoscope. Anaesthesist (1995);44(6) 558-565.

[56] Piquet J. Turbulent Flows: Models and Physics. Berlin-Heidelber-New York: Springer Verlag; (2001).

[57] Halder G. Introduction to chemical engineering thermodynamics. New Dehli: Book Vistas, PHI:learning; (2009).

[58] Winterbone D.E. Advanced Thermodynamics for Engineers; Oxford: Butterworth Heinemann; An imprint of Elsevier Science (2002).

[59] Leiter R, Aliverti A, Priori R, Staun P, Lo Mauro A, Larsson A, Frykholm P. Comparison of superimposed high-frequency jet ventilation with conventional jet ventilation for laryngeal surgery. Br J Anaesth. (2012);108(4):690-698.

[60] Lanzenberger-Schragl E, Donner A, Grasl M, Zimpfer M, AloyA. Superimposed High-Frequency Jet Ventilation for Laryngeal and Tracheal Surgery. Arch Otolaryngol Head Neck Surg. (2000);126:40-44.

[61] Rezaie-Majd A, Bigenzahn W, Denk DM, Burian M, Kornfehl J, Grasl MCh, Ihra G, Aloy A. Superimposed high-frequency jet ventilation (SHFJV) for endoscopic laryngotracheal surgery in more than 1500 patients. Br J Anaesth. (2006);96(5):650-9. Epub 2006 Mar 30.

[62] Nowak A, Langebach R, Klemm E, HellerW. Percutaneous dilational tracheostomy (PDT) and prevention of blood aspiration with superimposed high-frequency jet ventilation (SHFJV) using the tracheotomy-endoscope (TED): results of numerical and experimental simulations. Biomed Tech, Berlin. (2012);57(2):107-111.

[63] Aloy A, Schachner M, Spiss CK, Cancura W. Tube-free translaryngeal superposed jet ventialtion. Anaesthesist. (1990);39(10) 493-498.

[64] Lanzenberger-Schragl E, Donner A, Grasl MC, Zimpfer M, Aloy A. Superimposed high-frequency jet ventilation for laryngeal and tracheal surgery. Arch Otolaryngol Head Neck Surg. (2000);126(1) 40-44.

[65] Rezaie-Majd A, Bigenzahn W, Denk DM, Burian M, Kornfehl J, Grasl MCh, Ihra G, Aloy A. Superimposed high-frequncy jet ventilation (SHFJV) for endoscopic laryngotracheal surgery in more than 1500 patients. Br J Anaesth. (2006);96(5) 650-569.

[66] Jaquet Y, Monnier P, Van Melle G, Ravussin P, Spahn DR, Chollet-Rivier M. Complications of different ventilation strategies in endoscopic laryngeal surgery. A 10-year review. Anaesthesiology. (2006);104(1) 52-59.

[67] Rampii IJ. Anaesthesia for laser surgery. In Miller RD, ed. Miller`s Anesthesia. 7 th ed. Philadelphia: Chruchill Livingston; (2010); p2405-2418.

[68] Wöllmer W, Schade G, Kessler G. Endotracheal tube fires still happen – a short overview. Med Laser Appl. (2010);25(2) 118-25.

[69] Burian K, Höfler H. On microsurgical treatment of vocal cord carcinomas with CO2-laser. Laryngol Rhinol Otol. (1979);58(7) 551-556.

[70] Strong MS. Laser excision o fcarcinoma of the larynx. Laryngoscope. (1975); 85:1286-1289.

[71] Steiner W, Ambrosch P. Laser microsurgery for laryngeal carcinoma. In: Steiner W, Ambrosch P. (ed.) Endoscopic Laser Surgery of the Upper Aerodigestive Tract. New York: Thieme; (2000); p47-82.

[72] Thurnher D, Erovic BM, Frommlet F, Brannath W, Ehrenberger K, Jansen B, Selzer E, Grasl MC. Challenging a dogma--surgery yields superior long-term results for T1a squamous cell carcinoma of the glottic larynx compared to radiotherapy. Eur J Surg Oncol. (2008);34(6) 692-698.

[73] Grasl M.C, Donner A, Schragl E, Aloy A. Tubeless laryngotracheal surgery in infants and children via jet ventilation laryngoscope. Laryngoscope. 1997;107(2) 277-281.

[74] Aloy A, Schachner M, Cancura W. Tubeless translaryngeal superimposed jet ventilation. Eur Arch Otorhinolaryngol. (1991);248(8):475-478.

[75] Ossoff RH, Tucker JA, Werkhaven JA. Neonatal and pediatric microsubglottiscope set. Otol Rhinol Laryngol. (1991);100(4) 325-326.

[76] Bourgain JL, Desruennes E, Fischler M, Ravussin P. Transtracheal high frequency jet ventilation for endoscopic airway surgery: a multicentre study. Br J Anaesth. (2001); 87(6) 870-875.

[77] Ravussin P, Bayer-Berger M, Monnier P, Savary M, Freeman J. Percutaneous transtracheal ventilation for laser endoscopic procedures in infants and small children with laryngeal obstruction: report of two cases. Can J Anaesth. (1987);34(1) 83-86.

[78] Depierraz B, Ravussin P, Brossad E, Monnier P. Percutaneous transtracheal jet ventilation for paediatric endoscopic laser treatment of laryngeal and subglottic lesions. Can J Anaesth. (1994);41(12) 1200-1207.

[79] Ross-Anderson D.J, Ferguson C, Patel A. Transtracheal jet ventilation in 50 patients with severe airway compromise and stridor. Br J Anaesth. (2011);106(1) 140-144.

[80] Grasl M.C, Donner A, Schragl E, Aloy A (1997) Tubeless laryngotracheal surgery in infants and children via jet ventilation laryngoscope. Laryngoscope. (1997);107(2) 277-281.

[81] Mausser G, Friedrich G, Schwarz G. Airway mangement and anesthesia in neonates, infants and children during endolaryngotracheal surgery. Paediatr Anaesth. (2007); 17(10) 942-947.

[82] Ihra G, Hieber C, Adel S, Kashanipour A, Aloy A. Tubeless combined high-frequency jet ventilation for laryngotracheal laser surgery in paediatric anaesthesia. Acta Anaesthesiol Scand. (2000);44(4) 475-479.

[83] Tan SS, Dhara SS, Sim CK. Removal of a laryngeal foreign body using high frequency jet ventilation. Anasthesia. (1991);46(9) 741-3.

[84] Derkay CS, Faust RA. Recurrent respiratory papillomatosis. In: Flint PW, Haughey BH, Lund VJ, et al. eds. Cummings Otolaryngology: Head & Neck Surgery. 5 th ed. Philadelphia: Mosby; (2010); p2884-2885.

[85] Derkay CS. Recurrent respiratory papillomatosis. Laryngoscope. (2001);111(1) 57-69.

[86] Weisberger EC, Miner JD. Apneic anaesthesia for improved endoscopic removal of laryngeal papillomata. Laryngoscope. (1988);98(7) 693-697.

[87] Drenger B, Zidenbaum M, Reifen E, Leitersdorf E. Severe upper airway obstruction and difficult intubation in cicatricial pemphigoid. Anaesthesia (1986);41(10) 1029-1031.

[88] Hallenborg C, Rowe LD, Gamsu G, Boushev HA, Golden JA. Severe upper airway obstruction caused by bullous pemphigoid: diagnostic usefulness of the flow-volume curve.Otolaryngol Head Neck Surg. (1982);90(1):20-24.

[89] Monniere Ph, editor. Pediatric Airway surgery. Management of laryngotracheal stenosis in infants and children. New York: Springer; (2011).

[90] Schragl E, Donner A, Kashanipour A, Gradwohl I, Ullrich R, Aloy A. Anesthesia in acute respiratory tract obstructions caused by high grade degree laryngeal and tracheobronchial stenosis. Anaesthesiol Intensivmed Notfallmed Schmerzther. (1994); 29(5) 269-277.

[91] Schragl E, Donner A, Grasl MC, Kashanipour A, Aloy A. Beatmung während einer Tracheotomie bei langstreckiger 90% iger laryngealer Stenose mittels superponierter

Hochfrequenz Jet-Ventilation über das Jet-Laryngoskop. Laryngorhinootologie. (1995);74(4) 223-226.

[92] Cotton RT. Management of subglottic stenosis. Otolaryngol Clin North Am (2000); 33(1) 111-130.

[93] Aloy A, Kimla T, Schragl E, Donner A, Grasl M. (1994) Tubeless superimposed high frequency jet ventilation in high grade laryngeal stenosis. Laryngorhinootologie (1994);73(8) 405-411.

[94] Olak J, Rosenberg S. Simple technique for sizing and positioning tracheal stents. Ann Thorac Surg. (2000);70(4) 1389-1390.

[95] Wassermann K, Eckel HE, Michel O, Mueller RP. Emergency stenting of malignant obstruction of the upper airways: long-term follow-up with two types of silicone prosteses. Ann Otol Rhinol Laryngol (1998);107(2) 149-154.

[96] Saito Y, Imamura H. Airway stenting. Surg Today (2005);35(4) 265-270.

[97] Wood DE. Airway stenting. Chest Surg Clin N Am (2001);11(4) 841–860.

[98] Shin JH. Interventional management of tracheobronchial strctures. World Journal of Radiology. (2010);2(8) 323-328.

[99] Bourgain JL, Desruennes E, Fischler M, Ravussin.Transtracheal high frequency jet ventilation for endoscopic airway surgery: a multcenter study. Br J Anaesth (2001); 87(6) 870-875.

[100] Aloy A, Donner A, Strasser K, Klepetko W, Schragl E, Taslimi R, Rotheneder E, Kashanipour A. Jet ventilation superimposed on a special jet laryngoscope for endoluminal stent insertion in the tracheobronchial system. Anaesthesist. (1994);43(4) 262-269.

[101] Eckel HE, Berendes Sh, Damm M, Klusmann JP, Wassermann K. Suspension laryngoscopy for endotracheal stenting. Laryngoscope (2003);113(1) 11-15.

[102] Baraka AS, Siddik SS, Taha SK, Jalbout MI, Massouh FM. Low frequency jet ventilation for stent insertion in a patient with tracheal stenosis. Can J Anaesth (2001);48(7) 701-704.

[103] Brodsky JB. Anesthesia for pulmonary stent insertion. Curr Opin Anaesthesiol. (2003);16(1) 65-67.

[104] Klepetko W, Müller MR, Grimm M, Aloy A, Kashanipour A, Wisser W, Eckersberger F, Wolner E. doluminale Schienung (Stenting) bei Stenosen des Tracheobronchialsystems. Acta Chirurgica Austriaca. (1991);23(3)124-129 .

[105] Choudhury M, Saxena N. Total intravenous anaesthesia for tracheobronchial stenting in children. Anaesth Intensive Care (2002);30(3) 376-379.

[106] Wassermann K, Eckel HE, Michel O, Mueller RP. Emergency stenting of malignant obstruction of the upper airways: long-term follow-up with two types of silicone prostheses. J Thorac Cardiovasc Surg (1996);112(4) 859-66.

[107] Ernst A, Majid A, Feller-Kopman D, Guerrero J, Boisele P, Loring SH, O`Donnel C, Decamp M, Herth FJ, Gangadharan S, Ashiku S. Airway stabilisation with silicone stents for treating adult tracheoronchomalacies. Chest (2007);132(2) 609-916.

[108] Montgomery WW. T-tube tracheal stent. Arch Otolaryngol (1965);82(5) 320-321.

[109] Grillo HC. Surgery of the trachea and bronchi. London: B.C. Decker Inc.; (2004).

[110] Froese AB, Bryan AC, High frequency ventilation. Am Rev Respir Dis (1987);135(6) 1363-1374.

[111] Baum M, Benzer H, Geyer A, Haider W, Mutz N, Forced diffusion ventilation (FDV). Bases and clinical application. Anaesthesist. (1980);29(11) 586-591.

[112] Baum M, Benzer H, Mutz N, Pauser G, Tonczar L. Inversed ratio ventilation (FDV). Role of the respiratory time ratio in artifcial respiration in ARDS. Anaesthesist (1980); 29(11) 592-596.

[113] Slutsky AS, Drazen JM, Ventilation with small tidal volumes. N Engl J Med (2002); 347(9) 630-631.

[114] Krishnan JA, Brower RG. High-frequency ventilation for acute lung injury and ARDS. Chest (2000);118(3) 795-807.

[115] Shimaoku M, Fujino Y, Taenaka N, Hiroi T, Kiyono H, Yoshiya II. High frequency oscillatory ventilation attenuates the activation of alveolar macrophages and neutrophils in lung injury. Crit Care (1998);2(1) 35-39.

[116] Lunkenheimer PP, Redmann K, Krebs S, Gleich C, Brasselet M, Scheld HH. Ventilation by high frequency oscillations in adults. An experimental study of conditions and methods.Can Anesthesiol (1994);42(3): 303-314.

[117] Chang HK. Mechanisms of gas transport during ventilation by high-frequency oscillation J.App.Physiol. (1984) 56(3):553-563.

[118] El-Baz N, Penfield Faber L, Doolas A. Combined high-frequency ventilation for management of terminal respiratory failure: a new technique. Anesth Analg. (1983);62(1) 39-49.

[119] Yeston NS, Grasberger RC, McCormick JR. Severe combined respiratory and myocardial failure treated with high-frequency jet ventilation. Crit Care Med. (1985);13(3): 208-209.

[120] Keszler M, Donn SM, Spitzer AR. High-frequency jet ventilation in respiratory distress syndrome. J Pediatr. (1991);119(2):340-341.

[121] Boynton BR, Mannino FL, Davis RF, Kopotic RJ, Friederichsen G. Combined high-frequency oscillatory ventilation and intermittent mandatory ventilation in critically ill neonates. J Pediatr. (1984);105(2):297-302.

[122] Barzilay E, Kessler D, Raz R. Superimposed high frequency ventilation with conventional mechanical ventilation. Chest. (1989);95(3):681-682.

[123] Borg UR, Stoklosa JC, Siegel JH, Wiles CE 3rd, Belzberg H, Blevins S, Cotter K, Laghi F, Rivkind A. Prospective evaluation of combined high-frequency ventilation in post-traumatic patients with adult respiratory distress syndrome refractory to optimized conventional ventilatory management. Crit Care Med. (1989);17(11):1129-1142.

[124] Jousela I, Mäkeläinen A, Linko K. The effect of combined high frequency ventilation with and without continuous positive airway pressure in experimental lung injury. Acta Anaesthesiol Scand. (1992);36(6):508-512.

[125] McLuckie A, Editorial II: High-frequency oscillation in acute respiratory distress syndrome (ARDS). Brit J Anaesth (2004);93(3) 322-324.

[126] Ha DV, Johnson D. High frequency oscillatory ventilation in the management of a high output bronchopleural fistula: a case report. Can J of Anesth (2004);51(1) 78-83.

[127] Mehta S, Lapinsky SE, Hallett DC, Merker D, Groll RJ, Cooper AB, MacDonald RJ, Stewart TE. Prospective trial of high-frequency oscillation in adults with acute repiratory distress syndrome. Crit Care Med (2001);29(7) 1360-1369.

[128] Derdak S, Metha S, Steward T, Smith T, Rogers M, Buchmann T, Carlin B, Lowson S, Granton J and the multicenter oscillatory ventilation for acute respiratory distress syndrome TRIAL (MOAT) study investigators. High frequency oscillatory ventilation for acute respiratory distress syndrome in adults. Am J Respir Crit Care Med (2002);166(6) 801-808.

[129] Ferguson ND, Chiche JD, Kacmarek RM, Hallett DC, Metha S, Findlay GP, Granton JT, Slutsky AS, Stewart TE, Combining high-frequency oscillatory ventilation and recruitment maneuvers in adults with early acute respiratory distress syndrome: the treatment with oscillation and an Open Lung Strategy (TOOLS) trial pilot study. Crit Care Med (2005);33(3): 479-486.

[130] Cortiella J, Mlcak R, Herndon D. High frequency percussive ventilation in pediatric patients with inhalation injury. J Burn Care Rehabil (1999);20(3) 232-235.

[131] Kraincuk P, Körmöczi G, Prokop M, Ihra G, Aloy A. Alveolar recruitment of atelectasis under combined high-frequency jet ventilation: a computed tomography study. Intensive Care Med (2003);29:1265-1272.

Chapter 11

Diagnostic and Therapeutic Approaches in Respiratory Endoscopy

R. Peric, M. de Mol, N. van Walree and J.G. Aerts

Additional information is available at the end of the chapter

1. Introduction

The field of respiratory endoscopy has developed over the last decade. Endoscopy is now used for early detection, diagnostic procedures, endoscopic ultrasound and endobronchial interventions. Bronchoscopy is a standard procedure for endoscopists but recently new techniques like autofluoresence bronchoscopy have been introduced. It is not known how these techniques should be incorporated in standard clinical care. Autofluorescence bronchoscopy can be used for detection of premalignant lesions but it is known that the used histological classification does not correlate to biological behaviour. Premalignant lesions may regress or very early abnormal lesions may progress into tumor. Therefore the work up of these lesions is not known. To overcome this problem new techniques are introduced like optical coherence tomography or incorporation of spectroscopy. The value of these techniques for daily practice and research will be reviewed. We will discuss all the presently available techniques and there indications.

Endobronchial ultrasound is a new technique used for staging in lung cancer or diagnostics purposes. This technique offers impressive opportunities for endoscopists to perform minimal invasive staining of the mediastinum and lung lesions adjacent to the bronchus. However the exact role of the endobronchial ultrasound in staging of lung cancer has to be established. Also although quite limited the technique can have complications which should be kept in mind before performing this procedure. The indications and major drawbacks of this technique will be discussed.

Endobronchial interventions have proven to be of mostly palliative value for individual patients. As large randomised trials are lacking, lots of techniques are applied mostly depending on local habits. However from published data some guideline can be given. We will review the main endoscopic interventions and advise which technique to be used in which indication.

2. EUS and EBUS in non-small cell lung cancer

The development of transesophageal endoscopic ultrasound-guided fine needle aspiration (EUS-FNA) and transbronchial ultrasound real time guided needle aspiration (EBUS-TBNA) have drastically altered lung cancer staging algorithms. Both are minimally invasive techniques that enable ultrasound controlled tissue sampling in addition or as an alternative to surgical procedures. Tissue proof of presumed mediastinal spread is mandatory for accurate diagnosis and staging as well as treatment planning. Imaging modalities such as computed tomography (CT), positron emission tomography (PET) provide information regarding size and metabolic activity, respectively, but are not accurate enough to be used in clinical practice. Consequently, tissue diagnosis remains necessary. Mediastinoscopy is considered the standard method for mediastinal lymph node staging, however drawbacks are its invasiveness, requirement for general anesthesia, clinical admission and costs. The role of endosonography is evolving rapidly, the aim of the following is to present the status of E(B)US based on a literature survey.

2.1. EUS-FNA

Linear echo-endoscopes were originally developed for gastrointestinal diseases [1]. In 1995 it became apparent that a considerable part of the middle and posterior mediastinum could be reached and sampled [2] including lymph nodes paratracheal on the left (station 4L), in the aortopulmonary window (station 5), para-aortal (station 6), subcarinally (station 7), lower paraesophageal (station 8), pulmonary ligament (station 9), as well as the left adrenal gland. Levels 2 and 4R are not always accessible. Specific sonographic features of lymph nodes (short axis size >1cm, round shape, distinct margins, homogeneous echogenicity, absent central hilar structure, coagulation necrosis) are more likely to contain metastasis [3] for which EUS has a sensitivity, specificity, positive and negative predictive value of 78%, 71%, 75% and 79% respectively [4]. EUS in combination with FNA however is more accurate, with a pooled sensitivity of 83% and a pooled specificity of 97% [5]. Rapid on site evaluation by a cytopathologist (ROSE) has been shown to improve the diagnostic yield [6], if however on- site cytology isn't available, the optimal number of needle passes needed to obtain an optimal yield is three [7]. EUS-FNA is usually performed in an ambulatory setting under local anaesthesia and conscious sedation using midazolam. The procedure is considered safe as no serious complications have been reported. FNA of a cystic lesion, however, should be avoided due to the risk of mediastinitis [8, 9].

2.2. EBUS-TBNA

Sampling mediastinal lymph nodes through the tracheal carina using a rigid bronchoscope was first described in 1949 [10]. In 1983 Wang reported the use of TBNA for lung cancer staging [11]. The sensitivity varies between 39% and 78% depending on the prevalence of mediastinal metastasis [12]. Despite being an available technique for over 50 years, TBNA has been underused. The main reason for its limited use is the lack of real time needle visualization causing numerous false negative results and complications [13]. Radial endobronchial ultrasound first described in 1992 has been shown to increase the yield of TBNA, however, due to the nature of the probe it does not allow real time needle visualization [14]. Conversely, the linear endobronchial ultrasound developed in 2002 could reach and sample para-tracheal (stations 2 and 4), subcarinal (station 7), hilar and intrapulmonary nodes (stations 10 and 11) [15]. Specific sonographic features of lymph nodes (short axis size >1cm, round shape, distinct margins, homogeneous echogenicity, absent central hilar structure, coagulation necrosis) are more likely to contain metastasis [16] for which EBUS-TBNA has a pooled sensitivity of 88% and a pooled specificity of 100% [17]. Optimal results can be obtained in three aspirations per lymph node. When at least one tissue core aspiration is obtained, two aspirations per lymph node can be acceptable [18]. EBUS-TBNA is generally performed in a ambulatory setting under local anaesthesia and conscious sedation using midazolam. To date, no major complications have been reported.

2.3. Comparison of staging methods

Non-invasive methods such as CT and PET have limited sensitivity (57%) and specificity (82%), with a positive predictive value of only 79% for detection of mediastinal lymph node metastasis [4]. The combination of lymph node size and metabolic activity with PET/CT improves accuracy, but does not eliminate the need for invasive testing [19]. For primary mediastinal lymph node staging, the American College of Chest Physicians (ACCP) and the European Society of Thoracic Surgery (ESTS) consider mediastinoscopy the gold standard with a sensitivity of 78% and a negative predictive value of 88% [20, 21]. Although considered a standard, there are limitations to its diagnostic reach. Stations 5, 6, posterior part of 7, 8 and 9 are not accessible by cervical mediastinoscopy. Further limitations are the requirement for general anesthesia, clinical admission, costs, as well as a reported 2% risk morbidity [22]. Less invasive methods have emerged such as TBNA, EUS-FNA and EBUS-TBNA. TBNA has a variable yield, is a 'blind' technique, and the results depend on the size of the lymph node. In contrast, real-time ultrasound-guided nodal aspiration by EUS or EBUS has a higher sensitivity for mediastinal metastasis. In a comparison of EUS-FNA and mediastinoscopy, both methods are just as accurate (91% versus 90%), but due to their complementary reach, the combination of EUS-FNA and mediastinoscopy detect significantly more patients with lymph node metastasis than either method alone [23]. EUS-FNA prevented 50-70% of scheduled surgical procedures [24, 25]. Furthermore, in combining EUS-FNA and EBUS-TBNA a near complete minimally invasive mediastinal staging can be achieved with a higher sensitivity (93%) and negative predictive value (97%) compared with either method alone [26]. Strategies with an EBUS-TBNA bronchoscope placed first in the airway and then in the oesophagus can be just as useful with a sensitivity of 96% and a negative predictive value of 95% [27]. Finally, a staging strategy combining endosonography and surgical staging compared with surgical staging alone resulted in greater sensitivity (94% versus 79%) for mediastinal metastasis and fewer unnecessary thoracotomies [28]. Cost–minimization models for assessment of mediastinal nodal metastasis demonstrate that the pretest probability of nodal metastasis determines the most cost effective strategy. EUS alone or combined with EBUS is less costly compared with surgical staging [29]. In a strategy using PET, EUS-FNA reduced staging costs by 40% by preventing surgical staging [30]. Given that the sensitivity of EUS-FNA and EBUS-TBNA is similar to that of mediastinoscopy and that endosonography is less invasive, safe, and more cost- effective, endosonography is now regarded as the initial staging procedure of choice and incorporated in guidelines.

2.4. Conclusion

EUS-FNA and EBUS-TBNA enable complete ultrasound controlled mediastinal tissue sampling in addition or as an alternative to surgical procedures and as such have drastically altered lung cancer staging algorithms.

3. Therapeutic bronchoscopy in thoracic malignancies: Endobronchial interventions

In the last decades multiple endobronchial intervention techniques have been developed for the treatment of various pulmonary conditions and regaining airway patency. Especially in patients with pulmonary malignant diseases and significant partial airway obstruction, ensuring an open airway on a short notice is mandatory due to an increased risk of complete obstruction and suffocation. A surgical approach is usually not feasible in these patients, as it is mostly a palliative intervention. Also, significant comorbidities (i.e. COPD, heart failure) often do not permit a surgical approach as such a procedure is accompanied with an increased risk of severe complications. Therefore techniques are required that ensure a patent airway with a minimal risk of complications.

Obstruction of the airways in patients with thoracic malignancies is caused by three mechanisms: 1. endoluminal growth of neoplasms, 2. compression of the airway by a malignant process, and 3. a combination of these two. Interventions in patients are aimed at debulking of tumorous tissue and regaining an open airway. This can be best performed with rigid or flexible bronchoscopy and offers in most cases instant relief for the patient. Beneficial features of flexible bronchoscopy compared to rigid bronchoscopy are the lack of general anaesthesia and the easy access of the distal bronchi and the airways of the upper lobes. However, rigid bronchoscopy enables control of ventilation during the procedure, the removal of large fragments of tumorous tissue and stenting of the affected airways [31]. Examples of the applied techniques during these interventions are laser therapy, diathermia, argon plasma coagulation and the application of endobronchial stents. Application of brachytherapy, cryotherapy and photodynamic therapy are in most cases contraindicated for the treatment of lesions obstructing the airways, since they require time to achieve their effects.

We will discuss the different advantages and disadvantages of each technique and also their indications and contraindications. We will review their use in a palliative setting, but also evaluate their potential as a curative intervention.

3.1. Interventional techniques

3.1.1. Electrocautery

Electrocautery uses an electrical current to achieve its effects. The voltage difference between probe and target tissue generates a flow of electrons. Due to resistance of the target tissue for the electrons, heat is generated which is used for coagulation and tissue necrosis. The extend of the effect of electrocautery on the target tissue depends of several factors [32]. First, the smaller the contact area between probe and tissue, the more the current density is increased and thereby the effect on the tissue. Second, the time the electrons are allowed to flow through the tissue. Longer duration of application results in an increased effect. Third, the wattage or voltage difference between probe and tissue. An increased wattage corresponds with an increased flow of electrons and thus an increased effect. Reduction of the effect of electrocautery is due to the leakage of electrons via fluids and the metallic segments of the bronchoscope.

Compared with the YAG laser, electrocautery combines low costs [33] with easy to use features in daily practice and a lower risk of airway perforation [34]. Contact of the probe with the target tissue results in a similar effect as the YAG laser, although the extent of the effect is different. As with argon plasma coagulation (see below), the electrons do not reach the deeper tissue layers as compared with the photons of the YAG laser and therefore cause superficial necrosis. Due to these properties, electrocautery is very suitable for regaining airway patency in combination with mechanical debulking and stenting.

Since electrocautery causes superficial necrosis, it may be useful for the treatment of endobronchial carcinoma in situ and endoluminal superficial lung cancer [35]. Electrocautery should also be considered for the treatment of granulomatous tissue and various other benign lesions [36, 37].

Complications of electrocautery are endobronchial fires, especially when the fraction of inspired oxygen is more than 0.4 and high wattage settings are used, and perforation of the bronchial wall [34]. Contraindications for electrocautery are the same as for lasertherapy (see below) [32].

3.1.2. Argon plasma coagulation

Argon plasma coagulation allows coagulation without making contact with tissue. It uses ionised argon gas (plasma) to conduct electrons. These electrons do not reach the deeper layers of tissue, in contrast with the scattering photons emitted by the Nd-YAG laser, and thereby cause superficial coagulation/necrosis. A similar effect is achieved by the carbon dioxide laser. Argon plasma coagulation can be used for coagulation, vaporisation and cutting. In patients with airway obstruction by endobronchial tumour growth it should be combined with mechanical debulking. Since its effect is superficial, it minimizes the risk of bleeding in areas of the bronchial tree were major vessels rally just beneath the surface of the airway.

Due to its ability in achieving superficial necrosis, Argon plasma jet coagulation may be used in a curative setting for the treatment of superficial lungcancer [38, 39].

Complications of argon plasma coagulation are the same as with electrocautery. They include endobronchial fires and bronchial wall perforation [40]. Contraindications are comparable with the ones for laser surgery and electrocautery.

3.1.3. Laser resection

Laser resection of endobronchial lesions can be performed using rigid or flexible bronchoscopy. To date, the neodymium- yttrium aluminium garnet (Nd-YAG) laser is the most commonly applied laser. Toty et al were one of the firsts to describe the use of the Nd-YAG laser for patients with tracheal and bronchogenic cancer [41]. Since then several studies have evaluated its role as an instrument to relieve obstruction and achieve haemostasis [42, 43].

During procedures the power setting should be limited to 40 W to prevent complications [31]. The tumorous tissue is first devascularised after which it can be removed. In relatively small lesions a good strategy may be vaporisation of the whole lesion.

In contrast with the Nd-YAG laser the carbon dioxide laser has limited coagulation abilities. Its most important advantage lies in its quality as a precise cutting instrument.

When laser surgery is performed during flexible bronchoscopy, general anaesthesia is in most cases not required.

Advantages of the Nd-YAG laser are its ability to vaporise tissue and its excellence in coagulation. It disadvantages are the increased risk of perforation and the costs [33, 42]. Also localisation of the tumor, especially in the upper bronchi, has a negative influence on the success of the procedure [42].

Complications associated with endobronchial laser surgery are perforation, intraoperative ventilation problems, post and intraoperative bleeding, postoperative infections, fistula formation, endobronchial fire and even death [32, 42].

It is clear that laser therapy offers excellent opportunities for palliative care. Rapid relief of dyspnoea and haemoptysis can be achieved in patients with endobronchial growth of a malignancy. The only contraindication is external compression of the airways. Relative contraindications are coagulopathy and hypoxemia [32]. Laser surgery can also be considered in multiple non-malignant conditions [36]. Examples are stenosis due to trauma, sarcoidosis, radiation therapy, granulation tissue and benign tumors.

3.1.4. Endobronchial stenting

To date, endobronchial and tracheal stent placement is being performed for already multiple decades [44]. In these years various new stents have been developed ranging from bare metal stents to covered metal stents and silicone stents. Due to the high rate of complications associated with the use of bare metal stents, covered metal stents and silicone stents are now being preferred by most interventional pulmonologists [45]. Unfortunately, comparative data of the different stents is lacking. In almost all cases the choice of the applied stent is made by the personal experience of the performing interventional pulmonologist.

Some of the silicone stents, such as the Dumon stent [46], need to be placed by rigid bronchoscopy. This procedure requires general anestheisa. The self-expanding metal stents however, do not require general anaesthesia and can be inserted during flexible bronchoscopy.

Stents are being used for ensuring an open airway in cases with extrinsic compression due to neoplasms or after debulking of endobronchial malignancies. Furthermore, they can be applied to cover malignant fistulas or iatrogenic fistulas after surgery and for fistulas between the oesophagus and trachea.

Complications associated with endobronchial stenting are the increased production of mucoid secretions, migration of the stent, the development of granulation tissue and the increased chance of respiratory tract infections. Applying endobronchial stents is contraindicated if non-viable lung is present beyond the obstruction [45].

4. Conclusion

We summarised the different endobronchial interventional tools for patients with pulmonary malignancy. All the discussed methods have in common that they offer rapid relief of symptoms. Differences exist in the costs and the ease of use of the various methods. Unfortunately, no comparing data is available. Therefore the level of expertise of the interventional pulmonologist with a certain tool, the nature of the lesion and the associated risks should determine which tool to use. When not available and intervention is mandatory, patients should be referred to hospitals in which these procedures are being performed. It is clear that in the group of patients with malignancies, the risk of severe complications exists. Patients should be accordingly informed about these risks with in mind that in some cases time does not permit less radical interventions.

Author details

R. Peric, M. de Mol, N. van Walree and J.G. Aerts

Department of Pulmonary Diseases Erasmus MC Rotterdam and Amphia Hospital Breda, The Netherlands

References

[1] Wiersema MJ, Vilmann P, Giovannini M et al. Endosonography-guided fine-needle aspiration biopsy: diagnostic accuracy and complication assessment. Gastroenterology 1997; 112: 1087-1095

[2] Pedersen BH, Vilmann P, Milman N et al. Endoscopic ultrasonography with guided fine needle aspiration biopsy of a mediastinal mass lesion. Acta Radiol 1995; 36: 326-328

[3] Bhutani MS, Hawes RH, Hoffman BJ. A comparison of the accuracy of echo features during endoscopic ultrasound (EUS) and EUS-guided fine- needle aspiration for diagnosis of malignant lymph node invasion. Gastrointest Endosc 1997; 45: 474-479

[4] Toloza EM, Harpole L, McCrory DC. Noninvasive staging of non-small cell lung cancer: a review of the current evidence. Chest 2003; 123(Suppl): 137S-146S

[5] Micames CG, McCrory DC, Pavey DA et al. Endoscopic ultrasound-guided fine- needle aspiration for non-small cell lung cancer staging: a systematic review and metaanalysis. Chest 2007; 131: 539-548

[6] Tournoy KG, Praet MM, Van Maele G et al. Esophageal endoscopic ultrasound with fine-needle aspiration with an on-site-cytopathologist: high accuracy for the diagnosis of mediastinal lymphadenopathy. Chest 2005; 128(4): 3004-3009

[7] Leblanc JK, Ciaccia D, Al Assi MT et al. Optimal number of EUS-guided fine needle passes needed to obtain a correct diagnosis. Gastrointest Endosc 2004; 59: 475-481

[8] Annema JT, Veselic M, Versteegh MI et al. Mediastinitis caused by EUS-FNA of a bronchogenic cyst. Endoscopy 2003; 35:791-793

[9] Aerts J.G, Kloover J, Los J et al. EUS-FNA of enlarged necrotic lymph nodes may cause infectious mediastinitis. J Thorac Oncol. 2008; 3: 1191-1193

[10] Schieppati E. Mediastinal lymph node puncture through the tracheal carina. Surg Gynecol Obstet 1958; 107: 243-246

[11] Wang KP, Terry PB. Transbronchial needle aspiration in the diagnosis and staging of bronchogenic carcinoma. Am Rev Respir Dis 1983; 127: 344-347

[12] Holty JEC, Kuschner WG, Gould MK. Accuracy of transbronchial needle aspiration for mediastinal staging of non-small cell lung cancer: a meta-analysis. Thorax 2005; 60: 945-955

[13] Haponik EF, Sture D. Underutilization of transbronchial needle aspiration: experience of current pulmonary fellows. Chest 1997; 112: 251-253

[14] Hurter T, Hanrath P. Endobronchial sonography: feasibility and preliminary results. Thorax 1992; 47: 565-567

[15] Yasufuku K, Chiyo M, Sekine Y et al. Real-time endobronchial ultrasound-guided transbronchial needle aspiration of mediastinal and hilar lymph nodes. Chest 2004; 126(1): 122-128

[16] Fujiwara T, Yasufuku K, Nakajima T. et al. The utility of sonographic features during endobronchial ultrasound-guided transbronchial needle aspiration for lymph node staging in patients with lung cancer. Chest 2010; 138(3): 641-647

[17] Adams K, Shah PL, Edmonds L et al. Test performance of endobronchial ultrasound and transbronchial needle aspiration biopsy for mediastinal staging in patients with lung cancer: systematic review and meta-analysis. Thorax 2009; 64: 757-762

[18] Lee HS, Lee GK, Hwangbo B et al. Real-time endobronchial ultrasound-guided transbronchial needle aspiration in mediastinal staging of non-small cell lung cancer. Chest 2008; 134: 368-374

[19] Tournoy KG, Maddens S, Gosselin R et al. Integrated FDG-PET/CT does not make invasive staging of the intrathoracic lymph nodes in non-small cell lung cancer redundant: a prospective study. Thorax 2007; 62: 696-701

[20] Detterbeck FC, Jantz MA, Wallace MB et al. Invasive mediastinal staging of lung cancer: ACCP evidence based clinical practice guidelines (2nd edn). Chest 2007; 132: 202S-220S

[21] De Leyn P, Lardinois D, Van Schil PE et al. ESTS guidelines for preoperative lymph node staging for non-small cell lung cancer. Eur J Cardiothorac Surg 2007; 32:1-8

[22] Hammoud ZT, Anderson RC, Meyers BF et al. The current role of mediastinoscopy in the evaluation of thoracic disease. J Thorac Cardiovasc Surg 1999; 118(5):894-899

[23] Annema JT, Versteegh MI, Veselic M et al. Endoscopic ultrasound added to mediastinoscopy for preoperative staging of patients with lung cancer. JAMA 2005; 294: 931-936

[24] Tournoy KG, De Ryck F, Vanwalleghem LR et al. Endoscopic ultrasound reduces surgical mediastinal staging in lung cancer: a randomized trial. Am J Respir Crit Care Med 2008; 177: 531-535

[25] Annema JT, Versteegh MI, Veselic M et al. Endoscopic ultrasound guided FNA in the diagnosis and staging of lung cancer and its impact on surgical staging. J Clin Oncol 2005; 23: 8357-8361

[26] Wallace MB, Pascual JM, Raimondo M et al. Minimally invasive endoscopic staging of suspected lung cancer. JAMA 2008; 299: 540-546

[27] Herth FJ, Krasnik M, Kahn N et al. Combined endoscopic-endobronchial ultrasound-guided fine-needle aspiration of mediastinal lymph nodes through a single bronchoscope in 150 patients with suspected lung cancer. Chest 2010; 138: 790-794

[28] Annema JT, van Meerbeek JP, Rintoul RC et al. Mediastinoscopy vs endosonography for mediastinal nodal staging of lung cancer: a randomized trial. JAMA 2010; 304: 2245-2252

[29] Harewood GC, Pascual J, Raimondo M et al. Economic analysis of combined endoscopic and endobronchial ultrasound in the evaluation of patients with suspected non-small cell lung cancer. Lung Cancer 2010; 67: 366-371

[30] Kramer H, van Putten JW, Post WJ et al. Oesophageal endoscopic ultrasound with fine needle aspiration improves and simplifies the staging of lung cancer. Thorax 2004; 59: 596-601

[31] Du Rand IA, Barber PV, Goldring J, Lewis RA, Mandal S, Munavvar M, Rintoul RC, Shah PL, Singh S, Slade MG, Woolley A; British Thoracic Society Interventional Bronchoscopy Guideline Group. Britisch Thoracic Society guideline for advanced diagnostic and therapeutic flexible bronchoscopy in adults. Thorax, 2011; 66(3); iii1-21

[32] Bolliger CT, Sutedja TG, Strausz J, Freitag L.Therapeutic bronchoscopy with immediate effect: laser, electrocautery, argon plasma coagulation and stents. Eur Respir J, 2006; 27; 1258-1271

[33] Van boxem T, Muller M, Venmans B, Postmus P, Sutedja T, Nd-YAG laser vs bronchoscopic electrocautery for palliation of symptomatic airway obstruction : A cost-effectiveness study., 1999; 116(4):1108-12

[34] Tremblay A, Marquette C. Endobronchial electrocautery and argon plasma coagulation: A practical approach. Can Respir J, 2004; 11;305- 310

[35] Van Boxem T, Venmans BJ, Schramel FM, et al. Radiographically occult lung cancer treated with fiberoptic bronchoscopic electrocautery: A pilot study of a simple and inexpensive technique. Eur Respir J, 1998; 11; 169-172

[36] Marel M, Pekarek Z, Spasova I, Pafko P, Schutzner J, Betka J, Pospisil R. Management of benign stenoses of the large airways in the university hospital in Prague, Czech republic, in 1998-2003. Respiration, 2005; 72(6); 622-628

[37] Wahidi MM, Unroe MA, Adlakha N, Beyea M, Shofer SL. The use of electrocautery as the primary ablation modality for malignant and benign airway obstruction. J Thorac Oncol, 2011; 6(9); 1516-1520

[38] Sutedja TG, van Boxem AJ, Postmus PE. The curativepotential of intraluminal bronchoscopic treatment forearly-stage non-small-cell lung cancer. Clin Lung Cancer, 2001; 2; 264–270

[39] Mathur PN, Edell E, Sutedja G, Vergnon JM. Treatment of early stage non-small cell lung cancer. American College of Chest Physicians. Chest 2003; 123: Suppl. 1, 176S–180S

[40] Reichle G, Freitag H, kullmann J, Prenzel R, Macha HN, Farin G. Argon plasma coagulation in bronchology: A new method – alternative or complementary? J Bronchol, 2000; 7; 109-117

[41] Toty L, Personne C, Colchen A. Vourc'h G. Bronchoscopic management of tracheal lesions using the neodynium yttrium aluminium garnet laser. Thorax, 1981; 36(3); 175-178

[42] Hujala K, Sipilä J, Grenman R. Endotracheal and bronchial laser surgery in the treatment of malignant and benign lower airway obstructions. Eur Arch Otorhinolaryngol, 2003; 260(4); 219-222

[43] Han CC, Prasetyo D, Wright GM. Endobronchial palliation using Nd:YAG laser is associated with improved survival when combined with multimodal adjuvant treatment. J Thorac Oncol, 2007; 2; 59-64

[44] Montgomery WW. T-tube tracheal stent. Arch otolaryngol, 1965; 82; 320-321

[45] Bolliger CT, Mathur PN, Beamis JF, Becker HD, Cavaliere S, Colt H, Diaz-Jimenez JP, Dumon JF, Edell E, Kovitz KL, Macha HN, Mehta AC, Marel M, Noppen M, Strausz J, Sutedja TG; European Respiratory Society/American Thoracic Society. ERS/ATS statement on interventional pulmonology. European Respiratory Society/American Thoracic Society. Eur Respir J, 2002 Feb; 19(2) ; 356-73

[46] Dumon JF, Cavaliere S, Diaz-Jimenez JP, et al. Seven-year experience with the Dumon prosthesis. J. Bronchol, 1996; 3; 6-10

[47] References by our group related to the subject:

[48] Optical detection of preneoplastic lesions of the central airways. van der Leest C, Amelink A, van Klaveren RJ, Hoogsteden HC, Sterenborg HJ, Aerts JG.

[49] ISRN Oncol. 2012;2012:957835. Epub 2012 Mar 22

[50] Endoscopic ultrasound fine needle aspiration in the diagnosis of lymphoma. Creemers K, van der Heiden O, Los J, van Esser J, Newhall D, Djamin RS, Aerts JG. J Oncol. 2011;2011:785425. Epub 2011 Apr 10.

[51] Characterization of mediastinal lymph node physiology in vivo by optical spectroscopy during endoscopic ultrasound-guided fine needle aspiration. Kanick SC, van der Leest C, Djamin RS, Janssens AM, Hoogsteden HC, Sterenborg HJ, Amelink A, Aerts JG. J Thorac Oncol. 2010 Jul;5(7):981-7.

[52] Integration of single-fiber reflectance spectroscopy into ultrasound-guided endoscopic lung cancer staging of mediastinal lymph nodes. Kanick SC, van der Leest C, Aerts JG, Hoogsteden HC, Kascáková S, Sterenborg HJ, Amelink A. J Biomed Opt. 2010 Jan-Feb;15(1):017004.

[53] EUS-FNA of enlarged necrotic lymph nodes may cause infectious mediastinitis. Aerts JG, Kloover J, Los J, van der Heijden O, Janssens A, Tournoy KG. J Thorac Oncol. 2008 Oct;3(10):1191-3.

[54] Endoscopic ultrasound reduces surgical mediastinal staging in lung cancer: a randomized trial. Tournoy KG, De Ryck F, Vanwalleghem LR, Vermassen F, Praet M,

Aerts JG, Van Maele G, van Meerbeeck JP. Am J Respir Crit Care Med. 2008 Mar 1;177(5):531-5. Epub 2007 Oct 25.

[55] HIF1a expression in bronchial biopsies correlates with tumor microvascular saturation determined using optical spectroscopy. Aerts JG, Amelink A, van der Leest C, Hegmans JP, Hemmes A, den Hamer B, Sterenborg HC, Hoogsteden HC, Lambrecht BN. Lung Cancer. 2007 Sep;57(3):317-21. Epub 2007 May 7.

[56] Optical spectroscopy for the classification of malignant lesions of the bronchial tree. Bard MP, Amelink A, Skurichina M, Noordhoek Hegt V, Duin RP, Sterenborg HJ, Hoogsteden HC, Aerts JG. Chest. 2006 Apr;129(4):995-1001.

[57] Measurement of hypoxia-related parameters in bronchial mucosa by use of optical spectroscopy. Bard MP, Amelink A, Hegt VN, Graveland WJ, Sterenborg HJ, Hoogsteden HC, Aerts JG. Am J Respir Crit Care Med. 2005 May 15;171(10):1178-84.

[58] Improving the specificity of fluorescence bronchoscopy for the analysis of neoplastic lesions of the bronchial tree by combination with optical spectroscopy: preliminary communication.

[59] Bard MP, Amelink A, Skurichina M, den Bakker M, Burgers SA, van Meerbeeck JP, Duin RP, Aerts JG, Hoogsteden HC, Sterenborg HJ. Lung Cancer. 2005 Jan; 47(1): 41-7.

Section 4

Miscellaneous

Chapter 12

Endoscopy in Pregnant Patients

Nurten Akyurek Savas

Additional information is available at the end of the chapter

1. Introduction

Although gastrointestinal endoscopy is generally safe, its safety must be separately analyzed during pregnancy. Though it is prudent to postpone the investigation to the third trimester or rather to the postpartum period; in certain clinical situations where therapeutic intervention is necessary, it offers a relatively safe alternative to radiologic or surgical intervention. There are a number of potential risks associated with endoscopy during pregnancy [1]:

1. Oversedation may cause maternal hypotension and hypoxia, which in turn may lead to fetal hypoxia, with potentially fatal consequences.

2. The fetus may be exposed to potentially teratogenic drugs and radiaton.

3. Care must be taken with maternal positioning to avoid inferior vena caval compression by the pregnant uterus, which can lead to decreased uterine blood flow and fetal hypoxia.

The American Society for Gastrointestinal Endoscopy (ASGE) guidelines [2] list the following general principles guiding endoscopy in pregnancy (Table1).

Fetal risks from endoscopic medications are minimized by avoiding FDA category D drugs, minimizing endoscopic medications, and anesthesiologist attendance at endoscopy. Esophagogastroduedenoscopy (EGD) seems to be relatively safe for the fetus and may be performed when strongly indicated during pregnancy. Flexible sigmoidoscopy during pregnancy also appears to be relatively safe for the fetus and may be performed when strongly indicated. Colonoscopy may be considered in pregnant patients during the second trimester if there is a strong indication. Data on colonoscopy during the other trimesters are limited. Therapeutic endoscopic retrograde cholangiopancreatography (ERCP) seems to be relatively safe during pregnancy and should be performed for strong indications (for example, complicated choledocholithiasis). Endoscopic safety precautions during pregnancy include the performance of endoscopy in hospital by an expert endoscopist and only when strongly indicated, deferral of endoscopy to the second trimester whenever possible, and obstetric consultation.

1	Always have a strong indication, particularly in high-risk pregnancies
2	Defer endoscopy to second trimester whenever possible
3	Use lowest effective dose of sedative medications
4	Whenever possible, use category A or B drugs
5	Minimize procedure time
6	Position pregnant patients in left pelvic tilt or left lateral position to avoid vena cava or aortic compression
7	Presence of fetal heart sounds should be confirmed before sedation is begun and after the endoscopic procedure
8	Obstetric support should be available in the event of a pregnancy-related complication
9	Endoscopy is contraindicated in obstetric complications such as placental abruption, imminent delivery, ruptured membranes, or eclampsia

Table 1. General Principles guiding endoscopy in pregnancy (ASGE)

2. Fetal safety of endoscopic medications

One of the most important point in endoscopic procedures of pregnant patients is to avoid maternal hypoxia and hypotension which can cause placental hypoperfusion and potential fetal injury. Maternal oversedation with resulting hypoventilation or hypotension, or maternal positioning that might lead to inferior vena caval compression by the gravid uterus can lead to decreased uterine blood flow and fetal hypoxia. Other potential risks to the fetus include teratogenesis (both from medication given to the mother and radiation exposure from fluoroscopy) and premature birth [1-6]. To prevent hypoxia and hypotension during the intervention, pregnant patients should be positioned in the left lateral position, prompt intravenous hydration with normal saline or a similarly high osmolar solution should be made, use of analgesics and sedatives should be restricted if possible and in the case of necessity abortion of the endoscopic procedure should be considered [5,6].

Sedation in pregnancy has always been a challenge to anesthesiologists. No anesthetic drug, inhaled anesthetics, or local anesthetic has been proven to be teratogenic in humans. A notable exception is benzodiazepine group, which has been linked to congenital anomalies. All agents that are administered during pregnancy must be used with caution and vigilence. It is clear that anesthetic effects on placental perfusion and the placental transfer of depressant drugs may influence the fetus [5,6,7].

During the endoscopic procedures in pregnant patients, anesthesiologic asistance is recommended in the first and third trimester because of the increaed risk of teratogenecity and the risk of premature labor, respectively [5].

The US Food and Drug Administration (FDA) lists 5 categories of drugs with regard to safety during pregnancy [8] (Table 2).

Category	Risk	Description
A	Controlled studies show no risk	Adequate, well-controlled studies in pregnant women have failed to demonstrate a risk to the fetus in any trimester of pregnancy
B	No evidence of risk in humans	Adequate, well-controlled studies in pregnant women have not shown increased risk of fetal abnormalities despite adverse findings in animals or, in the absence of adequate human studies, animal studies show no fetal risk. The chance of fetal harm is remote, but remains a possibility
C	Risk cannot be ruled out	Adequate, well-controlled human studies are lacking, and animal studies have shown a risk to the fetus or are lacking as well. There is a chance of fetal harm if the drug is administered during pregnancy, but the potential bene fits may outweigh the potential risk
D	Positive evidence of risk	Studies in humans, or investigational or postmarketing data, have demonstrated fetal risk. Nevertheless, potential benefits from the use of the drug may outweigh the potential risk. For example, the drug may be acceptable if needed in a life-threatening situation or for serious disease for which safer drugs cannot be used or are ineffective
X	Contraindicate d in pregnancy	Studies in animals or humans, or investigational or postmarketing reports, have demonstrated positive evidence of fetal abnormalities or risk which clearly outweighs any possible benefit to the patient

Table 2. FDA categorization of drug safety during pregnancy

This categorization indicates general risks based on four components: individual experimental studies on drug risk in laboratory animals, number and quality of experimental studies, individual clinical studies on drug risk in humans, and number and quality of clinical studies. FDA categorization is, nonetheless useful in clinical practice. Category A drugs are safe during pregnancy. Category B drugs may generally be used during pregnancy. Category C drugs may often be used if required during pregnancy. Category D drugs are relatively contraindicated, and when used should be administered with extreme caution. Category X drugs are absolutely contraindicated during pregnancy [8].

There are no category A drugs used for endoscpy. For use during endoscopic procedures category B and, when necessary, category C drugs are recommended. Category D drugs may be used when benefits clearly outweigh the risks. These categories are of limited value for determining the safety of one- time use; therefore, consultation with an obstetrician regarding medication should be considered. For most procedures the level of sedation should be anxiolysis or moderate sedation. If deep sedation is necessary, it should be administered by an anesthesiologist [2].

Key data on safety of commonly used endoscopic medications are summarized in table 3.

Drug	FDA category in pregnancy	key points regarding drug safety
Narcotics		
Meperidine	B, but D at term	Repeated high dose and prolonged administration can cause respiratory depression and seizures.
Fentanyl	C	In low doses it is safe.
Propofol	B	Generally suggested to be used in difficult to sedate and complicated clinical situations.
General anesthetics		
Ketamine	B	Human data is limited; animal data suggests prolonged usage is unsafe.
Sedatives		
Diazepam	D	Some of congenital malformations and mental retardations are possibly associated with diazepam usage so its usage is discouraged during pregnancy.
Midazolam	D	As a benzodiazepine member, its usage is restricted during pregnancy especially in first trimester.
Reversal agents		
Naloxone	B	It is probably safe and should be used only in respiratory depression, systemic hypotension or unresponsiveness in a closely monitored pregnant after endoscopy.
Flumazenil	C	Its fetal risks are largely unknown, it should be given in small doses carefully.

Table 3. Safety of anesthetics commonly used in gastrointestinal endoscopy

Meperidine, an opiate analgesic, was commonly used for gastrointestinal endoscopy in the general population, but has been replaced by short-acting analgesics due to theoretical concerns about toxicity, manifested as respiratory depression and seizures. Meperidine is rapidly transferred across the human placenta after intravenous administration, after that metabolized to normeperidine which has a long half-life. Repeated high dose and prolonged administration of meperidine can cause progressive accumulation of normeperidine, and produce toxic effects of maternal respiratory depression and seizures. Meperidine is rated a category B drug during pregnancy, but rated category D when used for prolonged periods (>36 h) at high doses at term. Meperidine use should be limited to 50–75 mg during routine endoscopy during pregnancy [4,5,9].

Fentanyl is a potent narcotic agonist with a rapid onset of action and a shorter patient recovery time than meperidine. It is an FDA category C drug during pregnancy. It appears safe when given in low doses (<125 mg) in patients undergoing endoscopy during pregnancy [2,4,5].

Benzodiazepines (diazepam and midazolam) are commonly administrated before gastrointestinal endoscopy to reduce anxiety, induce brief amnesia, and produce muscle relaxation. Prolonged use of diazepam during early pregnancy has been associated with cleft palate malformations [4,11] but several large studies have not shown this association [12,13]. Some studies have raised possible associations between diazepam administration and mental retardation or neurologic defects,[14] cardiac defects [11] and Mobius syndrome (sixth and seventh nerve palsies) [15]. Diazepam is rated a category D drug during pregnancy, because of these potential associations its use during pregnancy is discouraged, particularly in the first trimester. Clinical data concerning fetal safety of midazolam are limited; however, the drug has not been associated with oral cleft palates. Administration of midazolam during labor has been reported to transiently depress neonatal neurobehavioral responsiveness [16,17]. Although rated a category D drug, since it has not been reported to be associated with congenital abnormalities, midazolam is the preferred benzodiazepine when meperidine is inadequate. Due to a similar mechanism of action as diazepam, midazolam use should be restricted during pregnancy, especially during the first trimester [1,2,4,5].

Propofol is increasingly used for anesthesia at endoscopy in the general population. It is short –acting with a recovery period much shorter than with standard agents. However, as a result of a relatively narrow therapeutic index (defined as a ratio given by average toxic dose divided by average therapeutic dose) and the potential for respiratory depression which can cause respiratory arrest and even death if improperly monitored, it is generally administrated by anesthesiologists. Endoscopy socities have recommended the usage of this agent for difficult to sedate and complicated clinical situations. Propofol is rated a category B drug and it is considered relatively safe to use during pregnancy, although its safety during the first trimester is inadequately studied [4,5,18].

Ketamine is useful for endoscopy in patients who are expected to experience insufficient sedation from propofol. Like propofol, ketamine has a rapid onset of action and a short duration of effect. Although rated a category B drug during pregnancy, ketamine carries the caveats that fetal safety during the first trimester is unstudied and unknown in humans, and an extremely high dose or prolonged administration of it during pregnancy may be unsafe [4,19].

Naloxone, a rapidly acting narcotic antagonist, crossing the placenta within 2 minutes of intravenous administration, is occasionally administered during endoscopy to reverse narcotic overdose [2,4,20]. The drug is rated a category B drug during pregnancy. It should only be used in respiratory depression, systemic hypotension or unresponsiveness in a closely monitored setting during or after endoscopy. It should be administered during pregnancy in small, graded doses titrated to the desired effect. It should not be routinely administered after endoscopy during pregnancy,since one neonatal fatality has been attributed to its use [21]. Naloxone is contraindicated in pregnant patients who are dependent on narcotics because it can precipitate opiate withdrawal syndrome [22]. Flumazenil, a benzodiazepine antagonist, is used to reverse oversedation from benzodiazepines administered during endoscopy. It is rated a category C drug during pregnancy. The drug should only be used to reverse benzodiazepine overdose during pregnancy because its fetal risks are largely unknown, with only few case reports of use during pregnancy. Flumazenil overdose can cause maternal seizures, particularly when administrated to patients who are chronically habituated to benzodiazepines. This overdose can be prevented by careful and slow titration and administration of minimal dosage of benzodiazepines required for endoscopy. [4,19,20,23].

3. Upper gastrointestinal endoscopy

Although it would be ideal to postpone all endoscopic procedures until after delivery, pregnant patients can develop conditions that require urgent upper endoscopy. The most common indications for EGD in pregnant patients are significant or continued gastrointestinal hemorrhage, dysphagia and refractory nausea and vomiting (Table 4). In a multicenter retrospective study of 83 pregnant women on safety and clinical efficacy of EGD in pregnant patients; endoscopy indications included gastrointestinal bleeding, abdominal pain and vomiting in decreasing order [24]. The Mallory-Weiss tear was an important cause of upper gastrointestinal bleeding in 14% of patients, the peptic ulcer was also responsible for 14% of gastrointestinal bleeding in those patients which is significantly lower than the reported frequencies in non pregnant patients. The diagnostic yield for upper gastrointestinal bleeding was 95% and there was no cases of premature labour or congenital fetal malformation. Labor was not induced in any of the patients and 95% of the patients gave birth to healthy infants. The four fetal deaths in the study were in all high risk patients and were unrelated to EGD. The mean Apgar scores of live born infants were not significantly different than control groups.

In an other study conducted by Debby et al [25], 60 pregnant women underwent EGD for recurrent and intractable nausea and vomiting in their first trimester. In that study only 11 patients had the upper gastrointestinal bleeding, the other majority had only intractable nausea and vomiting. The diagnostic yield of EGD in those patients appeared higher for gastrointestinal bleeding than for intractable vomiting but the difference was not statistically significant. Since the endoscopic findings only minimally changed the clinical management of patients with nausea and vomiting the authors suggested the necessity of EGD for upper gastrointestinal bleeding but not nausea and vomiting or hyperemesis gravidarum. A mailed survey of over 3000 members of the American College of Gastroenterology, which included information over 73 upper endoscopies performed during pregnancy. Endoscopic diagnoses from these procedures included esophagitis, gastritis, ulcers, Mallory-Weis tears and normal findings in descending order. This survey reported no significant complications adversly affecting pregnancy [26].

The relationship between hyperemesis gravidarum and Helicabacter Pylori (H.Pylori) infection is estimated by Bagis et all, in their study, H Pylori infection was histologically demonstrated in 95% of pregnant patients with hyperemesis gravidarum and 50% of control patients. In that study patients with hyperemesis gravidarum had more severe H. Pylori infection compared to controls with H.Pylori infection, as measured histologically by density of bacterial infiltration. Authors suggested the usage of H.Pylori diagnostic tests to be part of hyperemesis gravidarum investigation [27]. Upper gastrointestinal complaints, especially nause and vomiting, are very common in pregnants. During pregnancy with the effect of progesteron and estrogen and with a lesser effect of motilin hormone the lower esophageal sphincter (LES) tone, gastric and intestinal motility decrease, causing gastroesophageal reflux disease (GERD) symptoms. As pregnancy progresses, the frequency of and intensity of GERD symptoms increase which is caused by gastrointestinal motility changes during pregnancy and with a small contribution of physical effects of gravid uterus [28,29]. So as a conclusion endoscopy is rarely helpful and rarely indicated for nausea and vomiting, or even hyperemesis gravidarum, during pregnancy. In the presence of significant upper gastrointestinal bleeding or severe nause and vomiting accompanied by abdominal pain or refractory to medical treatment or signs of gastroduedenal obstruction, EGD may be appropriate to exclude significant peptic ulcer, gastric outlet obstruction or to treat bleeding site. According to the results of studies endoscopically the pregnant women has lower rate of peptic ulcer diseases but higher rate of reflux esophagitis compared to non pregnant patients, and the diagnostic yield of EGD for upper gastrointestinal bleeding during pregnancy is similar to that of EGD performed for the same indication in the general population of about 95% [30].

Acute nonvariceal upper GI bleeding (NVUGB) is a common clinical emergency leading to 50-160 hospitalizations per 100000 adults. Mortality may be as high as 10-14%, although this appears to be decreasing in many countries [31]. Endoscopy for the nonvariceal upper GI bleeding (NVUGB) allows assesment of the risk of rebleeding and enables therapeutic hemostasis that reduces bleeding, the need for surgery, and mortality. The largest analysis of pregnant women for NVUGB is conducted by Geoffrey et al [32] in a population based study including 1210 pregnant women with NVUGB and 6050 nonpregnant women with NVUGB. Mallory-Weis tear was the most common identified cause of NVUGB in pregnant women, in contrast peptic ulcer diesase and gastritis were the predominant etiologies for NVUGB in nonpregnant patients. Pregnant women were less likely to require blood transfusion and were less likely to present with hypovolemic shock compared to nonpregnant women. EGD was performed substantially less frequently in pregnant women compared with nonpregnant women. The proportion of EGD's that led to therapeutic intervention was similar between pregnant and nonpregnant women, 8.9% vs 7.2% respectively. The mean interval from admission to EGD was longer for pregnant women compared with nonpregnant women. There were no in-hospital deaths among pregnant women with NVUGB, the proportions of pregnant and nonpegnant women requiring surgery for upper GI bleeding were not statistically different. Average hospital lenght of stay was shorter among pregnant women compared with nonpregnant women. Although the rates of maternal mortality and fetal loss were well below 1% in both groups, fetal distress/complications were lower in the pregnant group admitted with NVUGB, as was premature delivery. It can be concluded as; it is quite appropriate to defer endoscopy in a significant proportion of cases, who remain hemodynamically stable with self-limited NVUGB.

The indications of endoscopy in pregnacy is shown in table 4 [2].

1	Significant or continued bleeding
2	Severe or refractory nausea and vomiting or abdominal pain
3	Dysphagia or odynophagia
4	Strong suspicion of colon mass
5	Severe diarrhea with negative evaluation
6	Biliary pancreatitis, choledocholithiasis, or cholangitis
7	Biliary or pancreatic ductal injury

Table 4. Indications for endoscopy in pregnancy (ASGE)

4. Therapeutic endoscopy

4.1. Endoscopic hemostasis for variceal bleeding

Patients with cirrhosis are not likely to become pregnant due to endocrine and metabolic imbalances. On the other hand, women with non-cirrhotic portal hypertension have normal fertility rates. The incidence of variceal bleeding during pregnancy may reach up to 45% with a mortality rate of 18-50% The variceal bleeding frequently occurs during the last two trimester of gestation. The possible explanation for the high severity of variceal bleeding in pregnancy seems to be related to the increase in water retention and cardiac output, typical of both pregnancy and cirrhosis. Women with esophageal varices or severe liver disease should be advised, in case of planning the pregnancy, about the high risk of both variceal bleeding and hepatic decompensation during pregnancy. Also patients who have esophageal varices should be informed about the benefits of β-adrenergic receptor antagonist therapy during pregnancy to reduce portal pressure.

Both endoscopic injectional sclerotheraphy (EIS) and endoscopic band ligation (EBL) either prophylactic or urgent seem to be safe procedures during pregnancy. When bleeding is not arrested endoscopically in cirrhotic patients, an emergency transjugular intrahepatic portosystemic shunt (TIPS) is indicated, but data regarding pregnant cirrhotic women are scarce [33-39]. Since there are only a few case reports regarding the treatment options for this clinical condition, the management of esophageal varices and their major life-threatining complication – hemorhage during pregnancy is still under evaluation. In the early 80's EIS was generally accepted as the first line treatment procedure for bleeding esophageal varices. Despite this fact, only few cases of EIS with conventional sclerosants (polidocanol, absolute alchocol, sodium tetradecyl sulphate) were reported during pregnancy [36,38,39]. There are no studies regarding the effect of the conventional sclerosants on the fetus published in the literature, although the procedure is considered safe and effective to control active variceal bleeding. Vasoactive drugs used to achieve hemostasis are contraindicated during pregnancy, since these (vasopressin and terlipressin) may induce labor or fetal malformations [36]. Recently EBL was reported as an effective treatment option for active variceal hemorrhage as well as prophylaxis of this severe complication during pregnancy [36-39].

In early 90's EBL has been proven effective in controlling active hemorrhage and in long term prevention of recurrent bleeding. There are several case reports that describe successful hemostasis without fetal complications [40,41]. When EBL is used there is no risk of migration of a toxic substance to placenta. Studies of EBL versus EST in nonpregnant patients have shown improved reduction in rebleeding and mortality with EBL [40,42]. But there are no studies directly comparing EBL to EST in pregnant patients.

In a study conducted by Aggarwal et al, 17 patients with noncirrhotic portal hypertension caused by extrahepatic portal vein obstruction or portal fibrosis, underwent EIS with either absolute alcohol or sodium tetradecyl sulphate for acute variceal bleeding without complications during pregnancy. In that retrospective analysis pregnancy outcomes included six healthy full-term infants, two preterm deliveries, three stillbirths, one neonatal death, and five voluntary abortions. In that report two patients required EBL after failure of EIS to obliterate esophageal varices [43].

In an another report 10 patients underwent EIS with absolute alcohol, 5 patients for active variceal bleeding and another 5 patients for the profilaxis of variceal bleeding. Hemostasis was achieved in 5 actively variceal bleeding patients. All 10 patients delivered healthy infants [44]. According to the reported studies as in the nonpregnant population, EBL seems to be a reasonable option for acute variceal bleeding as well as for the profilaxis of variceal bleeding. EIS could be a secondary choice for the acute variceal bleeding due to the probable effects on fetal safety.

When the endoscopic and pharmacological theraphy fails; TIPS may be a rescue procedure in pregnant women with recurrent and difficult-to treat variceal bleeding. Several papers confirm the utility and efficacy of TIPS for variceal bleeding unresponsive to endoscopic and pharmacological treatment, however since adequate controlled trials are lacking, it should be limited to a selected group of patients. TIPS placement is associated with radiation exposure of both the patient and the medical staff, it usually requires prolonged fluoroscopy. In the literature there is a few case of TIPS placement in pregnancy in which between 5.2 mSv and 2.1 mGy fetal dose of radiation reported [35,45,46]. So pregnancy is not an absolute contraindication for TIPS placement in the treatment of relapsing bleeding varices and may be a rescue procedure when medical and endoscopic treatments have failed.

4.2. Endoscopic hemostasis for nonvariceal bleeding

Endoscopic hemostatic techniques for nonvariceal bleeding include injection therapy with saline, with adrenaline, sclerosants, thrombin, fibrin, cyanoacrilate, ablative therapy with thermocoagulation, electrocoagulation, photocoagulation, argon plasma coagulation, and mechanical compression with hemoclips, detachable snares, graspers, or sutures [47]. In spite of these numerous techniques, there are a few case reports on fetal safety of endoscopic hemostasis for NVUGB. In those case reports adrenalin injection, thermocoagulation and electrocoagulation was used for hemostasis. In only one of the pregnant patient the hemostatic procedures were unsuccesful so patient required surgery. The fetal outcomes were healthy infants without fetal malformations [24,25,47,48,49].

Adrenalin is category C drug and can cause a decrease in uterine blood flow. Although there is limited data of case reports, no advers events from adrenaline injection were reported, in this case the benefits (cessation of hemorhage, prevention of rebleeding) would seem to outweigh the risks [1,2,29,50].

Amniotic fluid can conduct electrical current to the fetus. During the electrocoagulation the grounding pad should be placed in such a position that the uterus is not between the electrical catheter and grounding pad. Bipolar electrocautery should be used to minimize the risk of 'stray' currents going through the fetus. Electrocautery is relatively safe when used for hemostasis[2]. Due to the limited data on hemostasis for nonvariceal bleeding in pregnant patients, the therapeutic technique choice is based on expert opinion and generally made according to the results of clinical studies of nonpregnant patients.

4.3. Percutaneous endoscopic gastrostomy

During pregnancy, optimal nutrition is essential in order to minimize maternal and neonatal morbidity [51]. Nause and vomiting are seen in 80% of pregnancies but usually symptoms are mild and self limited. In case of severe hyperemesis gravidarum with dehydration and ketonuria, patients should be hospitalized and receive intravenous hydration and anti-emetic agents. When the hospitalization duration prolongs without oral intake then supportive nutrition with enteral feeding or total parenteral nutrition should be considereed [29]. Long term nasogastric feeding is limited by patient intolerability and nasal septal necrosis. Side effects of long term total parental nutrition limit its usage during pregnancy[52]. Thus percutaneous endoscopic gastrostomy (PEG) becomes an important option for long term enteral feeding. However, concerns about uterine damage, fetal injury, premature labor, and infections have restricted the application of PEG tube placement in pregnant women. There were no major complications with PEG tube placement in the several reported cases in the literature [53-61]. PEG enteral nutritional support was provided for an average of 14 weeks in the literature. During the pregnancy PEG tube placement is a feasible procedure for optimal enteral nutrition in the critical care setting. It is also feasible to perform PEG tube placement in the third trimester of pregnancy. A potential problem with PEG during pregnancy is puncture of uterus or fetus instead of the stomach during transabdominal neddle insertion. This risk is reduced by demarcating the upper border of uterus before PEG by abdominal ultrasonography and by inserting the PEG needle ≥5cm cephaled.

PEG tube placement should be reserved only for severe refractory cases where the nutrition of the mother and the fetus is at risk. The pregnant should be informed about the risks of the procedure and potential placental injury. If possible less invasive alternative techniques as nasoenteric feeding tube or peripherally inserted catheter for parenteral nutrition should be attempted if this is not succesful or is refused by the patient, PEG tube placement should be considered.

4.4. Percutaneous endoscopic gastrojejunostomy

Percutaneous endoscopic gastrojejunostomy(PEGJ) is a feeding tube placement in to the jejenum via a gastrostomy. This placement enables food to be delivered more distally to decrease the sensation of nausea, vomiting and risk of aspiration. PEGJ indications are similar to PEG indications with additional risk of aspiration. In case of refractory nause and vomiting in the presence of PEG tube feeding, PEG tube can be converted to PEGJ. There are only few case reports of PEGJ for hyperemesis gravidarum and one patient with coma from massive stroke [62-65]. As in the PEG, PEGJ can be considered in very severe hyperemesis gravidarum refractory to medical treatment and the other noninvasive treatment modalities.

5. Sigmoidoscopy/ colonoscopy

Most pregnant patients are young, healthy women and the gestational period is only 40 weeks in duration, because of that; it is unusual for them to need flexible sigmoidoscopy or colonoscopy during pregnancy. Lower endoscopy should be avoided for weak indications during pregnancy and should be deferred until after the first trimester, or if possible, until the postpartum period [66].

Although flexible sigmoidoscopy will be sufficient for most pregnant women, colonoscopy may be required when there is life-threatening colonic bleeding and when a cause has not been established by sigmoidoscopy. In late pregnancy, patients should not be placed in the decubitus or prone position during colonoscopy. External abdominal pressure should generally be avoided; if pressure is required, it should be minimal and directed away from the uterus.

All avilable evidence suggests that sigmoidoscopy is safe during pregnancy and the indications include rectal bleeding, chronic diarrhea, abdominal pain and rectal pain. Guidelines for colonoscopy in pregnancy are not readily available due to insufficient data, although studies which have been done demonstrate safety and efficacy of the procedure provided that obstetrical consultation and close monitoring take place. Colonoscopy is indicated for suspected colon cancer, uncontrolled severe hemorrhage or when necessary before colonic surgery in pregnant women as well as in general population [67,68].

The safety and efficacy of the flexible sigmoidoscopy during pregnancy has been studied in one case-controlled study of 45 patients undergoing 48 sigmoidoscopies [69]. The most common clinical indication was hematochezia in 29 patients, diarrhea was the indication in 10 patients and abdominal pain was in 4 patients. The most common sigmoidoscopic diagnosis included reactivated or newly diagnosed inflamatory bowel disease, bleeding internal hemorroids and other colitis. Among the 29 patients with hematochezia, 8 patients were de novo diagnosis or flare of ulcerative colitis, 7 patients were de novo diagnosis or flare of Crohn's disease, 3 patients with acute proctosigmoitidis, 2 patients were bleeding internal hemorrhoids, 1 patient was pseudomembraneous colitis, and 1 patient was sigmoid adenoma. Hematochezia gave the highest diagnostic yield compared with the other clinical indications. Excluding one unknown pregnancy outcome and four voluntary abortions, 38 (93%) of 41 pregnant patients who underwent sigmoidoscopy delivered healthy infants, including 27 at term. The mean Apgar score of live-born infants in this study was not statistically different from the mean national Apgar score of live born infants.

Therapeutic changes because of the sigmoidoscopic findings occured in 24 patients, including changing or instituting medication for inflamatory bowel disease in 15 patients, steroid enemas for nonspesific proctitis in two patients, avoiding surgery in two patients, and hemorrhoidal treatment in two patients.

Other than this study there are individual case reports of sigmoidoscopy performed during pregnancy and a mailed survey study [26, 70-74]. Multiple case reports describing flexible sigmoidoscopy in pregnant patients showed the safety of this procedure. In the mailed survey study; after contacting 3300 gastroenterologists, their responses indicated that there were no endoscopic complications in 13 pregnant women who underwent flexible sigmoidoscopy. In addition all pregnancies resulted in healthy infants. Common themes among these reports include a relatively high diagnostic yield of flexible sigmoidoscopy when performed during pregnancy for strong indications, clinically important changes in therapy resulting from sigmoidoscopic diagnosis, a relatively high rate of favorable fetal outcomes, poor fetal outcomes generally occuring only in very sick mothers and unrelated to sigmoidoscopy etiologically or temporally, and a low rate of congenital anomalies.

Studies suggested that sigmoidoscopy during pregnancy does not induce labor or cause congenital malformations, it is not contraindicated, and should be considered in medically stable patients with important indications. Sigmoidoscopy should be performed with maternal monitoring by electrocardiography and pulse oximetry, after obstetrical consultation and after medical stabilization. Medical stabilization may require blood transfusions and supplemental oxygenation [4,66,68]. Sigmoidoscopy is not recommended during pregnancy for indications of a change in bowel habits, abdominal pain, a family history of colon cancer, and routine screening or surveillance. In these cases, sigmoidoscopy is best deferred until at least 6 weeks postpartum [67, 68].

Little is known about the safety or otherwise of bowel cleansing agents during pregnancy. Studies have shown that the systemic absorbtion of Polyethylene glycol is minimal and the problems with abdominal bloating and gas are less common as compared to other laxatives [75] But since polyethylene glycol solutions have not been studied during pregnancy, therefore it is a category C drug during pregnancy. Sodium phosphate solutions (also category C) may cause fluid and electrolyte disturbance, and therefore probably best avoided during pregnancy. Also it was published that newborns were shown to manifest bone demineralization and bone growth failure because of maternal phosphate overload [76], although a one time use in pregnancy has not shown to be detrimental. Another consideration when using phosphosoda preperations is the risk of phosphate nephropathy [77] which has been reported in selected cases. As for bowel preperation for flexible sigmoidoscopy, phosphate enemas should be relatively safe, but have not been studied in pregnancy. Tap water enemas may be sufficient. In a study [78] of the preference of gastroenterologist and obstetricians of bowel cleansing agent for sigmoidoscopy and colonoscopy in the same hospital, it was shown that 50% of gastroenterologist prefer to use polyethylene glycol solutions and 50% avoid use of fleet phosphosoda. Twent percent of obstetricians seem to prefer fleet phosphosoda, and 26% avoid polyethylene glycol solutions which is exact opposite of gastroenterologist. Both groups prefer fleet enema the most (51%), while magnesium citrate is used least often (38%).

6. Colonoscopy

There are insufficient data regarding the safety of performing colonoscopy during pregnancy. The largest case control study of 20 patients [79]; there were 20 pregnant patients undergoing colonoscopy and 20 pregnant controls who were matched for colonoscopy but who did not undergo colonoscopy. Colonoscopy indications in the study patients included diarrhea, hematochezia, bloody diarrhea, abdominal pain, and other reasons. Colonoscopy was performed in the second trimester in the majority of patients (n=16) with only 4 patients undergoing the procedure in the first and third trimester. Colonoscopic diagnoses were; ulcerative colitis, ischemic colitis, Crohns colitis, and lymphocytic colitis. Colonoscopy led to significant therapeutic changes in 7 (35%) patients. Two mothers experienced minor colonoscopic complications of mild, transient hypotension. Study patients had relatively favorable fetal outcomes: 18 relatively healthy infants, 1 involuntary abortion, and 1 infant born with a congenital defect (septum secundum cardiac defect).

In a mailed survey of 3300 gastroenterologists 13 colonoscopies were performed without complications [26]. This study was retrospective, and subject to biases relating to recall and dependence on voluntary reporting. In an other study Cappell and co workers [69] retrospectively examined eight pregnant women undergoing colonoscopies at 10 different medical centers. Excluding one elective abortion and one fetal demise unrelated to the colonoscopy occuring 4 months later, six healthy infants were born. There was no difference in outcomes based on the trimester during which colonoscopy was performed.

There are several case reports about colonoscopy during pregnancy [80-88], fetal outcomes after colonoscopy included 8 healthy babies, 2 stillbirth unrelated to the colonoscopy (in mothers with either metastatic colon cancer or massive lower gastrointestinal hemorrhage requiring emergency colonic surgery), and one unknown fetal outcome.

Given the limited data on its safety and the potential to cause significant adverse events, colonoscopy should be reserved to strong indications or life-threatining emergencies during second trimester. But in case of suspicion of colon cancer, evaluation of colonic mass or colonic stricture of unknown etiology, for severe uncontrolled colonic hemorrhages, for colonic pseudoobstruction when the alternative is surgical decompression and when required before urgent colonic surgery, colonoscopy should be considered even in the first and third trimester. Colonoscopy should generally be deferred in any trimester of pregnancy until after delivery for elective indications, such as surveillance for prior history of colon cancer or colonic polyps.

7. Therapeutic colonoscopy

Therapeutic colonoscopy includes hemostasis of lower gastrointestinal bleeding, colonoscopic polypectomy, and colonic stenting. As mentioned in the hemostasis for NVUGB section,injection therapy with saline, with adrenaline, sclerosants, thrombin, fibrin, cyanoacrilate, ablative therapy with thermocoagulation, electrocoagulation, photocoagulation, argon plasma coagulation, and mechanical compression with hemoclips, detachable snares, graspers, or sutures are used during lower gastrointestinal bleeding [47].

Epinephrine is commonly used to treat gastrointestinal bleeding and achieves hemostasis through its vasoconstrictive effects. There are numerous studies about the fetal safety of epinephrine administration during labor which established its fetal safety so it is commonly added to spinal epidural anesthesia. Although in the report of Briggs and colleagues' [10], there was no congenital defect in 35 infants with first trimester in utero exposure of epinephrine, there is a case report of fatal intracranial hemorrhage in an infant during childbirth after excessive in utero epinephrine [89]. Because of the epinephrine's α adrenergic effect of decreasing uterine blood flow, it is a category C during pregnancy and its dosage should be kept low during pregnancy.

Electrocautery is also another method of providing hemostasis during lower gastrointestinal bleeding, also used for performing polypectomy or hot biopsy. Using electrocautery to lesions may occasionally be required during pregnancy and has been safely performed without detectable advers effcts to fetus. However, because amniotic fluid has been demonstrated to conduct electrical current, externally placed grounding pad should be placed close to the electrical catheter, devices should use bipolar currents. Polyp removal if not bleeding, should be postponed after pregnancy [4, 5, 66].

Colonic tattooing is done with Indian ink and methylene blue in nonpregnant patients. Indian ink has been shown to persist for the entire life of patient. There have ben no reports of long term complications of Indian ink tattooing. Methylene blue tattooing during pregnancy is not been studied but there are reports of examination of Metylene blue during amniocentesis and in detection of ruptured membranes. In these reports fetal death, jejunal atresia, is reported which labels Metylene blue as teratogenic. Although safety of colonic injection is not studied; its usage should be avoided during pregnancy [66, 90, 91].

8. Enteroscopy

Enteroscopy takes a very long time of procedure with a long time of anesthesia. There is no case report of enteroscopy during pregnancy, so the fetal safety of enteroscopy could not be predicted.

9. Video capsule endoscopy

Video capsule endoscopy (VCE) represents a significant advance in the investigation of small bowel diseases. The main indications are obscure gastrointestinal hemorrhages, Crohn's disease, celiac disease, small bowel tumors and polyposis syndromes. The main contraindications are known or suspected gastrointestinal obstruction, strictures, fistulas, cardiac pacemakers and swallowing disorders [92]. During pregnancy the growing gravid uterus pushes and compresses the gastrointestinal tract, and gastrointestinal motility decreases due to inhibition of intestinal smooth muscle by gestational progestin. These effects raise the theoretical concerns regarding capsule impaction during pregnancy [4,93]. Although according to the FDA, pregnancy is a relative contraindication for VCE [92]; there is a report of VCE usage in a young acute bleeding pregnant patient in whom endoscopy and colonoscopy revealed no lesion other than fresh blood exiting the terninal ileum. On VCE an actively bleeding jejunal lesion was shown of which pathology was jejunal carcinoid tumor. Patient and fetus did well after surgery [94]. From this report, it can be concluded that VCE may be considerable during pregnancy for strong indications, it is not absolutely contraindicated during pregnancy. But it is more likely to be incomplete when done during pregnancy because of slowed intestinal transit time during pregnancy.

9.1. Endoscopic retrograde cholangiopancreatography

Pregnancy is associated with an increased risk of gallstone formation. Fortunately, complications due to cholelithiasis, such as cholecystitis, choledocholithiasis and pancreatitis are relatively uncommon and in many cases can be managed conservatively. However occasionally patients develop complications related to gallstones that require intervention during pregnancy. Although there are no precise estimates of the incidence, several reports have found that biliary tract disease (most commonly cholecystitis) represented one of the most frequent indications for non-obstetrical surgery during pregnancy [95-99].

A subset of patients requires ERCP, most commonly for choledocholithiasis or presumed gallstone pancreatitis. Opinions regarding the safety of ERCP during pregnancy differ in various reports, reflecting the relatively limited data. Major concerns surround issues related to radiation exposure to the fetus and the risk of procedure on pregnancy outcome.

A general principle in the care of the women with an acute biliary tract disorder during pregnancy is to provide the most conservative management possible with the hope of delaying intervention until after pregancy or until the second trimester, when surgical intervention is relatively safer. There are numerous reports about ERCP during pregnancy especially for the last ten years.

The largest series in the literature included 65 pregnant patients [100]; the most common indications for ERCP during pregnancy were recurrent biliary colic, abnormal liver function tests, and a dilated bile duct on ultrasound. Sixty eight ERCP was performed on 65 pregnant patients, 17 pregnants were in the first trimester, 20 pregnants were in the second trimester and 31 pregnants were in the third trimester. The median fluoroscopy time was 1.45 minutes. Almost all patients underwent a therapeutic procedure. Post ERCP pancreatitis developed in 11 patients (16%), none of whom had a severe course. Most patients achieved a term pregnancy (89%), there were no fetal deaths, perinatal deaths, or evident congenital malformations. Only 5 babies (8%) were born prematurely or with low birth weight.

Another series of 23 patients included 20 of whom underwent a therapeutic ERCP while three underwent a diagnostic ERCP only [101]. One patient developed post ERCP pancreatitis (after each of her three ERCP). There was one spontaneous abortion and one neonatal death 26 hours after delivery. The neonatal death and post-ERCP pancreatitis were in the same patient who undergone three ERCPs (twice during the first and one during the third trimesters) with pancreatic duct stenting for stenosis of pancretaic orifice after a previous surgical sphincteroplasty.

Shelton et al in a retrospective series of 21 cases of ERCP with sphincterotomy reported successful extraction of stones in 14 women and successful removal of sludge in 7 women. There was one maternal complication of pancreatitis. There were 17 healthy babies delivered at term; One preterm, low birth weight baby, and 3 unknown fetal outcomes [102].

Another series described long term follow up of 18 pregnant women who underwent biliary sphincterotomy for common bile duct stones during pregnancy (first trimester 4, second 6, third 8) [103]. Despite short term complications (one with postsphincterotomy bleedings, one with mild post ERCP pancreatitis and preterm labor), no long term maternal complications were seen after a median of six years (range 1-11 year). Only 11 of the 18 families were retrospectively contacted; all 11 babies were healthy on follow up at a mean of 6 years postpartum. Only one mother had preterm delivery.

Kahaleh et al reported a total of 17 pregnant patients underwent ERCP; of which 15 had radiation dosimetry measured. Mean fluoroscopy time was 14 seconds (1-48seconds), mean estimated fetal radiation exposure was 40mrad (1-180mrad). Complications were reported as; postsphincterotomy bleeding in one patient, which was controlled by placement of hemoclip, and post-ERCP pancreatitis in one patient. All infants delivered had Apgar scores of 8 or greater. Thirteen of 15 patients who delivered were contacted, and they confirmed that their child was in good health. [104].

In an another series of 15 patients, the incidence of complications (7%) was no different than the rate of complications observed in nonpregnant patients. [105]. There were no serious adverse outcomes to the fetus or mother.

Different from the aforementioned reports, Farca et al reported a prospective study ≥10 therapeutic ERCP during pregnancy [106]. In this study a single 10F stent was placed without sphincterotomy, all patients had uncomplicated pregnancies and delivered healthy infants. All underwent ERCP with sphincterotomy and stent extraction postpartum; 8 had stones extracted. In two patients, the single 10F stent remained in place for 7 and 8 months, respectively; no one developed cholangitis.

During the ERCP in pregnancy the perceived risk of radiation exposure is much greater than the actual risk, but a full explanation of these risks to the pregnant patient and her family is more credible if given prior to exposure. Patients should be fully informed, background population risks for miscarriage, congenital anomalies, genetic disease, and the growth restriction are approximately 20, 4, 10 and 10 percent, respectively. Potential radiation exposure risks to the fetus can be divided into four categories: intrauterine fetal death, malformations, disturbance of growth and development, mutagenic and carcinogenic effects.

Ionizing radiation is measured in special units, rad (radiation absorbed dose) and rem (radiation equivalent man) and in the international units, gray (Gy) and sievert (Sv)

(1 rad = 1rem = 0.01Gy = 0.01Sv). The avarage person in United States receives about 360 mrem of ionizing radiation annually, of which about 60 mrem comes from man-made sources, including medical exposures such as diagnostic radiographs. The rem is a unit used to measure the effect of radiation on the human body is referred to as the ' effective dose equivalent'. Fetal radiation exposure can result in developmental abnormalities, particularly if exposure is during the first trimester when organogenesis occurs. High radiation exposure may result in fetal wastage. Although estimates vary, it is recommended that fetal radiation exposure not exceed 100mrem during the first trimester [104].

Data from studies of animals and nuclear bomb survivors suggest that the period of major organogenesis, between the 8th and 15th weeks of gestation, is the most sensitive for growth retardation, which may be observed with exposures of 200-250mrem. Exposures greater than 100mrem occuring later, during neuron development and migration, may be associated with microcephaly, seizures, decline in mental ability, and childhood cancer [107]. During the whole of gestation, the maxium permitted dose of ionizing radiation to the fetus is 500rems [108].

Lead shielding should be used to minimize radiation exposure to the uterus. The lead apron shield must be placed underneath the patient and not draped over the abdomen since the radiation source is underneath the patient when using the standard fluoroscopy C-arm [109]. External shielding can not elimineta fetal exposure due to internally scattered radiation. Even though the fetus can be shielded, efforts should be made to avoid performing ERCP during the first trimester. While harmful effects of radiation exposure are unlikely to develop below a certain threshold of radiation dose, the threshold associated with a risk of childhood cancers such as leucemia is not known precisely.

Though a majority of investigators have reported no immediate complication in newborn, because of low dose radiation exposure, no one has looked 10-20 years after the exposure, from that point; ERCP without fluoroscopy is investigated.

ERCP without fluoroscopy has been reported in some studies [102,111] in the last years. Sharma and Maharshi [110] described a two step procedure with biliary sphincterotomy and stenting without fluoroscopy or ultrasound (US) asistance as a first step and definitive ERCP with stone extraction after delivery. In another series [102] it is described as; endoscopist controls wire –guided cannulation first; then the cannule is not advanced in to the duct unless the endoscopist is confident that the bile duct has been cannulated, as assesssed by the presence of bile flowing around the wire from the papillary orifice. Once biliary cannulation is confirmed, a standard wire-guided biliary sphincterotomy is performed using the papillotome. While the bile is not seen flowing around the guidewire, instead of advancing the catheter to aspirate fluid, a 5F 2 cm stent is inserted over the wire and the drainage from the stent is observed. The color of draining fluid is used to assess whether the stent is in the bile duct or the pancreatic duct. If the stent reveals bile flow, a stent –guided biliary sphincterotomy using a needdle-knife is performed. The stent is removed after biliary sphincterotomy.

Even though the introduction of ERCP without fluoroscopy, ERCP should be avoided for weak indications such as preoperative cholangiography in patients with a low probability of having choledocholithiasis. Women of childbearing age should be asked about the possibility of pregnancy and a pregnancy test should be ordered based on clinical history. Other methods of diagnosis that do not involve radiation should be considered, magnetic resonance cholangiopancreatography (MRCP) can provide diagnostic information for a variety of hepatobiliary conditions while endoscopic ultrasonography (EUS) is highly sensitive and spesific for choledocholithiasis. MRCP for the detection of common bile duct stone and subsequent extraction without using fluoroscopy has been reported in some newly published case reports. In a study conducted by Oto et al [111], the role of MRCP in the evaluation of pregnant patients with acute pancreaticobiliary disease is investigated; 18 pregnant patients underwent MRCP for the indications of right upper quadrant pain, cholangitis, jaundice and pancreatitis. Fifteen of the 18 patients were also evaluated with abdominal US. Biliary dilatation was detected in 8 patients with US, but the cause of biliary dilatation could not be determined by US in 7 patients. MRCP demonstrated the etiology in four of these patients (choledocholithiasis, Mirizzi syndrome, choledochal cysts, and intrahepatic biliary stones) and excluded obstructive pathology in the other four patients. MRCP was unremarkable in the 7 patients who had no biliary dilatation on US. Three patients underwent only MRCP; two had choledocholithiasis, and one had cholelithiasis and pancreatitis. While this study suggests that MRCP may be very helpful diagnostically for acute pancreatobiliary disease in the pregnant population, this study does not give any information about the fetal outcomes, including the incidence of congenital amlformations after MRCP during pregnancy.

So, in the case of choledocholithiasis, biliary pancreatitis, cholangitis and findings of coledochal dilatation on abdomianl US with abnormal serum liver function tests and known gallstones, ERCP with / without fluoroscopy should be made.

9.2. Electrocautery and hemostasis

Using cutting and cauterizing current to lesions may occasioanlly be required during pregnancy and has been safely performed without detectable adverse consequences to the developing fetus. However, because amniotic fluid has been demonstrated to conduct electrical current [112], a number of precautions are appropriate. These include ensuring that the externally placed graunding pad is placed close to the interventional electrical catheter so that the uterus does not lie between them. Devices using only bipolar currents should be used to minimize this risk of 'stray' currents going through the fetus. Electrocautery is relatively safe when used for sphincterotomy and hemostasis[2,5].

Epinephrine is category C drug during pregnancy and causes a decrease in uterine blood flow. Its safety, when used as an endoscopic injectant, has not been studied, although, when given in low dose combinations for analgesia, it is safe. Its use for hemostasis should balance the benefits with the potential risks [2].

10. Endoscopic ultrasonography

Endoscopic ultrasonography (EUS) is a widely accepted modality for the diagnosis of gastrointestinal and pancreatobiliary diseases. EUS has been shown to reduce unnecessary interventions in patients with low or moderate probabilities for choledocholithiasis. It is a safe alternative to fluoroscopy for the evaluation of biliary disorders during pregnancy. However, there are only case reports on EUS for pregnant patients in the literature. The largest series consist of 6 cases of EUS performed for suspected choledocholithiasis in pregnant patients [102]. EUS findings revealed choledocholithiasis in two patients, biliary sludge in two patients and nonsignificant findings in two patients.

All six patients were underwent ERCP after EUS, there were no maternal complications. Fetal outcome was favorable for 5 infants but one infant outcome was unknown. In another report, EUS was performed for acute pancreatitis of unknown etiology in 3 pregnant patients. Biliary pancreatitis without common bile duct stones found in 2 patients and pancreatitis due to unspecified pancreatic anomaly was found in one pregnant patient. There were no reported maternal complications in this study with 2 healthy infants but one fetal death 10 weeks after EUS probably due to recurrent cholangitis [113].

One may argue that EUS will prolong the overall time for a procedure. However, when EUS is normal, ERCP interventions can be avoided. In addition, EUS may provide other useful information. In experienced hands, the added time for EUS can be only a few minutes. So further studies are required to assess the role of EUS in the management of pregnant patients. However, it would seem acceptable to perform EUS when choledocholithiasis is a possible but unproven diagnosis and MRCP is an undesirable alternative.

11. Endoscopic spyscopy

The SpyGlass system is a recently developed system for performing cholangioscopy, pancreatoscopy. The main advantage over standard ERCP is that with the SpyGlass system the scope can be inserted directly into the bile duct and the pathology can be directly visualized, rather than using radiographs to visualize the bile ducts. This direct visualization allows the endoscopists to obtain a targetted biopsy, if needed, or to use electrohydraulic lithotripsy to crush stones under direct vision. This technique has been applied to 7 pregnant patients in the literature, five patients underwent choledochoscopy using spyscopy after ERCP, sphincterotomy, and balon sweeps; this procedure confirmed the removal of all choledochal stones in those patients. In one patient this technique is used to show residual 2 mm common bile duct stones after balon sweeping at ERCP, and in the remainig patient it has been used to show the sludge coming from the cystic duct. Choledochoscopy produced no maternal complications in those reports. This technique allows for the limitation or elimination of ionizing radiation through direct intraductal visualization and stone clearence confirmation. The diagnostic and therapeutic capability of ERCP is increased in a manner that contributes to patient safety and hopefully better maternal and fetal outcomes. So more studies are needed of this technique during pregnancy to asses the fetal outcomes [4, 114-116].

12. Endoscopic cystogastrostomy

Endoscopic cystogastrostomy with or without endosonographic guidance for drainage of pseudocyst has been demostrated to be an acceptable alternative to radiologic or surgical drainage. For the pregnant patient who has a pancreatic pseudocyst, this technique would be ideal because it would eliminate the risk of radiation incurred by a radiologic drainage and would involve less risk to the fetus than an intraabdominal surgical procedure. There are only two cases of endoscopic cystogastrostomy procedure applied to pregnant patients. In one patient it was successful; the pseudocyst was punctured percutaneously under conventional ultrasound guidance, than it is aspirated and filled with contrast agent. Then endoscopically a cystogastrostomy was created and a stent was inserted. The patient got well and gave birth to a healthy infant. In the second patient unfortunately the stent was migrated making the procedure partially unsuccessful, but with other techniques patient again got well and gave birth to a healthy infant too. So according to these two cases endoscopic cystogastrostomy is still a little bit experimental during pregnancy, it should be considered in pregnants who have symptomatic pseudocysts and cannot delay the procedure until delivery [4,29,116-118].

Author details

Nurten Akyurek Savas

Baskent University, Department of Gastroenterology, Istanbul Hospital, Turkey

References

[1] O'Mahony S. Endoscopy in pregnancy. Best Practice & Research Clinic Gastroenterol. 2007; 21 (5): 893-9.

[2] ASGE Guideline: guidelines for endoscopy in pregnant and lactating women Gastrointest Endoscopy 2005; 61 (3):357-62.

[3] Kammerer WS. Non-obstetric surgery during pregnancy. Med Clin North Am 1979; 63: 1157-64.

[4] Cappell MS. Risks versus benefits of gasrointestinal endoscopy during pregnancy. Nat Rev Gastroenterol Hepatol 2011; 8: 610-34.

[5] 5.Gilinsky NH, Muthunayagam N. Gastrointestinal endoscopy in pregnant and lactating women: Emerging Standard of care to guide decision-making. Obstet and Gynecol Survey 2006;61: 791-9.

[6] Glosten B. Anesthesia for Obstetrics. Miller RD (ed) Anesthesia Churchill Livingstone. New York. 2000; 2025-68.

[7] Morgan GE, Mikhail SM, Murray JM. Clinical anesthesiology . McGrow-hill, New York 2000; 819-46.

[8] Food and Drug Administration. Federal Register 1980; 44: 37434-67

[9] Jiraki K. Lethal effects of normeperidine. Am J Forensic Med. Pathol. 1992; 13(1): 42-3.

[10] 10. Briggs GC, Freeman RK, Yaffe SJ. Drugs in pregnancy and lactation: a reference guide to fetal and maternal risks, 8th edn (Lippincott, Williams & Wilkins, Philadelphia, 2008)

[11] Rothman KJ, Fyler DC, Goldblatt A, Kreidberg MB. Exogenous hormones and other drug exposures of children with congenital heart disease. Am J Epidemiol 1979; 109: 433-9.

[12] Ornoy A, Arnon J, Shechtman S, Moerman L, Lukashova I. Is benzodiazepine use during pregnancy really teratogenic? Reprod Toxicol. 1998; 12: 511-5.

[13] Czeizel A. Lack of evidence of teratogenicity of benzodiazepine drugs in Hungary. Reprod. Toxicol. 1987; 1(3): 183-8.

[14] Laegreid L, Olegard R, Walström J& Conradi N. Teratogenic effects of benzodiazepine use during pregnancy. J Pediatr. 1989; 114: 126-31.

[15] Arduini D, Rizzo G, Dell'Acqua S, Mancuso S, Romanini C. Effect of naloxone on fetal behavior near term. Am J Obstet Gynecol. 1987; 156: 474-8.

[16] Bland BA, Lawest EG, Duncan PW, Wanell I, Downing JW Comparison of midazolam and thiopental for rapid sequence anesthetic induction for elective cesarean section. Anesth Analg. 1987; 66(11): 1165-8.

[17] Ravlo O, Carl P, Crawford ME et al. A randomized comparison between midazolam and thiopental for elective cesarean section anesthesia: II. Neonates Anesth Analg. 1989, 68, 234-7.

[18] Lazzaroni M, Bianchi Porro G. Preparation, premedication, and surveillance. Endoscopy 2005; 37 (2): 101-9.

[19] Cappell MS. Sedation and analgesia for gastrointestinal endoscopy during pregnancy. Gastrointest Endosc Clin N Am 2006; 16: 1-31.

[20] Fassoulaki A, Theodoraki K, Melemeni A. Pharmacology of sedation agents and reversal agents. Digestion 2010; 82: 80-3.

[21] Goodlin R.C. Naloxone and its possible relationship to fetal endorphin levels and fetal distress. Am J Obstet Gynecol. 1981; 139: 16-9.

[22] Gibbs J, Newson T, Williams J, Davidson D.C. Naloxone hazard in infant of opioid abuser. Lancet. 1989; 2 (8655): 159-160.

[23] Brogden RN, Goa KL. Flumazenil. A reappraisal of its pharmacological properties and therapeutic efficacy as a benzodiazepine antagonist. Drugs1991; 42:1061-89.

[24] Cappell MS, Colon VJ, Sidhom O A. A study at eight medical centers of the safety and clinical efficacy of esophagogastroduedenoscopy in 83 pregnant females with follow-up of fetal outcome and with comparison to control groups. Am J Gastroenterol 1996; 91: 348-54.

[25] Debby A, Golan A, Sadan O, Glezerman M, Shirin H. Clinical utility of esophagogastroduodenoscopy in the management of recurrent and intractable vomiting in pregnancy. J Reprod Med. 2008; 53: 347-51.

[26] Frank B. Endoscopy in pregnancy. In: Karlstadt RG, Surawicz CM, Croitoru R., editors. Gastrointestinal disorders during pregnancy. Arlington, VA: American College of Gastroenterology:1994. 24-9.

[27] Bagis T, Gumurdulu Y, Kayaselcuk F, et al. Endoscopy in hyperemesis gravidarum and Helicobacter pyleri infection. Int J Gynacol Obstetr 2002; 79:105-9.

[28] Baron TH, Ramirez B, Richter JE. Gastrointestinal motility disorders during pregnancy. Ann Intern Med 1993;118 (5):366-75.

[29] Bruno JM, Kroser J. Efficacy and safety of upper endoscopy procedures during pregnancy Gastrointest Endoscopy Clin N Am 2006; 16: 33-40.

[30] Chak A, Cooper GS, Lloyd LE, et all. Effectiveness of endoscopy in patients admitted to the intensive care unit with upper GI hemorrhage. Gastrointest Endosc. 2001; 53:6-13.

[31] Barkun AN, Bardou M, Kuipers EJ, et al. International consensus recommendations on the management of patients with nonvariceal upper gastrointestinal bleeding. Ann Intern Med 2010; 152(2): 101-13.

[32] Nguyen GC, Dinani AM, Pivovarov K. Endoscopic management and outcomes of pregnant women hospitalized for nonvariceal upper GI bleeding: a nationwide analysis. Gastrointest Endoscopy 2010; 72: 954-9.

[33] Russell MA, Craigo SD. Cirrhosis and portal hypertension in pregnancy. Semin perinatol 1998; 22: 156-65.

[34] Homburg R, Bayer I, Lurie B. Bleeding esophageal varices in pregnancy. A report of two cases. J. Reprod Med 1988, 33: 784-6.

[35] Lodato F, Cappelli A, Montagnani M, et al. Transjugular intrahepatic portosystemic shunt: A case report of rescue management of unrestrainable variceal bleeding in a pregnant woman. Digestive and Liver Dis 2008; 40: 387-90.

[36] Starkel P, Horsmans Y, Geubel A. Endoscopic band ligation: a safe technique to control bleeding esophageal varices in pregnancy. Gastrointest Endosc 1998; 48: 212-4.

[37] Dhiman RK, Biswas R, Aggarwal N, Sawhney H, Chawla Y. Management of variceal bleeding with endoscopic variceal ligation and N-butyl-2 cyanoacrylate: report of these cases. Gastrointest Endosc 2000; 51: 91-3.

[38] Iwase H, Morise K, Kawase T, Horiuchi Y. Endoscopic injection sclerotherapy for esophageal varices during pregnancy. J. Clin Gastroenterol 1994; 18: 80-3.

[39] Ghidirim G, Mishin I, Dolghii A, Lupashcu A. Prophylactic endoscopic band ligation of esophageal varices during pregnancy. J Gastrointestin Liver D. 2008;17: 236-7.

[40] Stiegmann GV, Goff JS, Michaletz-Onady PA, ET AL.. Endoscopic sclerotherapy as compared with endoscopic ligation for bleeding esophageal varices. N eng J Med 1992; 326: 1527-32.

[41] Gimson AE, Ramage JK, Panos MZ, et al. Randomised trial of variceal banding ligation versus injection sclerotherapy for bleeding esophageal varices. Lancet 1993; 342: 391-4.

[42] de la Pena J, Rivero M, Sanchez E, etal. Variceal ligation compared with endoscopic sclerotherapy for variceal hemorrhage: prospective randomized trial. Gastrointest Endosc 1999; 49: 417-23.

[43] Aggarwal N, Sawhney H, Vasishta K, Dhiman RK, Chawla Y. Non-cirrhotic portal hypertension in pregnancy. Int J Gynaecol Obstet. 2001; 72: 1-7.

[44] Kochhar R, Kuma S, Goel RC., et al. Pregnancy and its outcome in patients with non-cirrhotic portal hypertension. Dig Dis Sci 1999; 44:1356-61.

[45] Sanyal AJ, Freedman AM, Luketic VA, et al. Transjugular intrahepatic portosystemic shunts for patients with active variceal hemorrhage unresponsive to sclerotherapy. Gastroenterolgy 1996; 111: 138-46.

[46] Tesdal IK, Filser T, Weiss C, et al. Transjugular intrahepatic portosystemic shunts: adjunctive embolotherapy of gastroesophageal collateral vessels in the prevention of variceal rebleeding. Radiology 2005; 236: 360-7.

[47] Cappell MS. Therapeutic endoscopy for acute upper gastrointestinal bleeding. Nat Rev Gastroenterol Hepatol. 2010; 7: 214-29.

[48] Brunner G, Meyer H, Athmann C. Omeprazole for peptic ulcer disease in pregnancy. Digestion 1998; 59; 651-4.

[49] Macedo G, Carvalho L, Ribeiro T. Endoscopic sclerotherapy for upper gastrointestinal bleeding due to Mallory-Weiss syndrome. Am J Gastroenterol. 1995; 90, 1364-5.

[50] Marcus MA, Vertommen JD, Van Aken H, Wouters PF. Hemodynamic effects of intravenous isoproterenol versus epinephrine in the chronic maternal-fetal sheep preperation. Anesth Analg 1996; 82: 1023-6.

[51] Villar J, Merialdi M, Gülmezoğlu AM, et al. Nutritional interventions during pregnancy for the prevention or treatment of maternal morbidity and preterm delivery: an overview of randomized controlled trials. J Nutr 2003; 133: 1606-25.

[52] Wong M, Apodaca CC, Markenson MG, Yancey M. Nutrition management in a pregnant comatose patient. Nutr Clin Pract.1997; 12: 63-6.

[53] Koh ML, Lipkin EW. Nutrition support of a pregnant comatose patient via percutaneous endoscopic gastrostomy. JPEN J Parenter Enteral Nutr 1993; 17: 384-7.

[54] Shaheen NJ, Crosby MA, Grimm IS, Isaacs K. The use of percutaneous endoscopic gastrostomy in pregnancy. Gastrointest Endosc 1997; 46: 564-5.

[55] Godil A, Chen YK. Percutaneous endoscopic gastrostomy for nutrition support in pregnancy associated with hyperemesis gravidarum and anorexia nervosa. JPEN J Parenter Enteral Nutr 1998; 22: 238-41.

[56] Serrano P, Velloso A, Garcia-Luna PP, et al. Enteral nutrition by percutaneous endoscopic gastrojejunostomy in severe hyperemesis gravidarum: a report of two cases. Clin Nutr 1998; 17: 135-9.

[57] O'Connell MP, Wilson OF, Masson EA, Lindow SW. Pregnancy outcome in a patient with chronic malnutrition. Hum Reprod 2000; 15: 2443-5.

[58] Wejda BU, Soennichsen B, Huchzermeyer H et al. Successful jejunal nutrition therapy in a pregnant patient with apallic syndrome. Clin Nutr 2003; 22: 209-11.

[59] Irwing PM, Howell RJ, Shidrawi RG. Percutaneous endoscopic gastrostomy with a jejunal port for severe hyperemesis gravidarum. Eur J Gastroenterol Hepatol 2004, 16: 937-9.

[60] Ceccaldi PF, Bazin A, Gomis P, et al. Persistent vegatative state with encephalitis in a pregnant woman with successful fetal outcome. BJOG. 2005 ; 112(6): 843-4.

[61] Senadhi V, Chaudhary J, Dutta S. Percutaneous endoscopic gastrostomy placement during pregnancy in the critical care setting. Endoscopy 2010; 42: E358-359.

[62] Pereira JL Velloso A, Parejo J, et al. Percutaneous endoscopic gastrostomy and gastrojejunostomy. Experience and its role in domiciliary enteral nutrition. Nutr Hosp 1998; 13:50-56. .

[63] Saha S, Loranger D, Pricolo V, Degli-Esposti S. Feding jejunostomy for the treatment of severe hyperemesis gravidarum: a case series. JPEN J Parenter Enteral Nutr. 2009 33(5):529-34. .

[64] Belda O, Serrano P, Bozada JM, et aI. Percutaneous endoscopic gastrostomy. Reality in the intra and extra community clinical nutritional practice. Rev Clin Esp 2005; 205: 472-7.

[65] Schrag SP, Sharma R, Jaik NP, et al. Complications related to percutaneous endoscopic gastrostomy (PEG) tube. A comprehensive clinical review. J Gastrointestine Liver Dis 2007; 16: 407-18.

[66] Siddiqui U, Proctor D.D. Flexible sigmoidoscopy and colonoscopy during pregnancy. Gastrointest Endoscopy Clin N Am. 2006; 16: 59-9.

[67] Cappell MS, Sidhom O. Multicenter, multiyear study of safety and efficacy of flexible sigmoidoscopy during pregnancy in 24 females with follow-up fetal outcome. Dig Dis Sci 1995; 40: 472-9.

[68] Cappell MS. The fetal safety and clinical efficacy of gastrointestinal endoscopy during pregnancy Gastroenterol Clin North Am 2003; 32: 123-179.

[69] Cappell MS, Colon VJ, Sidhom OA A study at 10 medical centers of the safety and efficacy of 48 flexible sigmoidoscopies and 8 colonoscopies during pregnancy with

follow up of fetal outcome and with comparison to control groups. Dig Dis Sci 1996; 41:2353-61.

[70] Huang WS, Lin PY, Wang JY, Chin CC, Hsieh CC. Urgent colectomy and cesarean section of a pregnant familial adenomatous polyposis: a case report. Int J Colorectal Dis 2007; 22: 847-8.

[71] Ishijima N, Ojima E, Tonouchi H, Suzuki H, Fukunishi S. Delivery of a normal newborn after intensive medical treatment for an acute exacerbation of ulcerative colitis during pregnancy; a case report. Surg Today 1999; 29:1257-9.

[72] Minter A, Malik R, Ledbetter L, et al. Colon cancer in pregnancy. Cancer control 2005; 12: 196-202.

[73] Mirza M S, Mulla M., Hall RI, Large bowel obstruction in pregnancy: a rare entity, an unusual case. Arch. Gynecol. Obstet.2009; 279: 171-178.

[74] Seubert DE, Puder K, Goldmeier P, Gonik B. Colonoscopic release of the incarcerated gravid uterus. Obstet. Gynecol. 1999; 94: 792-4.

[75] Prather CM. Pregnancy-related constipation. Curr Gastroenterol Rep 2004; 6: 402-4.

[76] Rimensberger P, Schubiger G, Willi U. Connatal rickets following repeated administration of phosphate enemas in pregnancy: a case report. Eur J. Pediatr 1992; 151: 54-6.

[77] Desmeules S, Bergeron MJ, Isenring P. Acute phosphate nephropathy and renal failure. N Eng J Med 2003; 349: 1006-7.

[78] Vinod J, Bonheur J, Korelitz BI, Panagopoulos G. Choice of laxatives and colonoscopic preperation in pregnant patients from the viewpoint of obstetricians and gastroenterolgists. World J Gastroenterol 2007; 13 (48): 6549-6552.

[79] Cappell MS, Fox SR, Gorrepati N. Safety and efficacy of colonoscopy during pregnancy: an analysis of pregnancy outcome in 20 patients. J Reprod Med 2010; 55: 115-23.

[80] Bashir RM, Montgomery EA, Gupta PK, et al. Massive gastrointestinal hemorrhage during pregnancy caused by ectopic decidua of the terminal ileum and colon. Am J Gastroenterol 1995; 90: 1325-7.

[81] Gonsoulin W, Mason B,Carpenter RJ. Colon cancer in pregnancy with elevated maternal serum alpha-fetoprotein level at presentation. Am J Obstet Gynecol. 1990; 163: 1172–3.

[82] Rojansky, N. Shushan A, Livni N, et al. Pregnancy associated with colon carcinoma overexpressing p53. Gynecol. Oncol. 1997; 64: 516–20.

[83] Van Voorhis, B, Cruikshank, D P. Colon carcinoma complicating pregnancy. A report of two cases. J Reprod Med. 1989; 34: 923–7.

[84] Woods, JB, Martin JN, Ingram FH, et al. Pregnancy complicated by carcinoma of the colon above the rectum. Am J Perinatol. 1992; 9: 102–10.

[85] Chan, YM, Ngai SW, Lao T T Colon cancer in pregnancy. A case report. J Reprod Med. 1999; 44: 733–6.

[86] Montes H, Wolf J. Cecal volvulus in pregnancy. Am J Gastroenterol. 1999; 94: 2554–6.

[87] Rausch, ME, Troiano NH, Rosen T. Use of neostigmine to relieve a suspected colonic pseudoobstruction in pregnancy. J Perinatol. 2007; 27, 244–6.

[88] Rozen, P., Schreiber, L. & Brazowski, E. Endometriosis, pregnancy, and colonoscopy. Endoscopy 2003; 35: 975

[89] Entmann SS, Moise KJ. Anaphylaxis in pregnancy. South Med J.1984; 77: 402.

[90] Kidd SA, Lancaster PA, Anderson JC, et al. A cohort study of pregnancy outcomes after amniocentesis in twin pregnancy. Pediatr Perinat Epidemiol 1997; 11: 200-13.

[91] Cragan JD. Teratogen update: metylene blue. Teratology 1999; 60: 42-8.

[92] Waterman M, Eliakim R. Capsule enteroscopy of the small intestine. Abdom Imaging 2009; 34: 452-8.

[93] Lawson M, Kern F, Jr, Everson GT. Gastrointestinal transit time in human pregnancy: prolongation in the second and third trimesters followed by postpartum normalization. Gastroenterology 1985; 89: 996-9.

[94] Hogan RB, Ahmad N, Hogan RBIII, et al. Video capsule endoscopy detection of jejunal carcinoid in life threatening hemorrhage, first trimester pregnancy Gastrointest Endosc 2007; 66: 205-7.

[95] Glenn F, McSherry CK. Gallstones and pregnancy among 300 young women treated by cholecystectomy. Surg Gynecol Obstet 1968; 127: 1067-72.

[96] Printen KJ, Ott RA. Cholecystectomy during pregnancy. Am Surg 1978; 44: 432-4.

[97] Amos JD, Schorr SJ, Norman PF, et al. Laparoscopic surgery during pregnancy. Am J Surg 1996; 171: 435-7.

[98] Curet MJ, Allen D, Josloff RK, et al. Laparoscopy during pregnancy. Arch Surg 1996; 131: 546-50.

[99] Graham G, Baxi L, Tharakan T. Laparoscopic cholecystectomy during pregnancy: a case series and review of the literature. Obstet Gynecol Surv. 1998; 53: 566-74.

[100] Tang SJ, Mayo MJ, Rodriguez –Frias E, et al. Safety and utility of ERCP during pregnancy. Gastrointest Endosc 2009; 69: 453-61.

[101] Jamidar PA, Beck GJ, Hoffman BJ, et al. Endoscopic retrograde cholangiopancreatography in pregnancy. Am J Gastroenterol 1995; 90: 1263-7.

[102] Shelton J, Linder JD, Rivera-Alsina M. E., Tarnasky P.R. Commitment, confirmation, and clearence: new techniques for nonradiation ERCP during pregnancy. Gastrointest. Endosc. 2008; 67: 364-368.

[103] Gupta R, Tandan M, Lakhtakia S , et al. Safety of therapeutic ERCP in pregnancy-an indian experience. Indian J Gastroenterol 2005; 24: 161-3.

[104] Kahaleh M, Hartwell GD, Arseneau KO, et al. Safety and efficacy of ERCP in pregnancy. Gastrointest Endosc. 2004; 60: 287-292.

[105] Tham TC, Vandervoort J, Wong RC, et al. Safety of ERCP in pregnancy. Am JGastroenterol 2003; 98: 308-11.

[106] Farca A, Aguilar ME, Rodriquez G, de la Mora G., Arango L. Biliary stents as temporary treatment for choledocholithiasis in pregnant patients. Gastrointest. Endosc. 1997; 46: 99-101.

[107] Wagner L, Lester R, Saldana L. Exposure of the pregnant patient to diagnostic radiations: a guide to medical management. 2nd ed. Madison (WI): medical Physics Publishing. 1997.

[108] Campbell N, Sparrow K, Fortier M, Ponich T. Practical radiation safety and protection for the endoscopist during ERCP. Gastrointest. Endosc 2002; 55: 552-7.

[109] Barthel JS, Chowdhury T, Miedema BW. Endoscopic sphincterotomy for the treatment of gallstone pancreatitis during pregnancy. Surg Endosc 1998; 12: 394-9.

[110] Shelton J, Linder JD, Rivera Alsina ME, Tarnasky PR. Commitment, confirmation, and clearence: new techniques for nonradiation ERCP during pregnancy. Gastrintest Endosc 2008; 67: 364.

[111] Oto A, Ernst R, Ghulmiyyah L, et al. The role of MR cholangiopancreatography in the evaluation of pregnant patients with acute pancreatobiliary diesase. The Br J Radiol. 2009; 82: 279-85.

[112] Einarson A, Bailey B, Inocencion G, et al. Accidental electric shock in pregnancy; a prospective cohort study. Am J Obstet Gynecol 1997; 176: 678-81.

[113] Roumieu F, Ponchon T, Audra P, Gaucherand P. Acute pancreatitis in pregnancy: place of the different explorations (magnetic resonance cholangiopancreatography, endoscopic ultrasonography) and their therapeutic consequences. Eur J Obstet Gynecol Reprod Biol 2008; 140: 141-2.

[114] Draganov P. The SpyGlass Direct Visualization system for cholangioscopy. Gastroenterol & Hepatol 2008; 4: 469-70.

[115] Uradomo L, Pandolfe F, Aragon G, Borum ML. SpyGlass cholangioscopy for management of choledocholithiasis during pregnancy. Hepatobiliary Pancreat Dis Int 2011; 10: 107-8.

[116] Girotra M, Jani N. Role of endoscopic ultrasound / SpyScope in diagnosis and treatment of choledocholithiasis in pregnancy. World J Gastroenterol 2010; 16: 3601-2.

[117] Ryan ME. Endoscopic management of a pancretaic pseudocyst during pregnancy. Gastrointest Endosc 1992; 38: 605-8.

[118] Gyokores T, Topa L, Marton I, Pap A. Endoscopic cystogastrostomy during pregnancy. Gastrointest Endosc 2001; 53: 516-8.

Chapter 13

Endoscopy in Pregnancy

Paul Mitrut, Anca Oana Docea,
Cornelia - Daniela Calina and Liliana Streba

Additional information is available at the end of the chapter

1. Introduction

In most of gastrointestinal disorders, endoscopy has a major diagnostic and therapeutic role, but though its clinical efficacy and safety have been established, it is not that well known when performing it in pregnant patients, due to the potential harm of the foetus like hypoxia, teratogenesis, trauma, placental abruption or induction of premature labor.

Endoscopy is generally considered to be a low risk procedure, the most frequently being performed at the patient`s request in ambulatory but also in hospitals [1]. Nevertheless, the safety and effectiveness of gastrointestinal endoscopy in particular circumstances at the pregnant woman has not been yet well studied. During the pregnancy the risks for the fetus and mother are various and the magnitude of this risk is different, according to the trimester. Taking into consideration the difficulties in the performance of those studies to pregnant women these risks have not been enough evaluated.

The main concern is the fetal safety and endoscopic medication and use of sedative and analgesics represent a significant risk if they are not chosen properly. It is strongly indicated the presence of an anesthesiologist and an obstetrician, in selected cases when a pregnancy-related complication is most probable. Before the procedure, the pregnant patient should be well evaluated by the gastroenterologist, anesthesiologist and obstetrician and should be informed about the potential risks of sedation and analgesia.

Because of the fact that there are potential risks for the fetus and for the pregnant woman, the indications of endoscopy to pregnant women limit to superior gastrointestinal hemorrhages, dysphagia, uncontrolled nausea/vomits, rectal bleeding, diarrhea, biliary lithiasis or biliary pancreatitis [2]. For that matter, endoscopy for pregnant women is considered to be a very rare procedure; in USA only 19000 pregnant women do this type of annual investigation [3].

It is being performed during the pregnancy only when there are no other ways of diagnosis or therapy less invasive, the indications for the procedure are clear and as much as possible the gastroscopy should be postponed until third trimester.

The safety of gastrointestinal endoscopy during the pregnancy was evaluated by Cappell et al [4] who performed esophago-gastro-duodenoscopies on a lot of 83 pregnant women and concluded on the fact that the procedure is safe and does not induce birth or congenital malformations. The same authors investigated the safety of sigmoidscopy to 46 patients and established the safety of the procedure to the pregnant women who had small gastrointestinal bleeding and avoided to induce early labor and the appearance of congenital malformations. Nevertheless, as a result of data which are rather limited and incomplete in what concerns the safety of the procedure, fetal risk to endoscopy in the pregnancy has not been completely excluded. In that effect, in Qureshi`s work et al. which has been approved by the American Society of Endoscopic Gastrointestinal Endoscopy (ASGE, 2005) there had been distinguished the principles that the doctor must comply with when he decides to make endoscopies to a pregnant woman [5].

2. Physiological modifications in the pregnancy and the endoscopy

Pregnant women are susceptible to gastrointestinal reflux disease, biliary tract complications and gastrointestinal bleeding, thus needing to be performed upper endoscopy, ERCP or colonoscopy. For example, only in the United States, upper endoscopy was necessary in over 12,000 pregnant patients per year and colonoscopy or sigmoidoscopy in more than 6000 pregnant patients per year. ERCP is also needed, as cholelithiasis has a 12% incidence in pregnant patients. Latest studies suggest that, if having good indication (upper gastrointestinal bleeding, refractory nausea or vomiting), upper endoscopy is relatively safe in pregnant patients.

Increase in size of pregnant uterus determines the lift of stomach along with the modification of intra abdominal segment of esophagus that gets into the thorax. As a result it is being reduced the tonus of the inferior esophagian sphincter and increases intragastric pressure which predisposes to gastroesophageal reflux. Even if gastric volume and acidity of gastric juice does not modify during the pregnancy, the pregnant women show a regurgitating risk through the decrease of pressure barrier of inferior eshophageal sphincter. This risk justifies the pharmacological methods of reduction of gastric secretion. 50-80% from the pregnant women show "retrosternal burning-pyrosis" which is the clinical correspondent of gastroesophageal reflux. On those grounds, the pregnant women are considered as having a full stomach [6].

During the last months of pregnancy, the pregnant uterus modifies anatomic relations between abdominal and pelvic organs. These modifications can extend the time of performance of the procedure, they can increase the quantity of anaesthesic medicines that are being administered and the air quantity inoculated in order to facilitate the intraluminal visualization. In order to diminish the compression of vena cava by the pregnant uterus there should be adopted the lying down position of the pregnant woman, position that was used in a normal way for colonoscopy. For those grounds, the endoscopist must be accustomed with endoscopic procedures to pregnant women and fully evaluate anatomic and pathological modifications of superior and interior gastrointestinal tract.

Biliary oversaturation and biliary hypomotility are as well frequently seen as physiological modifications that appear during the pregnancy. Unfortunately, this can lead to the formation of biliary sludge and biliary calculi, which at their turn can widen biliary colics, cholecystitis and even pancreatitis.

Airway mucosa is edematiated during the pregnancy, showing a reduction of airways. Moreover, there is a compensatory increase of ventilation on each minute in order to answer to demands of maternal and fetal oxygen. Nevertheless, pulmonary capacity is reduced as a result of ascension of the diaphragm.

As well, during the pregnancy there appear hemodynamic modifications. Cardiac frequency increases from 90 to 100 beats a minute. Systolic arterial pressure can increase. Pregnant women cannot often tolerate the supine position, especially after 30 pregnancy weeks, given reduced arterial pressure because of big weight of the uterus.

3. Endoscopy indications during pregnancy

Endoscopy should be performed during pregnancy only when the indication for the procedure is clear and there are no less invasive or therapeutical diagnosis ways. In order to perform this operation it is necessary the patient`s informed consent. It should be taken into account that the procedure should be postponed until second trimester. The specific indications for endoscopy during pregnancy, as ASGE recommends are the following:

- Significant or continued GI bleeding
- Severe or refractory nausea and vomiting or abdominal pain
- Dysphagia or odynophagia
- Strong suspicion of colon mass
- Severe diarrhea with negative evaluation
- Biliary pancreatitis, choledocholithiasis, or cholangitis
- Biliary or pancreatic ductal injury

Also, there are a few principles (ASGE) to respect:

- have a strong indication
- preferably perform endoscopy during the second trimester of pregnancy
- use lowest effective dose of sedative drugs and of category A or B, if available

- minimize procedure time
- position pregnant patients in left pelvic tilt or left lateral position to avoid vena cava or aortic compression
- presence of fetal heart sounds should be confirmed before sedation is begun and after the endoscopic procedure
- obstetric support should be available in the event of a pregnancy-related complication
- endoscopy is contraindicated in obstetric complications such as placental abruption, imminent delivery, ruptured membranes, or eclampsia.

The decision of performing an endoscopy to a pregnant patient must be taken by a team: obstetrician – endoscopist – anaesthesist, because there must be analyzed: the implications for the fetus, for the mother, the emergency of the situation and the possibility of therapeutical alternatives in order to solve the issue in safety conditions or postponement after labor [7]. An obstetrician must be available during the procedure if there are complications related to the pregnancy.

4. Fetal and maternal risks in endoscopic explorations

4.1. Endoscopic risks for the fetus

They can be: hypoxy given to oversedation, fetal hyperperfusion given to maternal position, teratogenity given to the medicines administration, uterine trauma along with the impact on the fetus through endoscopic trauma, preterm labor through uterine compression. That is why it is advisable to avoid the performance of endoscopies in first trimester, excepting clinical emergency cases.

Among these risks, potential risk to dermine a malformation in fetal development through pills administration, early labor or giving mechanical uterine trauma seriously need evaluation when it is being analyzed an endoscopic procedure to pregnant people. Moreover, medical and ethical problems require a reticence for doctors and pregnant people in what concerns endoscopic studies and require the patient`s informed consent. Fetal normal status must be confirmed before starting the endoscopy and it must be revaluated as soon as possible after its completion.

There is no evidence that certifies increased fetal morbidity for pregnant women that are subject to endoscopic procedures in comparison with pregnant women that had not been subject at any investigations. On the contrary, a case control study that enclosed a number of 83 superior digestive endoscopies performed to pregnant women showed that there had not been any preterm labors and any new born children of these women had not different Apgar scores to birth in comparison with those women that had not performed these kind of investigations [4].

A survey performed by 300 specialist gastroenterologists doctors, which included information regarding 73 digestive superior endoscopies and 13 colonoscopies performed during the pregnancy, did not succeed to report any significant complication for those pregnancies [8]. Just as well, a series of groups from 10 medical centers reported an experience of 48 flexible sigmoidoscopies and 8 colonoscopies performed during the pregnancy [9] and dit not report any negative result that could affect the fetus and that could be assigned to those endoscopic procedures.

From the point of view of gestation development, fetal complications are: fetal abnormalities, labor induction, preterm labor that could be determined by endoscopic procedures, having the greatest risk to appear in the first trimester of pregnancy [10]. In general, the second trimester is considered to have the lowest risk for endoscopic interventions.

Even if the studies that had been performed did not seem to indicate a negative result for the fetus and which could have been assigned directly to endoscopy, the procedure itself requires a great caution from the doctors. Endoscopy, which has a diagnostic or therapeutical role must be taken into consideration only when, without its execution, the risks are higher. General rules are to postpone the procedure until labor or at least after first trimester of pregnancy. Pre-procedure training of the pregnant woman must include a special examination from the obstetrician and his availability in care of eventual complications. There will be monitored the fetal heart beats before starting the procedure that will be revaluated as soon as possible after the completion.

The risk of fetal hypoxy can be reduced through minimum sedation of the pregnant woman. The procedure is not performed with the mother in position of lying down, because the pregnant uterus can compress the aorta and/inferior vena cava that causes maternal hypotension and therefore it could interfere with the placental perfusion. Therefore it is advisable left lateral position. American Society for Gastrointestinal Endoscopy has recently published the guidelines that must be fulfilled for the endoscopy to pregnant women, based on available data and the consent of specialist doctors [11].

Fetal monitoring is made through the hearts beats with the help of a monitor and it allows to the doctor to detect any fatal suffering. This difficulty can be improved through the correction of maternal hypoxy or hypotension.

In 2009 ASA and American College of obstetrics and gynecology (ACOG) issued a common statement regarding the endoscopic interventions performed during pregnancy [12]. The document contains the following mentions:

- endoscopist must obtain a pre-operative examination together with the obstetrician before performing each endoscopic procedure. This must be achieved no matter the gestation age of the fetus.
- when the fetus is pre-viable, Doppler detection of fetal heart beats immediately before and after the procedure is enough.
- when the fetus is viable, continuous intra-operative monitoring of fetal heart beats and the presence of a gynecology surgeon is ideal, if it appears an emergency labor.

The decision to use a monitor for fetal heart beats should be individualized, according to the availability of resources.

4.2. Endoscopic risks for the pregnant woman

Endoscopic risks for the pregnant woman can be:

- precipitated aspiration through abdominal dystensia
- hypotension through the compression of inferior vena cava
- uterine trauma through the anatomic modification

Maternal hypotension appears through the compression of inferior vena cava and the reduction of venous return. That is why there must be avoided the supine position during the procedures.

Compression of abdominal organs by the pregnant uterus can modify the digestive lumen and therefore the duration of endoscopy can be extended, and for the vizualization it is necessary a higher amount of air breathed, the endoscope can jump-up (especially to colonoscopies) and it can appear an abdominal dystensia accompanied by a discomfort of the pregnant woman.

Endoscopy for pregnant women is made only in carefully selected cases. It can't be made an endoscopy in case of an imminent abortion or if there are some obstetrical problems. The procedure is better performed during day in a specialized endoscopy office. It can be administered oxygen, but it is not compulsory.

5. Sedative medication used for endoscopy in pregnancy

As well the mother and the fetus are subject to some potential risks in case of endoscopic sedation. These risks vary according to pregnancy trimester.

Sedative and analgesic agents should always be used in that smaller dose in order to minimize the potential risk of teratogenic effects. The highest risk for the fetus takes place during the first trimester when it is the most vulnerable to possible teratogenic effects.

As there are no well controlled studies regarding the safety of the fetus towards the pharmacological agents that are used for sedation in the pregnant women endoscopy, no medicine has been framed by FDA in class A, without teratogenity [13].

Data for safe medicines, not teratogenic, are reduced, because the clinical studies to pregnant women are very rarely performed, they are expensive and require long term monitoring [14]. This point of view led to the recommendation of sedative medicines for endoscopy during the pregnancy in very small quantities and only if it is strictly necessary.

A good cooperation between the pregnant woman and gastroenterologist should bring to the performance of a fast endoscopic procedure, simple and without sedation. But most of them are made in emergency situations and with therapeutical intentions. In these situations it is necessary the sedation, and the endoscopist should consult with obstetrician doctor and with anasthesist about the anesthesic medicines, taking into account the FDA classification of teratogenity of medicines. It is very important that the doctor be familiar with the stages of fetal development and teratogenesis. At two weeks from the conception, embrionary cells are subject to the law „all or nothing". In this period the exposure to toxic drugs will lead either to a normal and healthy fetus or the embryo will not be viable. In the next eight weeks and until the second trimester it appears the difference of cells and organogenesis. At the moment, the exposure to teratogenic medicines will have as a result severe congenital malformations. In the second and third trimester the medicines can still generate fetal toxicity, especially from the neurological point of view.

In order to classify their safety when using in pregnancy, drugs were divided by FDA into 5 categories:

1. category A – defined as adequate and well controlled studied in pregnant women;
2. category B - animal studies have revealed no evidence of harm to the fetus, but there are no adequate studies in pregnant women or animal studies have shown an adverse effect, but adequate studies in humans have failed to demonstrate a risk to the fetus;
3. category C - animal studies have shown an adverse effect, and there are no adequate studies in pregnant women or no animal studies have been conducted and there are no adequate studies in pregnant women;
4. category D - studies in pregnant women have demonstrated a risk to the fetus (however, the benefits of therapy may outweigh the risk);
5. category X - studies in both animals and humans have demonstrated evidence of fetal abnormalities; use is contraindicated in women who are or may be pregnant.

Because there are no well controlled studies regarding fetus safety when using pregnant patients sedation in endoscopy, no drug was classified as category A by the FDA.

Most of the drugs used in pregnant patients sedation are category B or C. Category D drugs should be avoided and used only when the benefit outweighs the risks, while category X it is not used at all. Sedation should be moderate or anxiolisis; in case of deep sedation is needed, it should be only under the surveillance of a specialised anesthesiologist. It should be used the lowest efficacious dose of sedation or, if possible, the endoscopy should be performed without any sedation: most upper endoscopies and sigmoidoscopies can be accomplished without sedation.

The most common medicines that are used for endoscopic sedation and analgesia are Meperidine, Fentanyl, benzodiazepines and Propofol. Meperidine (FDA category B) does not seem to be teratogenic. It is better than choosing Fentanyl during pregnancy. Fentanyl (FDA category C) as well, can be relatively safe in small doses, but there are few available data referring to its safety. The use of some benzodiazepines (FDA category D) is not yet controversial.

The use of Diazepam is not recommended during pregnancy. The use of Diazepam during pregnancy had been associated with split of the hard palate to new born infants, according to some old studies [15] but other two meta-analyses did not succeed to confirm these results [16]. Midazolam has not been associated with fetal malformations, but its use must be avoided in the first trimester. The safety of Propofol (FDA category B) has not yet been established, but taking into account the short duration of action, with minimum secondary effects, it could be a drug of choice when it is necessary a more profound sedation.

In the first trimester endoscopic procedures must rather be achieved without sedation or by using Meperidine all alone. In the second and third trimester Meperidine remains the first choice drug, but little doses of Midazolam can be added according to needs.

If it is necessary a more profound sedation, it is recommended the examination with the anaesthesist. The pregnancy in trimesters two and three represents a great challenge for endoscopies, taking into account the management of airways, sedation and monitoring cardiac and respiratory functions and the fluids balance. Approaching must be made by a team that includes the obstetrician, anaesthesist and the endoscopist working together in a hospital.

There are certain drugs commonly used in gastrointestinal endoscopy: meperidine, fentanyl, naloxone, benzodiazepines, pethidine, flumazenil, propofol, simethicone, glucagon, topical anesthetics, colon-cleansing agents that need to be discussed extensively, according to their category.

5.1. Meperidine (category B)

Of all opioidagonists that have teratogenic effects on animals, meperidine appears to be safe when being used for endoscopy in pregnant women[17; 18]. This is one of the standard drugs used for analgesia and sedation and is the preferred opiate during pregnancy. It does not cross the blood brain barriers or a pidasmorphineandis often used by obstetricians for analgesia during labor. However, using high doses close to birth time, may cause neonatal respiratory depression. Meperidine may also be responsible for transient fetal heart rate abnormalities, but in the absence of other fetal changes it can not be considered an indicator of poor prognosis in this situation[19].

To obtain the minimum sedation effect during endoscopy in pregnant women it should be used the lowest dose, limited to a maximum of 75 mg meperidine during routine exploration. In case of occasional occurrence of respiratory depression or hypotension secondary to opiate use, there can be used rapid acting opiate antagonists such as naloxone (B category) [20]. It crosses the placenta shortly after administered to the mother and was not shown to be associated with teratogenicity. It is preferred compared to fentanyl and morphine.

5.2. Fentanyl (category C)

It is considered that fentanyl is a safe opiate when used in low doses if administered during pregnancy. It has a faster onset of action than meperidine and is generally indicated in pregnant patients with a previous history of seizures. Although it was found as being embryocidal to rats, clinical experience in pregnant women was very similar to meperidine [21].

5.3. Naloxone (category B)

It doesn't seem to be teratogenic. It is contraindicatedin mothers who are dependent on opiates because it may precipitate opiate-withdrawal symptoms. It is being used only in cases of respiratory depression, hypotension, or lack of response and under strict monitoring. It should be noted that there is a risk of resedation due to metabolising the drug.

5.4. Flumazenil (category C)

It is a benzodiazepine antagonist, not very well studied, but it seems it might determine neurobehavioral changes in rats if exposed to it in utero.

5.5. Benzodiazepines (category D)

Diazepam accumulates rapidly into fetal circulation after maternal administration and was associated with congenital defects in mice. As concerning the occurrence of similar anomalies in humans, opinions are divided. The data suggest that administration of diazepam in early pregnancy appears to be a risk factor, although using it during the second and third trimester could theoretically determine neurobehavioral disorders in neonates [25]. Therefore, the conclusion is that diazepam should not be used during pregnancy.

Midazolam is the most commonly used sedative for endoscopic procedures. Although it crosses the placentaandcanbedetected to the fetus, unlike diazepam, it is not concentrated in the fetal circulation and was not associated with congenital defects. However, belonging to benzodiazepines, it has the neonatal respiratory depressant potential. Therefore it should be used in small doses, with great care under the supervision of ananesthesiologist, when sedation with meperidineisin sufficient [26].A meta-analysis of studies on the risks of anesthesia for gastroscopies during pregnancy concluded that the only potential problem is a slight increased incidence of abortion in the first or second trimester of pregnancy[27]. It is not recommended during the first trimester of pregnancy [28].

5.6. Propofol (category B)

Propofolis an increasingly used for endoscopy sedative drug, especially in the United States. It is short acting, with a much shorter recovery period than other sedative pharmacological agents[22]. However, following an arrow therapeutic index and potential respiratory depression, itis generally administered only by anesthesiologists. Gastroenterologists' medical societies have recommended that this agent should be reserved for deeper sedation and other complicated clinical situations in a highly monitored for vital functions environment [23]. It is considered relatively safe for use during pregnancy, although few data are available regarding its use in the first trimester of pregnancy[24].

5.7. Simethicone (category C)

It is frequently used in pregnant patients, with no reported addverse effects, but it is not extensively studied yet so it belongs to category C drugs.

5.8. Glucagon (category B)

It is a safe to use antispasmodic, especially in ERCP.

5.9. Topical anesthetics (category B)

Lidocaine is used to provide pharingeal anesthesia and it was reported as being safe to use even in the first trimester of pregnancy.

5.10. Colon cleansing-agents

Most of them are category C, due to lack of studies during pregnancy, and this is the case for PEG solutions (polyethylene glycol) and sodium phosphate solutions which can cause fluid disturbance. It is considered that for flexible sigmoidoscopy tap water enemas are sufficient.

6. Endoscopy and variceal bleeding in pregnancy

Variceal gastrointestinal bleedings during pregnancy are true emergencies. A delay in their treatment could lead to serious complications and even death of the mother and fetus. Therapeutic endoscopic procedures (sclerotherapy) are recommended as first line treatment. Effectiveness and relative safety of these approaches during pregnancy is documented in the literature [29]. Octreotide is used to treat variceal bleeding but its safety in pregnancy has not been established.Non-variceal gastrointestinal bleeding were successfully treated with endoscopic therapy during pregnancy using an epinephrine injection plus either placement of hemostatic clips or thermo-coagulation.

7. Endoscopic Retrograde Cholangiopancreatography (ERCP)

It is strongly recommended to be performed by very well trained endoscopists and is indicated in pregnant patients with pancreatitis, cholangitis, choledocholithiasis (complicated with jaundice, impacted or not). If possible, ERCP should be postponed from the first trimester to the second in order to minimize irradiation's potential teratogenic effect. There should be used a lead shielding for the patient's abdomen, a guidewire as opposed to injection of contrast and minimal use of fluoroscopy and spot radiographs.

8. Lower endoscopy

It is indicated in important lower intestinal bleeding, severe unexplained diarrhea and colon neoplasm suspicion. Colorectal cancer screening or change in bowel habits are indications that may be postponed for the postpartum period.

Most of the studies specify **sigmoidoscopy** as a safely procedure during pregnancy (in stable pregnant patients, having strong indication: sigmoid or rectal mass, severe diarrhea – prolonged and not responding to specific treatment, lower intestinal hemorrhage). It should be postponed until after birth for patients complaining abdominal pain or change in bowel habits. Sigmoidoscopy is not causing congenital abnormalities and isn't inducing labor, all studies performed so far reporting delivery of healthy new borns at term.

Colonoscopy safety during pregnancy is not yet properly studied, thus guidelines are not available. It is recommended only for life-threatening situations. Maneuvers like placing the patient in the prone position or exerting external abdominal compression should be avoided, especially in the third trimester of pregnancy.

9. Nonendoscopic imaging modalities of the digestive tract during pregnancy

There can be used endoscopic videocapsules which offer theoretical advantages of gastrointestinal mucosa inspection. They do not need sedation of the patient or mechanical pressure on the abdomen, but safety of their use during pregnancy is unknown. Originally designed to view the small intestine, a change in the original design is now available to inspect the esophagus. It remains to be seen if technical adjustments of this technology will allow future use for the colonas well.

Virtual colonoscopy by MRI is safer during pregnancy than using classic CT. Although still classified as "experimental", virtual technologies are increasingly used as a screening tool for colorectal neoplasia. However, its safety has not been studied in pregnancy although there are some reports showing the usefulness and lack of teratogenicity from abdominal MRI with gadolinium as contrast agent in different clinical situations during pregnancy [30; 31; 32].

10. Conclusions

Performing endoscopies in pregnant patients has not only to be done by a physician experienced in general gastroenterology and endoscopic procedures but also highly experienced in performing such procedures in pregnant women. It is not recommended for these endoscopies to be performed by a beginner, as they carry the unique issue of fetal safety. Endoscopic interventions in pregnancy must be performed quickly and with caution. The endoscopist should always be prepared to discontinue the action at any time for safety reasons. An anesthesiologist and an obstetrician must be part of the working team, especially ready for emergencies.

A number of studies concluded that esophagogastroduodenoscopy and sigmoidoscopy are not contraindicated during pregnancy. If for instance significant upper gastrointestinal bleeding is suspected, emergency esophagogastroduodenoscopy should be performed. Sigmoidoscopy is to be considered when the pregnant patient is stabilized, and only if strong indications for this procedure exist.

Even if no definitive data exist at the present time, ERCP should be performed when the possibility for a sphincterotomy exists. It should only be attempted by highly trained personnel, in a center with extensive experience and the resources to resolve all possible issues that may incur.

Author details

Paul Mitrut[1], Anca Oana Docea[2], Cornelia - Daniela Calina[2] and Liliana Streba[1*]

*Address all correspondence to: lilianastreba@gmail.com

1 Department of Internal Medicine, University of Medicine and Pharmacy of Craiova, Romania

2 Department of Pharmacology, University of Medicine and Pharmacy of Craiova, Romania

References

[1] Mitruţ P., Mitrut Anca Oana, Streba Liliana, Calina Daniela, Salplahta D. Sedation related to gastrointestinal endoscopy. In: Pascu O. (ed.) Gastrointestinal Endoscopy. InTech, 2011; 3: 23-44.

[2] O'MahonyS. Endoscopy in pregnancy. Best Pract Res ClinGastroenterol. 2007; 21: 893-899.

[3] Cappell MS. The fetal safety and clinical efficacy of gastrointestinal endoscopy during pregnancy. GastroenterolClin North A m 2003; 32: 123-179.

[4] Cappell MS, Colon VJ, SidhomOA . A study of eight medical centers of the safety and clinical efficacy of esophagogastroduodenoscopy in 83 pregnant females with follow up of fetal outcome with comparison control groups. A m J Gastroenterol 1996; 9: 348-354.

[5] Qureshi WA, Rajan E, Adler DG, Davila RE, Hirota WK, Jacobson BC, Leighton JA, Zuckerman MJ, Hambrick RD, Fanelli RD, Baron T , Faigel DO. American Society for Gastrointestinal Endoscopy. ASGE Guideline: Guidelines for endoscopy in pregnant and lactating women. Gastrointest Endosc 2005; 6: 357-362.

[6] Acalovschi I, Anestezie clinică, Ed. Clusium Cluj Napoca, 2001.

[7] Gilinsky NH, Muthunayagam N. Gastrointestinal endoscopy in pregnant and lactating women: emerging standard of care to guide decision-making. Obstetrical & Gynecological Survey 2006; 61:791-799.

[8] Frank B. Endoscopy in pregnancy. In: Karlstadt RG, Surawicz CM, Croitoru R, eds. Gastrointestinal Disorders During Pregnancy. American College of Gastroenterology, 1994: 24–29

[9] Cappell MS, Colon VJ, SidhomOA . A study at 10 medical centers of the safety and efficacy of 48 flexible sigmoidoscopies and 8 colonoscopies during pregnancy with follow-up of fetal outcome and with comparison to control groups. Dig Dis Sci 1996; 4: 2353-2361.

[10] Gupta R, Tandan M, Lakhtakia S, Santosh D, Rao GV, Reddy DN. Safety of therapeutic ERCP in pregnancy-an Indian experience. Indian J Gastroenterol 2005; 24: 161-163.

[11] American Society for Gastrointestinal Endoscopy. Guidelines for Endoscopy in Pregnant and Lactating Women. Gastrointestinal Endoscopy. Vol. 61, No. 3: 2005.

[12] American Society of Anesthesiologists (ASA) and the American College of Obstetricians and Gynecologists (ACOG) Statement on non obstetric surgery during pregnancy 10/2009.

[13] Meadows M. Pregnancy and the drug dilemma. FDA Consumer Magazine, May–June 2001. Available at: www.fda.gov/fdac/features/2001/301_preg.html.

[14] Powrie RO. Principles for drug prescribing in pregnancy. Editors: Rosene-Montella K., Keely E., Barbour LA., Lee RV. Medical care of the pregnant patient. 2nd ed. Philadelphia: ACP press. 2008.

[15] Safra MJ., Okley GP., Association between cleft lip with or without cleft palate and prenatal exposure to Diazepam. Lancet 1975; 2: 478-80.

[16] Dolovich LR., Addis A., Vaillancourt JM., et al. Benzodiazepine use in pregnancy and major malformations or oral cleft: metaanalysis of cohort and case-control studies. BMJ 1998; 317: 839-43.

[17] Briggs GG, Freeman RK, Yaffe SJ. Drugs in Pregnancy and Lactation: A Reference Guide to Fetal and Neonatal Risk, 7th ed. Philadelphia: Lippincott Williams & Wilkins, 2005.

[18] Briggs GG, Wan SR. Drug therapy during labor and delivery, part 1. Am J Health Syst Pharm 2006; 63: 1038–1047.

[19] Cunningham FG, Grant NF, Leveno KJ, et al. Analgesia and sedation. In: Cunningham FG, Grant NF, Leveno KJ, et al, eds. William's Obstetrics, 21st Ed. New York: McGraw-Hill, 2001: 537–563.

[20] Cappell MS. The fetal safety and clinical efficacy of gastrointestinal endoscopy during pregnancy. GastroenterolClin N Am 2003. 32: 123–179.

[21] Martin LV, Jurand A. The absence of teratogenic effects of some analgesics used in anesthesia: additional evidence from the mouse model. Anesthesia 1992. 47: 473-6.

[22] Lazear SE, Course 1055: Moderate sedation/analgesia. CME resources. P. 44.

[23] Augustyn D, Brill JV, Faigel D, et al. National Affairs: Three Gastroenterology Specialty Groups Issue Joint Statement on Sedation in Endoscopy. March 8, 2004. Available at: www.acg.gi.org/members/nataffairs/trisociety.asp.

[24] Gin T. Propofol during pregnancy. ActaAnaesthesiol Sin 1994;32:127–132.

[25] Ornoy A, Arnon J, Shechtman S, et al. Is benzodiazepine use during pregnancy really teratogenic? ReprodToxicol 1998; 12: 511–515.

[26] Hawkins JL. Anesthesia for the pregnant patient undergoing nonobstetric surgery. ASA 2005; 33: 137-144.

[27] Boiven JF. Risk of spontaneous abortion in women occupationally exposed to anesthetic gases: A meta analysis. OccupEnviron Med 1997; 54: 541-548.

[28] Kost M. Moderate Sedation/Analgesia: Core Competencies for Practice, 2nd Ed. St. Louis, MO: Saunders, St. Louis; 2004; 59.

[29] Starkel P., Horsmans Y., Geubel A. Endoscopic band ligation: a safe technique to control bleeding esophageal varices in pregnancy. GastrointestEndosc1998; 48: 212-214.

[30] Brown MA, Birchard KR, Seminelka RC. Magnetic resonance evaluation of pregnant patients with acute abdominal pain. Semin Ultrasound CT MR 2005; 26: 206–211.

[31] Pedrosa I, Levine D, Eyvazzadeh AD. MR imaging evaluation of acute appendicitis in pregnancy. Radiology 2006; 238: 891–899.

[32] Garcia-Bournissen F, Shrim A, Koren G. Safety of gadolinium during pregnancy. Can Fam Physician 2006; 52: 309–310.

Chapter 14

Modern Upper Urinary Tract Endoscopy

Puru Naidu, Jessica Packer,
Maheshi Samaraweera and John G. Calleary

Additional information is available at the end of the chapter

1. Introduction

Upper urinary tract endoscopy has come a long way from the first endoscopic examination performed in 1912 by Young and McKay. They used a 9.5 F rigid cystoscope in a patient with a very dilated ureter [1]. Current semi-rigid and flexible instruments are purposely designed to allow diagnostic and effective therapeutic interventions with minimal associated morbidity. The timeline of this evolution is perfectly described elsewhere [2].This chapter summarises the instrumentation available to the modern urologist, the basic principles behind their use and the major clinical outcomes now expected from their use.

2. Technology

This section will describe the endoscopes in modern use and the ancillary equipment we use for therapeutic indications. While some units still use a rigid ureteroscope these have been replaced in many units by semi-rigid and flexible ureteroscopes.

2.1. Endoscopes

2.1.1. Semi-rigid

The semi-rigid ureteroscope is the workhorse of endoscopic ureteric surgery. It was developed from the larger rigid ureteroscope primarily because of concerns about the inability of the rigid scope to access the upper ureter without causing significant damage to the urothelium. The "flexibility" and reduced size are primarily due to the introduction of fibre-optics.

The fibre-optic bundles (clad for image transmission, unclad for light transmission) are fixed at both ends which permits movement without loss of picture quality.

Modern scopes have either straight (Figure 1) or offset eyepiece. The only advantage of the offset eyepiece is that it allows the use of larger therapeutic instruments.The shaft is usually tapered so that the distal diameter (4.5 – 9 F) is less than the proximal (6.5-15F). The difference between proximal and distal diameter varies between manufacturers but is of the order of 2-4 F. The scope length is described as being "short" at approximately 30 cm or long at 40+ cm. Short scopes are useful for the lower ureter in males and lower and upper ureter in females. The long ureteroscope is best for visualisation and treatment in the upper ureter.Within the metallic sheath are the fibre-optic bundles and either one or two working channels. If two channels are being used, one tends to be larger to allow instrumentation and either continued of irrigation or a second working instrument.The distal end tends to be ovoid (figure 2). A variety of accessories are available to improve irrigation flow but the vast majority of procedures are done using gravity, either alone or using pressurised irrigation bags.

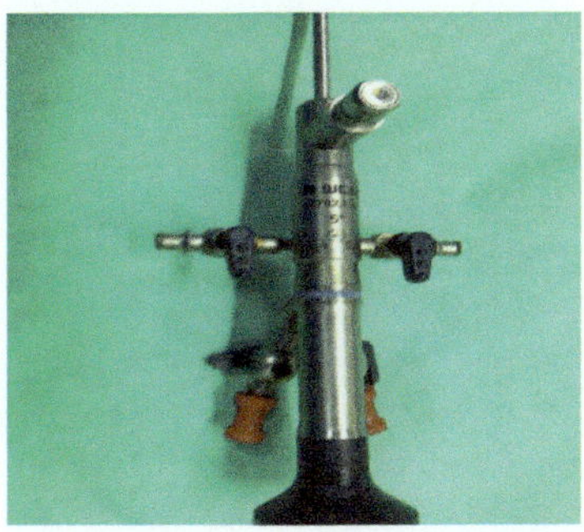

Figure 1. Headpiece of modern semi-rigid Ureteroscope. This model has a straight eyepiece with two working channels each with a red rubber seal. In this model both channels are equal in diameter.

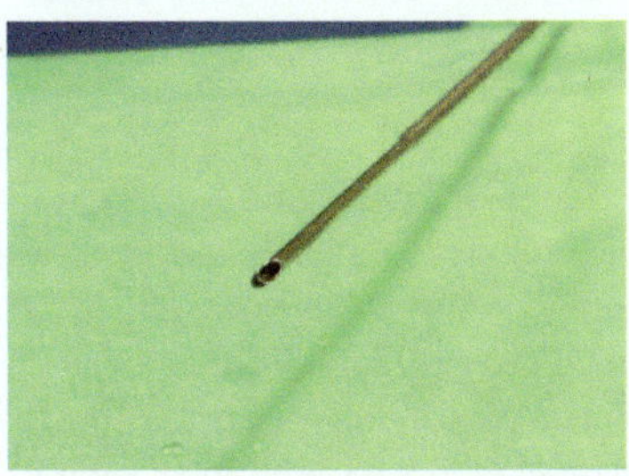

Figure 2. Distal tip of a semi-rigid ureteroscope showing the larger opening of the working channels (right side) compared to the optical opening. Note the stepped appearance as opposed to a more usually seen tapered tapered appearance. The lens is angled at 5 degrees to allow visualisation of the working instruments as they exit the channel.

Semi-rigid ureteroscopes are very durable instruments. The biggest reason for failure is improper use or maintenance. Factors associated with failure are age, shaft design (tapered < stepped) length (long > short) and diameter (narrow > wider). While the instruments flexibility has increased its therapeutic potential, it also increases its susceptibility to breakage and deflections above 5cm are said to be particularly damaging to the instruments [3-4].

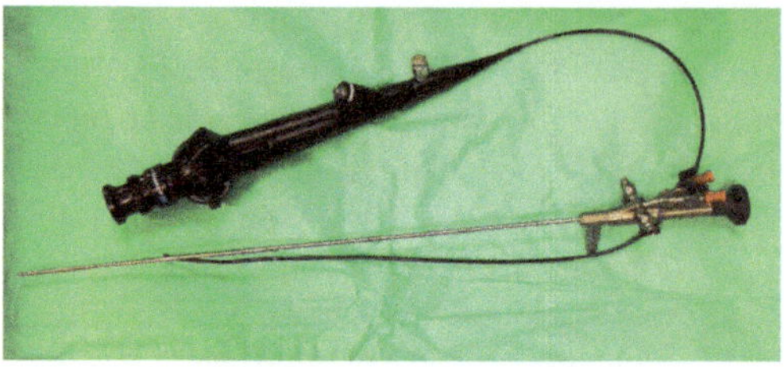

Figure 3. An Olympus flexible ureteroscope (single active deflection, one thumb handle) and Wolf semi-rigid ureteroscope.

2.1.2. Flexible ureteroscopy (figure 3)

2.1.2.1. Historical perspective

The first flexible ureteroscope was introduced through a ureterotomy at open surgery in 1960 [5]. The first trans-urethral instrument was used in 1962 to treat a stone in the lower ureter. This instrument and its immediate successor were diagnostic instruments which could not be manoeuvred. In addition they required forced diuresis to keep the ureter patent. A group from the University of Chicago pioneered the next major developments to incorporate a deflecting tip. This instrument still required insertion into the ureter through a rigid channel but was the first flexible ureteroscope to resemble a modern instrument [6]. The same group were the first to trial an actively deflecting flexible ureteroscope and introduced secondary passive deflection to produce the modern ureteroscope [7].

2.1.2.2. Modern design

The basic design of the instrument is similar to the semi-rigid instrument.Each uses non-coherently arranged light bundles for light transmission (flexi uses 1-2 only) and coherently arranged bundles for image transmission (flexi uses one). Likewise there is a working channel (one) which is usually 3.2 F diameter. In the flexible scope this is cylindrical and situated slightly off-center. This is because of the fibre-optics for image transmission.The degree of eccentricity of the working channel is greater with increasing diameter and results in a disproportionate larger loss of deflection when using instruments. A further loss of deflection ability comes from using "stiffer" instruments.The flexible ureteroscope is also hard wearing but rather than drawing its strength from steel column strength comes from composite polymeric materials. They also come in variable lengths (54 – 70 cm) and are tapered with a distal end of 4.9 – 11 F (most 5.3 – 8.7) and a proximal diameter of 5.8 – 11F(most 7.7-9.9).

2.1.2.3. Differences between semi-rigid and flexible ureteroscopes

The essential difference between the two types of ureteroscope are in terms of optics and ability to deflect. The fibre-optic bundles are smaller in the flexible scope. This usually does not adversely impact on light intensity because of the higher refractive index of the bundles. The angle of view is altered by fitting the distal bundles with an angled lens. Usually this is up to 10° and allows visualisation of instruments as they exit the working channel. The depth of view is less in the flexible scope due to fibre-optic technology, this is compensated for by magnification and focusing. This is a feature common for all flexible endoscopy.

The major difference between the two types of ureteroscope is in the degree of movement available with the flexible instrument. The initial range of deflection was up to 170°. This was based on the measurement of the maximum uretero-infundibular angle [8]. The most modern ureteroscopes can deflect to 270° both sides.

Deflection is sub-divided into active and passive deflection.Active deflection is controlled by a lever mechanism just behind the eyepiece. The basic principle behind this is that moving wires which pass through the scopes cladding and which are fixed to the distal tip causes the scope to bend. Where one lever is present this is called primary active deflection. The most modern scopes have a second active deflection mechanism (figure 4). Passive deflection is facilitated by a "softer" segment of the ureteroscope which on contact with the curves of the intra-renal collecting system allows the scope to be deflected. This allows inspection of and treatment in all parts of the collecting system.

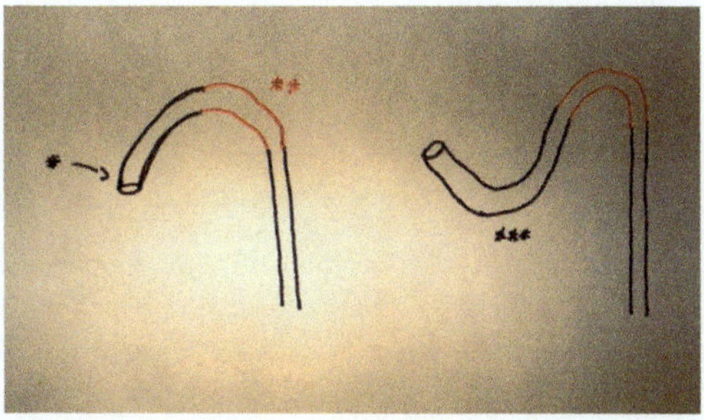

Figure 4. Cartoon depicting deflection in a flexible ureteroscope. The softer segment (**) is represented in red and is the point at which the flexible ureteroscope "bends" on contact with the urothelium. The single * represents the point of primary active deflection and the double ** represents the point of secondary active deflection.

Not surprisingly the flexible ureteroscope does not have the same longevity as the semi-rigid ureteroscope and the cost of repair is about twice that of a semi-rigid ureteroscope. The risk factors for damage are increasing length and decreasing diameter of flexible ureteroscope, instrument or laser damage to the working channel or overzealous deflection within the collecting system especially with an instrument in situ[4]. Pietrow et al have looked at factors to increase the lifespan of flexible instruments. The instrument should be stored with the headpiece upright and the tip dependent. At no time should the shaft be bent, as to do so risks damaging the light bundles. This damage is evident as black dots within the image. When inserting instruments it is best to ensure that the tip is straight and a laser should not be activated until the tip of the fibre is about two mm from the telescope. As repeated insertion can be damaging it is thought that access sheaths can prevent damage. The use of softer wires (eg Nitinol) and smaller calibre laser fibres can also help [9].

2.2. Ancillary technology

These are the instruments and technology which turn the instrument from a diagnostic tool into a potent therapeutic modality.

2.2.1. Tissue / stone destruction

There are four techniques for stone destruction in use in Urology. Of these two (laser and EHL) are most widely used in ureteric and intra-renal endoscopy.Electro-Hydrolic Lithotripsy (EHL) uses the cavitation bubble produced by an electrically induced spark to destroy calculi. This is achieved by the expansion of the bubble resulting in a shock wave, followed by its collapse and rebound off any surface with which it comes into contact. Using a 5F probe up to 90% of ureteral calculi can be successfully treated. The advantage of this technology is that it is relatively inexpensive with low running costs. The disadvantage is that, because of the uncontrollable nature of the shock wave, fragments are propelled forward. This is also the explanation for the ureteric perforation rates of up to 8.5% [10].For best results the probe should be held at a minimum distance of 1 mm from the stone and 1-2 mm from the ureteroscope and urothelium.

Ultrasound, pneumatic and EHL sources are useful only for treating calculi. Hence for treatment of upper tract lesions or haemostasis for biopsy other technologies are required. Contact diathermy probes are available but are limited by size to treating ureteric and renal pelvic lesions. Their use with a flexible ureterorenoscope limits deflection.

The primary energy method used in endourological management of both stones and small volume upper tract TCC is LASER. While many laser types have been used the main laser used is the Holmium: YAG laser (figure 5). The primary reason for this is that it is the only laser capable of destroying any stone type. The Holmium is a solid state pulsed laser with a wavelength of 2100 nm and delivers the enrgy through quartz fibres. The fibres range in size from 200 – 1000 μm. In our unit we use a 270 and 365 μm fibre both of which can be used through a semi-rigid and flexible ureteroscope. Most lasers use an acoustic shock wave (similar to EHL) generated by vaporising the fluid in front of the fibre creating a gas bubble.The Holmium laser does produce vaporisation but its primary effect is photo-thermal thus effectively evaporating the stone or tissue [11]. This produces tiny fragments of approximately the same size as the fibre. This is in contra-distinction to other energy forms which produce uneven larger fragments. However retro-pulsion of fragments can occur being seen most with larger fibres. Like EHL, the holmium laser can damage urothelium and perforate the ureter. However this requires direct contact with the urothelium as because of its high absorption in water the laser energy penetrates no more than 1 mm into hydrated tissue. It has been estimated that this contact time is of the order of two seconds [12].

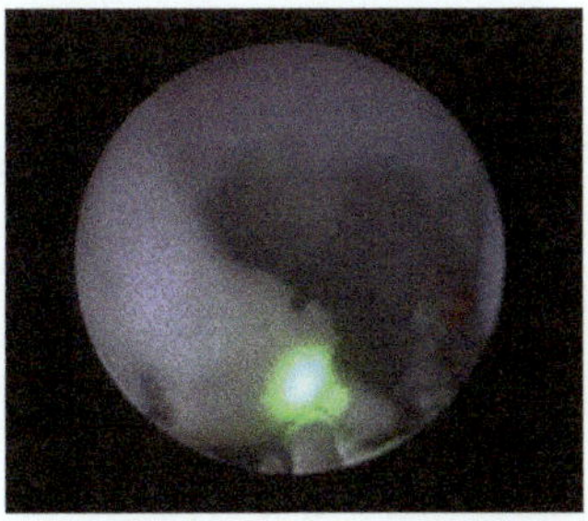

Figure 5. A holmium laser in use on an intra-renal stone at semi-rigid ureteroscopy.

2.2.2. *Anti-migration devices*

As indicated above one of the biggest problems withtreating stones in the ureter is retropulsion. There have been a number of approaches to reducing this migration. The most common approach is to place a device beyond the stone in a closed manner. Once past the stone the device is deployed to form a barrier to retrograde stone passage.The most used examples of this are the Stone cone © (Boston Scientific) (figure 6) and the N-Trap (Cook Medical). The Stone Cone is a Nitinol based wire with a length which is softer and forms a conical shaped when deployed. It is straightened by passing it over a wire and assumes its natural shape once the wire is removed. The N-Trap when deployed from its access sheath forms a basket. Laser lithotripsy is then performed and any fragments which migrate upwards do so into the Cone/Basket. At the end of the lithotripsy procedure, the Cone/Basket is gently removed under vision with the ureteroscope. Both devices are designed to release a stone fragment when a threshold level of pressure is reached. This prevents larger fragments impacting in the ureter at attempted removal.

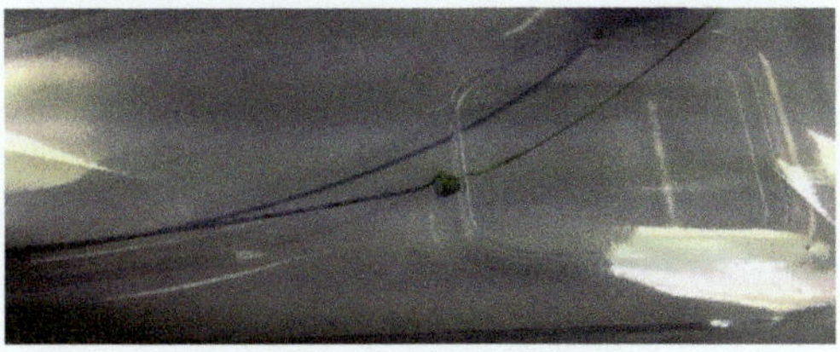

Figure 6. The Stone Cone (Boston Scientific) in its "cone" shape prior to use.

A newer approach is to inject a liquid polymer above the stone which on exposure to body temperature solidifies. This forms a seal or plug which prevents migration. Once the stone is destroyed cold saline irrigation is used which liquefies the gel. The polymers construction is such that any residual gel is degraded and gone from the ureter by two hours. The only commercially available model is the Backstop from Boston Scientific.

2.2.3. Baskets and graspers

These come in multiple shapes and sizes with the primary aim of grasping or trapping the stone fragments. This allows physical removal of the fragments. Graspers tend to have three prongs which facilitates extraction of "larger" fragments. They tend to have a co-axial design with inner and outer sheaths. Retrieval is facilitated by advancing the inner sheath. Baskets are designed to trap multiple small fragments within their Nitinol wires. There are various designs with varying features aimed at improving the stone free rate post lithotripsy. Tipless designs are said to reduce the risk of urothelial perforation. A recent trend is the basket in which laser lithotripsy can be performed with the laser fibre being introduced through the hollow shaft (eg Cook Flat wire stone extractor).

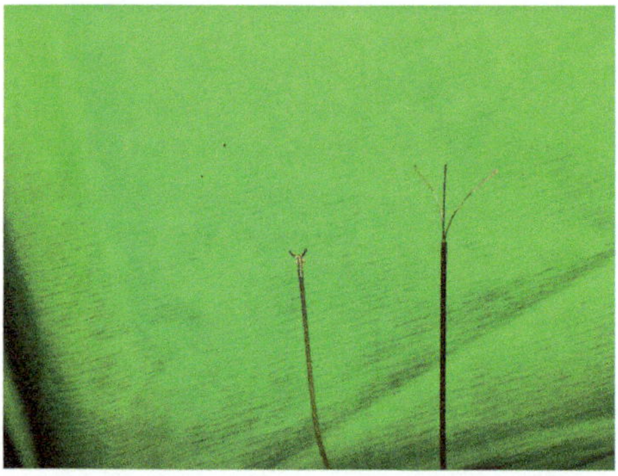

Figure 7. A re-usable ureteroscopic biopsy forceps (left) and a tri-radiate grasper (Captura, Cook medical)

2.2.4. Biopsy forceps

These instruments are a standard part of the endourologists arsenal. They are used for foreign body removal in the case of a migrated JJ stent. Also they are useful for biopsy of intra-ureteric lesions for histological evaluation. However because of size constraints resultant from the dimensions of the ureteroscope, they are very small and the biopsy sample attained is often too small for analysis. A solution to this was developed by Cook. They backloaded a larger biopsy forceps (Bigopty) through the ureteroscope and then connected it to the biopsy handle. The biopsy forceps thus enters the ureter before the ureteroscope and hence can be of greater size (figure 8).

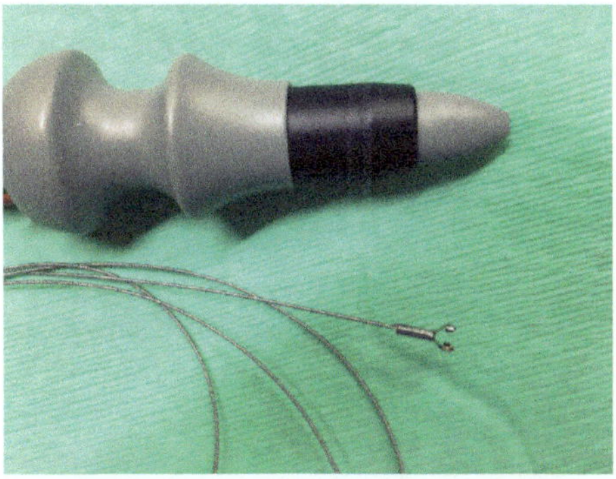

Figure 8. Bigopty (Cook Medical), a backloaded ureteric biopsy forceps,capable of taking large biopsy samples.

3. Ureteroscopy technique

All uretersocopy is preceded by a careful cystoscopy. A negative MSU or treatment with culture appropriate antibiotics is mandatatory. Active infection is the only absolute contra-indication to ureteroscopy. Relative contra-indications are ongoing anti-coagulation therapy or bleeding diatheses. Appropriate antibiotic prophylaxis is given at induction of anaesthesia. This has been shown to reduce infection rates from 13 to 2% [13].Ureteroscopy is usually under a general / spinal anaesthetic with the patient in the lithotomy position but can also be performed in the flank or prone positions.Some authors suggest that the ipsilateral leg be straightened to facilitate ureteral entry.A careful cystoscopy prevents bleeding from the bladder neck which can impair vision and identifies situations where ureteral access is more difficult such as the man with a median lobe or high bladder neck. The primary aim of the cystoscopy is to insert a 0.035 to 0.038 inches guidewire ("floppy" end first) into the relevant ureteric orifice which facilitates the safe introduction of the semi-rigid ureteroscope. This is placed into the renal pelvis under fluoroscopy so that the floppy end is seen to be coiled. This wire is typically called the "safety" wire. Should this prove difficult, the bladder should be emptied and a further attempt made. If it still proves difficult a ureteric catheter can be used to straighten the intra-mural ureter (figure 9). This usually allows the wire to pass. The bladder is emptied on completion to avoid distortion of the ureteric orifice and minimise kinking of the intra-mural ureter.

3.1. Semi-rigid ureteroscopy (AUA and EAU guidelines, ref 14-15)

The initial step is introducing the ureteroscope into the ureteric orifice. The tip of the scope can be passed under a "safety" guidewire to facilitate entry. If this does not permit entry then the scope should be rotated. Should this fail a second wire can be introduced and the tip of the scope passed between the two wires. This is called "rail-roading" (figure 10). If this does not work then the next step is dilatation of the ureteric orifice and should that fail then a JJ stent is placed. This results in dilation by loss of peristalsis. Interval ureteroscopy can then be performed after approximately two weeks.

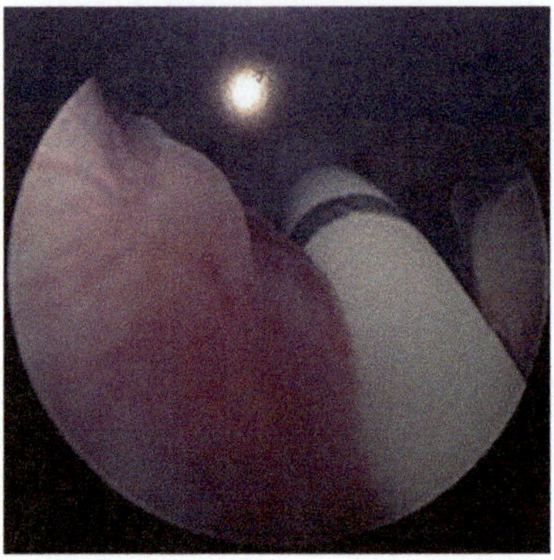

Figure 9. Use of a ureteric catheter (white tube) to facilitate entry into the left ureteric orifice in a man with a median lobe of prostate and a high bladder neck.

A longer ureteroscope is needed in males due to the combination of the longer urethra, the relatively immobile prostatic urethra and the better development of the Psoas muscle. The latter factor can make it difficult to negotiate the ureteroscope beyond the iliac vessels. A second wire can sometimes help straighten a tortuous ureter. However, excessive force should be avoided because of the risk to the ureter (mucosal damage, perforation) and to the ureteroscope because of shear forces.

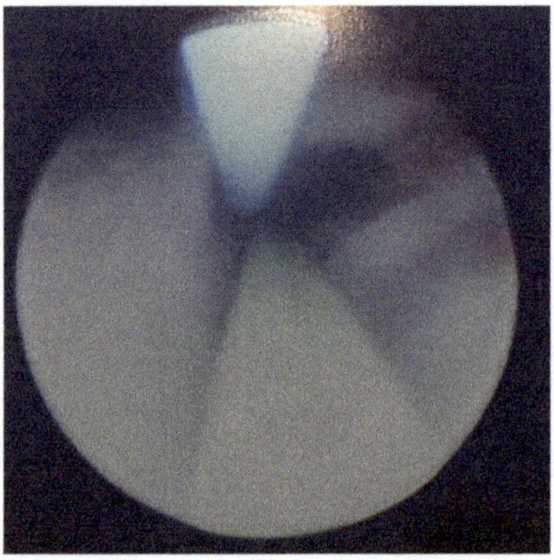

Figure 10. View from a ureteroscope as it is being inserted into the left ureteric orifice between two guidewires (rail-roading)

3.2. Flexible ureteroscopy (AUA and EAU guidelines ref 14-15)

Most flexible ureteroscopy is preceded by a semi-rigid examination of the ureter. This amongst other things dilates the ureteric orifice as well as allowing placement of a second guidewire. This second wire usually straightens out the ureter. There are two schools of thought on flexible ureteroscopic technique. One will introduce the flexible scope into the urethra and either beside or loaded along the guidewire into the ureteric orifice. The other will use a ureteric access sheath to allow repeated easy access to the ureter. A ureteric sheath (figure) is placed over a stiff guidewire under screening to the lower or mid ureter depending on the level at which the operator needs to work. The flexible ureteroscope is then placed through the sheath directly into the ureter. Where repeated insertions/removals are necessary, the access sheath reduces instrumentation time. The advantage of using the sheath is that it may reduce the intra-renal pressure during prolonged stone procedures hence minimising the risk of nephron loss.Once in the collecting system, the flexible ureteroscope can be manoeuvred to directly visualise all calyces. This is by a combination of torquing (twisting) the scope itself and active and passive deflection. Visualisation of the calyces is helped by retrograde contrast injection and radiological screening, thus outlining the whole system.

3.3. Complications of ureteroscopy (specific to ureteroscopy)

Ureteroscopy is performed in the lithotomy position. This position increases the risk of DVT and for this reason most endourologists use compression boots. The risk is small with modern series reporting a risk of 0.2%. The other risk of positioning is damage to nerves such as the common peroneal through inadequate padding. Thankfully the risk is very small and the damage is usually temporary.

Ureteric complications range in severity from bleeding to complete avulsion. Bleeding is usually self limiting and occurs following instrumentation. Its reported in 0-2.1 % of series and usually does not prevent procedure completion. The majority will settle with an indwelling JJ stent/ ureteric catheter for at most two weeks. More significant ureteric damage results in either a tear or perforation. A tear is defined as a breach in the urothelium. It is best to move any stone away fro the tear into dilated ureter to prevent further damage. Again they usually respond to a short period of stenting. Ureteric perforation occurs in one to five percent of modern studies. The rate is decreasing due to increasing experience and (more significantly) smaller calibre instruments.Stenting is the mainstay of management and it is in this situation that the safety wire really helps. The stent can be placed over the safety wire which has been pre-positioned into the renal pelvis. If the patient does not settle or develops an infected urinoma then a percutaneous nephrostomy may have to be placed.It is exceptional to require open repair of a perforation.

Ureteric intussusception (urothelium only, muscle in place) and avulsion are the most severe forms of ureteric injury. Both are due to overly aggressive attempts to remove stone fragments or to forcing a ureteroscope through a narrowed ureteric segment. The golden rule is to stop and re-evaluate. In the case of a ureter which will not accept a scope then the narrowed are can be dilated under radiological screening or a JJ stent can be left for a period of four weeks. The stent causes ureteric dilation and ureteroscopy can usually be completed at the time of stent removal. In the situation where a stone laden basket will not negotiate a narrowed area then it should be gently moved back up to dilated ureter and opened. This will release some fragments and permit a further attempt at removal. If this fails it means that the fragments are too large and further laser lithotripsy is warranted. If the basket will not open then it can be disassembled and laser lithotripsy performed to the fragments within the basket.If either avulsion or intussusception is suspected then an immediate retrograde examination is performed. If the renal collecting system is not outlined with contrast then the diagnosis is confirmed. Drainage of the collecting system is mandatatory and this is usually with a percutaneous nephrostomy. Open surgery is required and the technique used will depend on the site and extent of injury.

4. Upper tract stones

4.1. Introduction

Between 1200 and 1400 per 100,000 people will develop urinary stones each year with a male:female ratio of 3:1.The majority of stones are composed of calcium oxalate, often mixed with calcium phosphate, in both adults and children. The acute presentation is usually unmistakable with the classical history of loin to groin colicky pain. Evaluation with non-contrast CT is advisable for diagnosis. The immediate management usually involves analgesia and treatment of any infection present, and then determining definitive management [14]. Stones smaller than 5 mm will generally pass, but larger stones often require urological intervention [16]. For the purpose of this chapter, the management of upper urinary tract stones will be explored and outlined with the emphasis being on endourological management.

4.2. Management

The options available for the management of upper urinary tract stones include observation, Extra-Corporeal Shock wave Lithotripsy (ESWL), Ureteroscopy, Percutaneous Nephro-lithotomy (PCNL),laparoscopy and rarely open surgical removal. The appropriate modality for each individual patient will depend on the interaction between stone (size, location, appearance of the stone on imaging, composition),anatomical abnormalities, the presence of infection and concomitant co-morbidities which may affect the decision regarding appropriate anaesthetic time.There also is an increasing trend toward intervention because of technological improvements and a growing dissatisfaction with the overall success rates with extracorporeal shock wave lithotripsy [17].

Most stones less than 5mm in size will pass spontaneously.European Association of Urology guidelines state that active stone removal is recommended for renal stones >6-7mm in size [14]. However, those of less than 6mm in size, if symptomatic, can be considered for treatment [14-15].

4.2.1. Non invasive treatment of upper tract stones

ESWL is entirely non invasive, and it uses super sonic waves to fragment stones into small pieces that can be easily passed. Shortly after its introduction in 1983, it became widely accepted as the first line treatment modality for the majority of stones and rapidly replaced invasive surgical options. ESWL is effective for most renal stones less than 2 cm in size and ureteric stones less than 1 cm in size [18].In patients with normal anatomy, and with non lower pole renal stones < 20mm in size, ESWL is recommended as first line treatment. Lower pole stones have a higher failure rate with ESWL and so other treatment modalities should be sought (see below). In one study which compared stone free rates of ureteral stones of variable sizes and locations which were treated by ureteroscopy or extra-corporeal shock wave lithotripsy, ESWL was associated with a success rate of 64% (up to two treatments), as compared to 96% for ureteroscopy in a single treatment [17].

It is important to highlight that certain stone composition such as cystine or phosphate stones may be resistant to fragmentation.There are also multiple other contra indications to the use of ESWL which include pregnancy, bleeding diatheses, severe obesity, anatomical obstruction distal to the stone.

4.2.2. Invasive treatment of upper tract stones

Larger stones, particularly those composed of cystine or struvite, can be approached via establishing percutaneous access to the collecting system through a small flank incision. This would allow direct visualization and intra-corporeal lithotripsy for stone disruption, and removal of fragments known collectively as Percutaneous nephrolithotomy (PCNL).

PCNL has high success rates of around 90% however there are risks onvolved, and major intra-operative or post operative complication rates are often reported as 0.03% to 10% [19]. However, ureteroscopy is fast becoming the main form of treatment for upper urinary tract stone management and this is what will be discussed for the purpose of this chapter.

4.2.3. Selecting the treatment for a patient with stone management

Intra-renal calculi

Different stone sizes respond better to different therapies and success rates are variable for the size of stone. The European Urological Association recommends the following management plan for kidney stones in the renal pelvis or upper/middle calyx, categorised according to size:

Flexible ureteroscopy is used less as a first line treatment for stones > 1.5cm in size. However with ongoing improvements in newer generation flexible ureteroscopes, there is an increasing trend toward ureteroscopy and laser lithotripsy for intr-renal calculi of all sizes and compositions. In the available literature, there are very few reported studies on the use of semi rigid ureteroscopy to treat renal stones. A prospective analysis performed by Bryniarski and co-workers assessed the safety of PNCL and retrograde intrarenal surgery use semi rigid ureteroscopy for the management of renal stones of >2cm in size. Although stone free rates were superior in the PCNL group, the semi rigid ureteroscopy provides advantages for operating times, haemoglobin loss, post-operative visual analogue scoring by patients and reduced hospital stay [20]. The situation is slightly more complex in lower pole stones as the following table shows.

Stones <1cm in size	Stones 1-2cm in size	Stones >2cm in size
ESWL	ESWL or endourology	Endourology (PCNL / flexible ureteroscopy)
Flexible ureteroscopy		ESWL
PCNL		Laparoscopy

Table 1. European Association of Urology (EAU) recommendations for the treatment of Renal stones.

Treatment for renal calculi in the inferior calyx is also very dependent on size:

Stones <1cm in size	Stones 1-2cm in size	Stones >2cm in size
ESWL	Favourable factors for ESWL?	Endourology (PCNL or ureteroscopy)
Flexible ureteroscopy	No -> Endourology	
PCNL	Yes -> ESWL or endourology	

Table 2. EAU recommendations for the treatment of Lower pole stones.

Ureteric Calculi

The management of ureteric calculi is also dependent on the size of the stone involved. The table below outlines the European Urological Association guidelines for Stone management dependent on size of stone:

Location	Stone size	1st choice	2nd choice
Proximal ureter	<10mm	ESWL	Ureteroscopy
	>10mm	Ureteroscopy (retrograde or antegrade) or ESWL	Ureteroscopy (retrograde or antegrade) or ESWL
Distal ureter	<10mm	Ureteroscopy or ESWL	Ureteroscopy or ESWL
	>10mm	Ureteroscopy	ESWL

Table 3. EAU recommendations for the treatment of Ureteric stones

The outcomes of ureteroscopy

The European Association of Urology and the American Urological Association guidelines Panel have published stone free rates for different treatment modalities within their nephrolithiasis guidelines.In a cohort comparison group (early 1980s vs 1992) the success of ureteroscopic procedures rose from 86% to 96%. In addition, they observed an overall decrease in complications (20% to 12%) in ureteroscopy and 6.6% to 1.5% in ureteroscopic laser lithotripsy [21]. Partly, this was thought to be due to greater surgeon experience and that this is significantly correlated to higher success and lower complication rates in ureteroscopic laser lithotripsy with holmium laser [21].

Renal Calculi

The success rates (stone free or insignificant fragments) reported with PCNL are greater than 90% for renal stones >2cm. However, major complications during or after PCNL occur at reported rates of 0.03 % to 10% [22]. The success rates of retrograde intra-renal surgery have been reported as 75-95% for intra-renal stones >2cm after the first or second treatment, whereas the major or minor complications vary from 1.5 % to 12% [23].This is less frequent than rates in PCNL procedures. Major complications in ureteroscopy such as ureteric perforation or avulsion are extremely rare.

Ureteric Calculi

One study of a two year experience, highlighted that the success rates following ESWL were heavily influenced by stone size.The overall stone free success rate was 74.7% with one session. However, as the size of the stone increased, the success rate reduced. For stones <1cm the success ratewas 83.6%and when the stone size > 1cm the success rate reduced to 42.1%. The stone free rates also varied according to the site of the stone - 72.4% (proximal), 70% (mid ureter), and 82% (distal) after a single session [14-15].

In ureteroscopy, an overall stone –free rate of 87.8% was obtained irrespective of the size of the stone (88.9% for <1cm and 86.6% for >1cm). The success rates did slightly vary in relation to the stone site. The stone-free rates were 75% (proximal), 94.6% (mid ureter) and 84.6% (distal) [24].

The American Urological Association recent 2012 guidelines have published stone free rates for Shock Wave lithotripsy and ureteroscopy for the treatment of ureteric calculi and these are outlined in the tables below:

Proximal ureter:

Treatment	Overall	Stone size < 10mm	Stone size >10mm
ESWL	82%	90%	68%
Ureteroscopy overall	81%	80%	79%
Flexible ureteroscopy	89%	84%	

Table 4. Proximal Ureter; stone clearance comparison between Ureteroscopy and ESWL.

Mid Ureter:

The reduced success for stone free rates using ESWL in the mid ureter is likely explained by the anatomical changes at this site. The mid-ureter is closely related to the transverse processes of the lumbar verterbrae and focus of the lithotripsy beam is more difficult due to the anatomical relationships to the spine.

Treatment	Overall	Stone size < 10mm	Stone size >10mm
ESWL	73%	84%	76%
Ureteroscopy overall	86%	91%	78%
Flexible ureteroscopy	88%	Not documented	Not documented

Table 5. Mid Ureter; stone clearance comparison between Ureteroscopy and ESWL.

The reduced success for stone free rates using ESWL in the mid ureter is likely explained by the anatomical changes at this site. The mid-ureter is closely related to the transverse processes of the lumbar verterbrae and focus of the lithotripsy beam is more difficult due to the anatomical relationships to the spine.

Distal ureter:

Treatment	Overall	Stone size < 10mm	Stone size >10mm
ESWL	74%	86%	74%
Ureteroscopy overall	94%	97%	93%
Rigid ureteroscopy	94%	98%	94%

Table 6. Distal Ureter; stone clearance comparison between Ureteroscopy and ESWL.

The use of holmium laser lithotripsy via ureteroscopy is safe and effective in urinary stone management, particularly for larger calculi. It is associated with success rates of more than 90% and with complication rates as low as 10%.

In a study which described 300 procedures of ureteric stone lithotripsy with holmium laser, there was an overall complication rate of 10%. Their overall success rates were 90% and after the first episode, 86% were stone free [21]. In another series of 598 patients, the overall complication rate was 4%, with an overall the success rate of 97% and 94% after the first episode [25].

5. Upper tract Transitional Cell Carcinoma (TCC) / malignancy

Upper tract TCC accounts for approximately 10% of all renal tumors and 5% of all urothelial tumors. It is found to be more common in Caucasian, occurs more often in the sixth to seventh decade of life [26]. Worryingly there is evidence to suggest that the incidence of upper tract TCC is increasing [27]. The presentation is usually with haematuria and approximately 30% will have "ureteric colic" secondary to blood clot [28]. They occur more commonly in people with a history of bladder cancer.

CT Urography is the standard diagnostic tool. However non-visualisation of lesions has been reported in 20% of renal pelvis and 40% of ureteric tumors. Ureteroscopy (semi-rigid or flexible) has been used to improve this accuracy as well as provide histological confirmation (figure 11). Williams et al have shown that ureteroscopic biopsy accurately predicts final histology at Nephro-ureterectomy in 75% of cases and further increases accuracy when combined with exfoliative cytology (brushing the lesion with a brush passed endoscopically) [29]. Ureteroscopic technique is as outlined before with the exception of use of a safety wire. While a wire is used, it should be placed in the ureter under direct ureteroscopic vision. This is because wire related urothelial trauma can mimic TCC and such trauma does make cytological analysis more difficult.

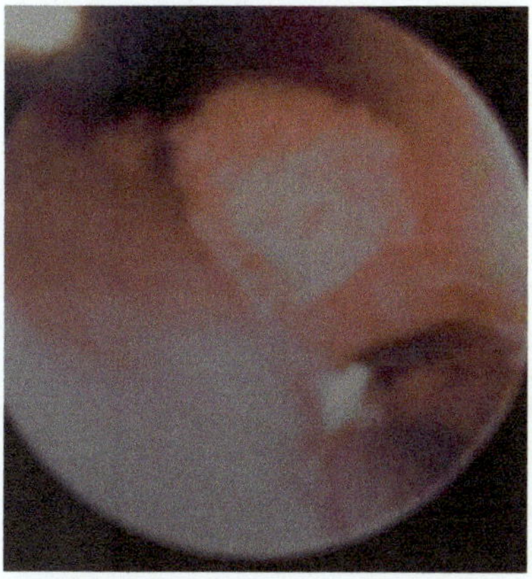

Figure 11. Bigopty ®(Cook Medical) forceps removing a superficial TCC from the ureter.

Radical nephroureterectomy with an ipsi-lateral bladder cuff is still the gold standard treatment for upper tract TCC. Endourological management was initially introduced for those in whom such radical procedure was not possible or who would have required dialysis post operatively. However, the indications for endourological management increased with increased experience [30]. Now endourological management can be considered as potentially curative for all bar those with high-grade or bulky lesions [31].

Because the indications for endoscopic management of upper tract TCC have expanded so rapidly it is difficult to evaluate its efficacy. Potential markers of success are the subsequent recurrence rate and the need for Nephro-ureterectomy.For tumors of the renal pelvis the recurrence rate is quite stable at 40%. This is not that dissimilar to bladder recurrences following endoscopic treatment of bladder TCC.However when looking at recurrences following treatment of ureteric tumors the rates have increased from 14 up to 25% with a corresponding rise in rates of nephro-ureterectomy from 4 up to 14%. It is unclear whether this reflects poor technique or the increasing expansion in use of ureteoscopy for upper tract TCC. As alluded to above the best tumors are those of low grade, solitary and small with a papillary appearance with negative cytology [32]. From the point of view of laser choice the Holmium is best for resection and Neodymium YAG is best for fulgaration.

6. Ureteric stricture / Pelvi-Ureteric Junction (PUJ) obstruction

PUJ obstruction is a functional blockage to antegrade flow of urine to the bladder from the upper tract due to a narrowing at the PUJ. Its classically treated by an open (or laterally laparoscopic) procedure by the name of Pyeloplasty. Retrograde endopyelotomy is a minimally invasive option.This is performed using a large calibre rigid ureterorenoresectoscope or using a Holmium laser. The laser procedure is more common and usually linked with subsequent balloon dilatation of the incised area. The incision is made laterally at the PUJ to minimise vascular injury. The incision is deepened until peri-ureteric fat is seen. Balloon dilatation up to 24 F is then performed and a special stent inserted (Tapered with greater diameter at the top end) for six weeks. Longterm success rates of up to 77% have been reported. Failure usually requires either open or laparoscopic pyeloplasty. A split function of less than 20% and redundant renal pelvis are factors predictive of failure.

Ureteric strictures can also be treated with laser incision. For distal strictures the success rates are of the order of 75% with an average follow-up of 3 years. Failures tend to occur early [33]. Similar results are reported for mid-ureteric and proximal ureteric strictures. The technique for ureteroscopic surgery is again incision to peri-ureteric fat but also includes incision into normal tissue either side of the stricture.

An alternative form of endo-urological stricture management is to use a combined balloon dilator and Monopolar electrode. Identification of the stricture is radiological as once the balloon is inflated with contrast, the stricture will be identified as an indentation on the balloon ie "waisting". As the procedure is not visualised an adequate incision is identified as contrast extravasation.

7. The future

There are now production models of video ureterorenoscopes. Their advantage is that they are smaller, more manoeuvrable with a better picture and fluid flow rate. These instruments use distal chip technology where the incoming light energy impacts on a digital chip. This energy transfer results in a charge which is transmitted along a single fibre to a processor which converts it into a usuable image.The better visual image is primarily due to less transmission loss. Energy (light) loss in fibreoptic ureteroscopes is multi-factorial but involves cladding damage, damage to the fibre-optic bundles, light lead / connection damage and camera head. It is primarily in the treatment of upper tract TCC where the improved imaging will be of most use. The increased magnification and resolution of the images together with technology such as Narrow Band Imaging should expand the place of ureteroscopy in the management of low grade upper tract TCC.

8. Conclusion

The use of endo-urological techniques in day to day urological practice is increasing. This is fuelled by many factors but amongst them is better technology, a greater number of trained individuals and a desire to improve patient experience while maintaining outcomes. The future will be even better as better image definition becomes more readily available as video-ureteroscopes become more durable.

Author details

Puru Naidu, Jessica Packer, Maheshi Samaraweera and John G. Calleary

*Address all correspondence to: johngcall@aol.com.

Department of Urology, Morth Manchester General Hospital, UK

References

[1] Young HH , McKay RE. Congenital valvular obstruction of the prostatic urethra Surg Gynecol Obstet 1929; 48:509-510)

[2] Payne DA, Keeley FX . Rigid and Flexible Ureteroscopes:Technical Features. In: Smith`s Textbook of Endourology, 3rd Ed. Eds Smith AD, Badlani GH, Preminger GM, Kavoussi LR. 2012 Blackwell Publishing

[3] Carey RI, Gomez CS, Maurici G et al. Frequency of ureteroscopic damage seen at a tertiary care center. J Urol 2006;176:607-610

[4] Sung JC, Springhart WP, Marguet CG et al. Location and aetiology of flexible and semi-rigid ureteroscope damage. Urology 2005;66:958-963

[5] Marshall VF, Fibreoptics in Urology J Urol 1964; 91: 110-114).

[6] Bagley DH, Ureteral endoscopy with passively deflectable, irrigating irrigating flexible ureteroscopes. Urology 1987;29:170

[7] Grasso M, Bagley DH A 7.5 / 8.2 actively deflectable ureteroscope: a new device for both diagnostic and therapeutic upper urinary tract endoscopy Urology 1994; 43:435-441

[8] Bagley DH, Rittenburg MH. Intrarenal dimensions. Guidelines for flexible uretero-pyeloscopes. Surg Endosc 1987;1:119-121

[9] Pietrow PK, Auge BK, DelvecchioFC et al Techniques to maxamise ureteroscope longevity. Urology 2003;62:218-222)

[10] Lingeman JE, Matlaga BR, Evan AP. Surgical management of upper urinary tract calculi. In: Wein AJ, Kavoussi LR, Novick AC, Partin AW, Peters CA eds. Campbell Walsh Urology, 9th ed Philadelphia: WB Saunders 2007, 1431-1506.

[11] Chan KF, Vasser GJ, Pfefer TJ, Teichman JM, Glickman RD, Weintraub ST, Welch AJ. Holmium: YAG laser lithotripsy. A dominant photothermal ablative mechanism with chemical decomposition of urinary calculi. Lasers Surg Med 1999; 25:22-37

[12] Santa-Cruz RW, Leveille RJ, Krongrad A. Ex vivo comparison of four lithotriptors commonly used in the ureter: what does it take to perforate? J Endourol 1998; 12:417-422)

[13] Knopf HJ, Graff HJ, Schulze H. Perioperative antibiotic prophylaxis in ureteroscopic stone removal. Eur Urol 2003; 44(1):115-118

[14] Turk F, Knoll T, Petrik A, Sarica K, Straub M, Seitz C. European Urology association guidelines on urolithiasis. http://www.uroweb.org/guidelines accessed 1st August 2012.

[15] AUA / EAU guidelines 2007, Ureteral calculi. http://auanet.org/content/clinical-practise/main-reports/Uretcal07 accessed 1st Aug 2012.

[16] Worcester E, Coe FL. Nephrolithiasis. Prim Care. 2008 June ; 35(2): 369–vii.

[17] Gerber Glenn S. Acharya Sujeet S. Management of ureteral calculi. Journal of endourology. Volume 24 number 6. June 2010. Pp 953-954

[18] Bach C, Buchholz N. Shock wave lithotripsy for renal and ureteric stones.European Urology Supplements. 2011.10 .423-432

[19] Atis Gokhan, Gurbuz Cenk, Arikan Ozgur, Canat Lutfi, Kiic Mert, Caskurlu Turhan. Ureteroscopic Management with Laser Lithotripsy of renal Pelvic Stones. Journal of Endourology. Volume 26. Number 00. 2012. pp 1-5

[20] Bryniarski P, Paradysz A, Zyczkowski M et al. A randomised control study to analyze the safety and efficacy of percutaneous nephrolithotripsy and retrograde intrarenal surgery in the management of stones more than 2cm in diameter. Journal of Endourology. 2012. Vol 26. Pp 52-57.

[21] Leijte Joost AP, Odeens Jorg R, Lock Tycho MTW. Holmiun laser lithotripsy for ureteric calculi: Predictive factors for complications and success. Journal of endourology. Volume 22. Number 23. February 2008. pp 257- 260

[22] Michel MS, Trojan L, Rassweiler JJ. Complications in percutaneous nephrolithotomy. European Urology. 2007. Volume 51. Pp 899 – 906

[23] Breda A, Ogunyemi O, leppert JT, et al. Flexible ureteroscopy and laser lithotripsy for single intra-renal stones 2cm or greater – is this the new frontier? Journal of Urology. 2008. Vol 179. Pp 981-984

[24] Park H, Park M and Park T. Two year experience with ureteral stones: Extracorporeal shock wave lithotripsy v Ureteroscopic manipulation. Journal of Endourology. Vol 12. Number 6. December 1998. Pp 501-504

[25] Sofer M, Watterson JD, Wollin TA, Nott L, Razvi H, Denstedt JD. Holmium: YAG laser lithotripsy for upper urinary tract calculi in 598 patients. Hournal of Urology. 2002. Volume 167. Pp 31-34

[26] Anderstrom C, Johansson SL, Pettersson S, Wahlqvist L. Carcinoma of ureter. J Urol 1989; 142:280.

[27] Munoz JJ et al.(2000) Upper tract urothelial neoplasms: incidence and survival during last two decades. J Urol 164: 1523-25

[28] Murphy DM, Zincke H, Furlow WI Management of high grade transitional cell cancer of the upper urinary tract. J Urol 1981; 125:25-29.)

[29] Williams SK, Denton KJ, Minervini AA, Oxley J, Khastigir J, Timoney AG, Keeley JR FX. Correlation of Upper –Tract Cytology, Retrograde Pyelography, Ureteroscopic appearance and Ureteroscopic biopsy with Histological Examination of Upper-Tract Transitional Cell Carcinoma. J Endourol 2008; 22:1, 71-76

[30] Elliot DS, Segura w, Lightner D, Patterson DE, Blute ML. Is nephroureterectomy necessary in all cases of upper tract transitional cell carcinoma? Long-term results of conservative endourological management of upper tract transitional cell carcinoma in individuals with a normal contralateral kidney. Urology 2001; 58 (2): 174-178.

[31] Painter DJ, Denton K, Timoney AG, Keeley FX. Ureteroscopic Management of Upper-Tract Urothelial Cancer: An exciting Nephron-sparing option or an Unacceptable Risk? J Endourol 2008; 22(8): 1237-1239).

[32] Bagley DH Ureteroscopic diagnosis and treatment of upper urinary trat neoplasms. In: Smith`s Textbook of Endourology, 3rd Ed. Eds Smith AD, Badlani GH, Preminger GM, Kavoussi LR. 2012 Blackwell Publishing

[33] Lane BR, Desai MM, Hegarty NJ, Streem SB. Long-term efficacy of holmium laser endoureterotomy for benign ureteral strictures. Urology 2006; 67: 894-897

Chapter 15

Innovative Uses and Emerging Technologies in Endoscopy

J. Van Den Bogaerde and D. Sorrentino

Additional information is available at the end of the chapter

1. Introduction

Endoscopy is a fast moving field, and new techniques are constantly emerging. In recent decades, gastrointestinal endoscopy has evolved and branched out from a visual diagnostic modality, using fibreoptic bundles, to enhanced video and computer assisted imaging, with impressive interventional capabilities. Some new endoscopic techniques will be too complex or expensive to make the leap into general gastroenterology practice, others already show major progress in the management of digestive diseases. In this chapter we will discuss some of the emerging techniques and technologies used to increase the diagnostic yield in the colon and small intestine including third eye retroscopes, colon capsule endoscopy, balloon and spiral enteroscopy and confocal laser endomicroscopy. We will also discuss over the scope clip (OTSC) devices, a relatively simple and inexpensive tool potentially capable of closing noninvasively intestinal perforations and allowing the removal of infiltrating tumors. Experimental modalities such as natural orifice translumenal endoscopic surgery (NOTES) will also be discussed, with emphasis on their future clinical use. We will also focus on endoscopic ultrasonography (EUS), which has moved from an experimental technique to a valuable established diagnostic modality which not only competes with modern imaging modalities such as MRI, but is also particularly useful in the interventional setting especially in pancreatic and hepatobiliary pathology. We will also discuss the importance of training endoscopists in the use of these new techniques and we will offer some speculation on which of them may become really useful in routine patient care or remain restricted to large teaching hospitals.

2. Improving adenoma detection rate during colonoscopy

The most important task of endoscopists is the early detection and timely removal of colonic polyps. After completing a colonoscopy, the endoscopist should be confident that all polyps have been removed, including proximal flat lesions. Polyps are however missed in up to 35% of colonoscopies, and proximal adenomas are more frequently missed [1]. Proximal sessile serrated adenomas are particularly difficult to diagnose, but are present in up to 13% of screening colonoscopies, and result in colorectal malignancies [2]. Variation in detection rates is related to endoscopic skill and training. Real life data show that colonoscopy reduced mortality from colorectal cancer by 65% [3]. Cancers developing 3 years after a colonoscopy almost certainly represent missed lesions, and as many as 14.4% of right sided neoplasms are not detected during conventional colonoscopy [4]. The data show that endoscopists should focus on improving detection of right sided colonic lesions, where missed lesions and reduction in mortality is not optimal [5,6].

2.1. Retroflexion in cecum

The folds of the colon hide neoplastic lesions, and the majority (93.3%) of undiagnosed polyps hide behind folds [7]. Endoscopists know that rectal lesions close to the anal verge are difficult to see, and experienced operators do a thorough rectal examination and retroflex in the rectum to avoid missing these lesions. According to these principles cecalretroflexion with withdrawal and evaluation of the folds of the ascending colon should also be useful. A recent report has documented that cecalretroflexion was safe, achievable in 94.4%, and increased adenoma detection rate by 9.8% [8]. The advantage of this technique is that conventional equipment is used, all competent endoscopists can perform this, and no perforations were documented in this study. The study is however uncontrolled and the authors report that similar results may be achievable by a careful antegrade second look of the ascending colon. The obvious difficulty of examining the proximal colon has resulted in the development of third eye retroscopes.

2.2. Third eye devices

Third eye retroscopes are thin fibreoptic probes that fit into the working channel of a colonoscope and can examine folds in the ascending colon, which are not easily visible with forward viewing instruments. In controlled studies adenoma detection rates were improved, with better detection of larger rather than smaller lesions [9-11]. Adenomas larger than 6 mm in size were detected at a 25% higher rate, and 10mm or larger lesions at 33.3% [9]. The reason for this preferential visualization of larger and therefore more important lesions with the retroscope was documented by other authors [10], and no clear explanation for this somewhat surprising finding has been advanced.

In expert hands, use of retroscopes increases withdrawal time from 7.58 to 9.52 minutes [11], but increased adenoma detection of approximately 20% seems worthwhile. A potential problem is that once a polyp has been detected the retroscope needs to be withdrawn, to make way for the polyp snare, thus losing sight of the polyp. Cost issues are crucial, and adding an expensive piece of equipment to every colonoscopy will increase costs. Indeed, cost issues may be the most important limiting factor in the universal acceptance of this promising new technology.

2.3. Mucosal enhancement techniques

Changing the appearance of the mucosa is now accepted as a method of increasing adenoma detection. Two methods exist: dye staining and equipment settings such as narrow band imaging. Blue dyes such as indigo carmine and methylene blue are useful in the colon, where mucosal definition and vascular pattern changes are emphasized. Lugol's iodine is useful in the esophagus, but can cause patient discomfort and allergic reactions.

Dye stains increase precision of diagnosis in Barrett's esophagus [12] and ulcerative colitis [13]. Chromoendoscopy using indigo carmine increased adenoma detection rate in a large and well designed study, from 36.3% to 46.2%, with a marginal increase in withdrawal times [14]. It is surprising that dye spray is not used more to increase adenoma detection. Personal experience and reports from working endoscopists suggest that the effort involved with dye spraying reduces enthusiasm for this technique as time goes by. Dye stains have the advantage of being cheap, but also dirty, time inefficient, and produce variable results [15].

Narrow band imaging (NBI) uses filters to emphasize blue coloured light, thus accentuating vascular structures. The touch button activation of this makes it user friendly, and NBI can accurately discriminate between hyperplastic and adenomatous polyps, according to pit patterns with a high sensitivity and specificity [16]. Dysplasia in ulcerative colitis [17] and early gastric cancer [18] are amenable to more precise analysis using NBI. In Barrett's mucosa, NBI has been shown to diagnose high grade dysplasia with a very high sensitivity (96%) and specificity (94%) [19].

The problem with NBI, is that the field depth is much reduced when compared to white light. Inevitably white light is used to see an abnormality, and then interrogation with NBI assists in confirming the pathology. It certainly is a "nice to have" technique for endoscopists who use it regularly, and training endoscopists to analzyse NBI enhanced mucosal pathology is not daunting [20]. Somewhat disappointingly there is little evidence that NBI increases adenoma detection rate, which is really the point of new equipment [21-24].

The diagnosis of difficult-to-see flat or depressed lesions will remain a challenge, In some studies flat lesions are documented in 9.4% of patients, and 33% of depressed lesions are malignant [25]. Endoscopist skill, training, and continued vigilance, in conjunction with ongoing technical advances will increase adenoma detection rate, and hopefully reduce right sided interval cancers.

2.4. CO^2 insufflation

One technical advance which has improved colonoscopy, both for patients and proceduralists is CO2 insufflation. Although described more than 30 years ago recent data have unequivocally shown superiority to room air insufflation [26-28]. In particular, patient recovery and distention after the procedure are markedly reduced. In our opinion, even the smallest unit should strive to change to CO^2 insufflation.

3. Colon capsule endoscopy

Although impressive advances have been made in colonic screening programs, the uptake of colonoscopy, which is the definitive screening tool is still disappointing [29,30]. In a large community based study the uptake of fecal occult blood testing was low (43%, 20.79% men), with obvious limitations of outcome [31].

The perception of what a colonoscopy is, and the perceived danger and invasiveness of the procedure contributes to poor patient uptake [32]. Other less invasive tests such as CT colonography have been suggested, but radiation and inability to detect flat polyps limit the usefulness of this study [33].

The establishment of small bowel capsule endoscopy has resulted in the development of colon capsule endoscopy (CCE), as an alternative to colonoscopy for diagnosis of colonic pathology.

CCE is technically more challenging than small bowel capsule evaluation, since the capsule has to travel through the small bowel, and then into the colon, which requires an increase in battery life. Lesions hidden in folds are difficult to visualize, as they are for conventional colonoscopy, and the bowel has to be even cleaner than for a normal colonoscopy, since mucosal washing is not possible [34].

Technical modifications of the original colon capsule, such as larger batteries, image capturing at both ends of the capsule, and increased image capture rate to accommodate faster colonic transit have improved diagnostic accuracy [35]. Sensitivity for polyp detection with second generation capsules is 89% [35], using colonoscopy as the gold standard.

Bowel preparation has to be rigorous [36], and some issues with capsule battery life remain challenging. Recent evidence-based guidelines for CCE have been produced by the European Society for Gastrointestinal Endoscopy [37].

CCE will probably be used in the same way as CT colonography, as an useful adjunct to colonoscopy. In patients who are at high risk for colonoscopy, or where completion of colonoscopy is not possible, evaluation by CCE may be useful. A small percentage of patients may be put off by colonoscopy and for them, the non invasiveness of CCE would be attractive. Cost comparisons would be essential in determining exactly where the future of CCE lies. Adenoma detection rates in colonoscopy screening populations approximate 50% or more [14,31], which suggests that successful screening procedures would necessitate colonoscopy in a majority of patients anyway, to remove visualized adenomas. Flat lesions remain a problem, regardless of the screening modality employed.

4. Small bowel evaluation and spiral enteroscopy

Small bowel evaluation has become precise and relatively easy with small bowel capsule evaluation. MR enterography has added excellent diagnostic capability, particularly in patients with Crohn'sdisease [38,39].

The different radiological and capsule techniques are complementary, and evaluation of the bowel wall and extraintestinal structures is a particular strength of MR enterography [40].

The challenge of the small bowel is intervention once pathology has been found. A patient with iron deficiency anemia may have small bowel vascular ectasia which are amenable to Argon plasma coagulation, or a polyp which can be removed endoscopically. In the last decade double balloon enteroscopy (DBE) has become an established technique with reported complete small bowel evaluation possible in 40 to 80 % [41]. Subsequently the single balloon enteroscopy (SBE) technique was introduced with lower rates of complete enteroscopy (up to 25% of cases) and a diagnostic yield of 40 - 60% [42,43]. Both DBE and SBE need up to 90 minutes to be completed and are demanding procedures. Complications include perforation (2.3% in SBE) and pancreatitis (0.3% in DBE) [42,43]. Interventions are sometimes difficult due to the unstable endoscope position.

Spiral enterography is a new technique whereby an overtube with a distal thread is placed over a conventional colonoscope and twisted into the small bowel [44]. The insertion time for spiral enterography appears to be shorter than double balloon enterography, but depth of insertion is considerably less [45]. Stent insertion and therapeutic maneuvers may be easier with the spiral technique due to overtubestabilization [46]. DBE uses a Fujinon platform, while the SBE uses an Olympus platform. Spiral enteroscopy has the advantage of using different endoscopic platforms, but its role has not been sufficiently defined to make recommendations yet.

Small bowel pathology is an important part of the work up in a substantial proportion of patients with an undefined iron deficiency anemia. The chosen diagnostic modality depends on availability and expertise, but small bowel capsule is probably the choice examination for the time being. Once pathology has been identified, the depth of the lesion in the small bowel determines which of the three interventional modalities is optimal. DBE is the established technology, but in more proximal small bowel lesions, particularly if stenting is required, spiral enterography may be the procedure of choice. The role of this technology outside teaching hospitals awaits good comparative studies.

5. ERCP and endoscopic ultrasound

Ironically the greatest advance in ERCP in the last 10 years is the development of MRCP, which has almost completely dispensed with the need for diagnostic ERCP. Techniques have not really changed in 10 years, although some useful stent modifications have occurred. Novel stenting devices include stents impregnated with radioactive seeds, which not only can palliatively drain obstructed common bile ducts, but also irradiate the contiguous pancreatic malignancy [47].

The interplay between endoscopic ultrasound (EUS) and ERCP in challenging patients is an interesting new development. ERCP drainage of malignant biliary strictures often fails, and EUS drainage bypassing the papilla is feasible, and in expert hands has a high success rate [48,49].

Patients with altered anatomy after surgery present a special challenge, and ERCP may be impossible. In expert hands EUS can assist in placing stents, but the authors of an authorative review point out that the technical difficulties and the specialized nature of these interventions are best left to experts in referral centres [50]. Certainly these technologies are not going to enter community based departments soon.

Exciting applications of EUS based interventions include the now standard celiac plexus blocks and drainage of pseudocysts, as well as inplantation of radioactive seeds and even viral vectors in tumours, ablation of cysts, variceal cyanoacrylate injection, and vascular coil placement [47,51-53]. Obviously these techniques are at the moment very far from mainstream gastroenterology.

6. Confocal laser endomicroscopy

Confocal laser endomicroscopy (CLE) is a technology which allows real time histology of the mucosa during upper and lower endoscopy. Laser illumination of the mucosa combined with fluorescent dye illumination enables immediate and precise "microscopic" evaluation of mucosal lesions [54]. Fluorescent dye injection is essential for this technique, and tissue uptake occurs within seconds of injection. There is a very extensive literature of fluorescent dye injection in ophtalmology, confirming its excellent safety profile. The limitation of fluorescein is that it highlights cells, connective tissue and vessels but not nuclear material. Topical application of acroflavine stains cell nuclei, and can be used separately or in addition to fluorescein.

Depth of view of the endoscopic CLE system is up to 250 μm, while the probe system which is inserted down the working channel of any endoscope has a more limited depth of view [55]. The area which can be examined is limited - no more than 700 μm^2 in the endoscopy based system and even less in the smaller probe based system so precise targeting is important. New generation probes can be placed through needles allowing novel approaches to endoultrasonographic tissue sampling, hepatobiliary assessment, and even laparoscopically assisted real time hepatic tissue histology [56].

CLE has been used extensively in evaluating Barrett's mucosa. It has also been used in patients with colonic neoplasia, gastric metaplasia, and celiac disease.

When used in combination with conventional endoscopy, CLE allows excellent prediction of high grade dysplasia and malignancy in Barrett's mucosa [57]. In addition to targeting biopsies, assessment of submucosal tissue, which may be particularly important in patients who have undergone ablation of Barrett's dysplasia can be performed. CLE predicted malignancy in Barrett's lesions with a specificity of 96%, and sensitivity of 88% [58]. CLE combined with four quadrant biopsies was twice as effective in detecting neoplasia, and the majority of patients in the CLE arm did not need biopsies at all [59].

Gastric metaplasia or malignancy are amenable to CLE evaluation, with high accuracy and reproducibility, and significantly better accuracy than conventional endoscopy [60-62].

During colonoscopy CLE polyp evaluation, when compared with standard histology produces sensitivity for adenoma of 97.3%, while high and low grade dysplasia was analyzed accurately in 96.7% [63]. CLE evaluation in patients with UC resulted in far higher detection of intra-epithelial neoplasia (4.75 fold), as well as reducing the number of biopsies by half [64].

The future focus of CLE is the use of specific labeled markers in a method similar to immunohistochemistry, to light up pre malignant or malignant mucosa [65,66] The application of this methodology beyond the research setting is however still unclear.

The concept of optical biopsies [67] has been well established for colonic and gastric neoplastic lesions, particularly by Japanese endoscopists assessing flat colonic lesions, but microscopic *in vivo* biopsies using CLE technology advances this concept to a new level. What has not been addressed is the medico legal issue related to this technique. How confident can an endoscopist be when making a diagnosis by CLE of high grade dysplasia in a patient with Barrett's esophagus, and use only this information to guide subsequent therapy? In these cases the gold standard will remain conventional histopathology, with its established and extensive guidelines.

Finally, this technology does not improve detection rate of suspicious lesions, but relies on conventional endoscopic evaluation to target the optical biopsy. As discussed at the beginning of this chapter, the greatest problem with endoscopy is the missed lesion. Although the reduced number of biopsies is mentioned as an advantage this is a tenuous advantage at most. The time taken to analyze tissue by CLE, would be easily spent taking more biopsies if clinically indicated. In a recent study the advantage of optical biopsy in patients on anticoagulation is brought forward as a reason to pursue *in vivo*histology [68] but current guidelines do not exclude patients on anticoagulation from undergoing biopsy [69].

Although CLE appears glamorous and exciting as a technology, it has been around for almost a decade, and has not really expanded its reach beyond the research setting. The time constraints, expense and technical difficulties probably will keep this as a "nice to have" technology in selected tertiary hospitals where enthusiasts will use it.

7. Over the scope clip devices

Colonic perforation remains an important complication of colonoscopy, with a large recent series reporting an alarming 0.33% rate [70].

Both diagnostic and therapeutic interventions can cause perforation, and even argon plasma coagulation (APC) can result in perforations. Even in the best hands, perforation occurs when complex polyps are removed, and indeed increased polyp detection and removal of increasingly large polyps will result in more rather than less colonic endoscopic complications [71].

Over the scope clip devices (OTSC) are pre armed on a transparent silicone cap, and are released by winding up a pre loaded thread similar to band ligators. A large pair of forceps is passed through the working channel to approximate the defect and pull the tissue into the cap, followed by release of the bear trap-like device. Even deep lesions penetrating into the serosa can be closed. OTSC devices have been successfully used in animal models to close full thickness perforations [72]. Perforation closure strength has been shown to approximate conventional surgical techniques [73].

In a small clinical case report study perforation closure was achieved in 6 of 7 cases, and avoidance of any surgery achieved in 4 of 7 [74]. Perforations of up to 20 mm were managed using these clips in a clinical setting [75], and surgery was performed in only one of 10 patients.

These clips have been shown to close colonic fistulae, without surgical intervention [76]. In another report, 11 of 12 patients were treated successfully for chronic fistulae and colonic perforations with no reported complications [77]. Placing clips is technically challenging, but a mean procedure time of 54 minutes for fistula closure is not dauntingly long when compared to other difficult endoscopic techniques [78].

Even refractory chronic duodenal fistula and esophageal anastomotic perforation after gastrectomy have been managed by OTSC devices [78,79].

The bear trap structure of these clips does however demands caution when placing, and very careful consideration of clip removal if placement is incorrect.

Large defects greater than 2.5 cm are not amenable to treatment with these clips, but application of more than one clip may be helpful. Severe fibrosis over a large area is also not amenable to clip application in patients with long standing ulcers or fistulae. Reports of complications are scarce. One paper reports no complications [77] but post clip pain may be due to grasping of visceral fat or peritoneum [75]. Strictures can also develop, particularly when large portions of mucosa are grasped and clipped.

In addition, when drawing back the mucosa with forceps, the clip must not grasp the forceps during deployment, since loosening of the clip is impossible. This then results in the clip and forceps being stuck in the channel of the endoscope, and stuck to the mucosa. Surgical removal is the only option: a true endoscopic nightmare.

OTSC devices can control bleeding in animal models [80]. A recent study of upper gastrointestinal bleeding documented a 13% re-bleed rate after initial endoscopy, and a mortality of 10% [81]. Although the study does not precisely detail the endoscopic appearance of peptic ulcers in re-bleeding patients, a substantial percentage of these patients probably had chronic fibrotic ulceration, with endoscopically difficult to control visible vessels in the ulcer base. It is well recognized that these patients often re-bleed and need surgical intervention. Placing conventionally available clipping devices on these vessels is challenging, dangerous and often unsuccessful. In theory, the OTSC device offers a far better approach to these patients, and this indication may actually become the most important of these devices.

7.1. OTSC and endoscopic submucosal dissection

Endoscopic submucosal dissection (ESD) allows *en block* removal of gastric and colonic neoplasia. Perforation rates of 4.1% in gastric [82] and as high as 20.4% in colon lesions have been reported [83]. OTSC devices may assist in closing some of the larger perforations in these patients. Full thickness endoscopic resection of tumours or polyps is possible with a combination of OTSC and snare devices [84]. In those patients where endoultrasonography has shown invasion of the muscular wall, and endoscopic mucosal resection (EMR) or endoscopic submucosal dissection (ESD) is not feasible, the OTSC device may offer a non surgical approach for removal of these neoplastic and invasive lesions in selected patients. In particular, this technique could be potentially useful in treating gastrointestinal stroma tumors, granulosa cell tumours, carcinoids, or any other slowly growing neoplasms which invade the muscular wall and are therefore not amenable to other endoscopic techniques.

7.2. NOTES

One of the problems of natural orifice translumenal endoscopic surgery (NOTES) procedures is the gastrostomy, which may be amenable to OTSC closure [85]. However, NOTES remains a modality that has yet to find its place outside the experimental sphere. The technical challenges of these procedures, with the relatively minimal gain of avoiding minor entrance wounds in laparoscopic surgery, would suggest that these techniques may not be going to become routine.

8. Endoscopic control of bleeding

Techniques for controlling bleeding have not substantially changed in the last decade, but a new method of nanopowder spray seems to be both effective and easy to apply [86,87]. This powder could be of potential benefit in difficult to control arterial bleeds, where visibility is an issue, or as a bridge to surgery. The major advantage of this would possibly be that less experienced endoscopists could obtain control of bleeding, without performing technically difficult procedures. In our opinion, most senior endoscopy consultants would appreciate this modality if it would mean that more junior consultants could safely handle emergency bleeds.

Author details

J. Van Den Bogaerde[1,2*] and D. Sorrentino[1,2,3]

*Address all correspondence to: Johan_van_den_Bogaerde@health.qld.gov.au

1 Department of Gastroenterology, Nambour General Hospital, University of Queensland, Australia

2 Sunshine Coast Clinical School, Australia

3 University of Udine Medical School, Udine, Italy

References

[1] Laiyemo AO, Doubeni C, Sanderson AK, Pinsky PF, Badurdeen DS, Doria-Rose VP, et al. Likelihood of missed and recurrent adenomas in the proximal versus the distal colon. GastrointestEndosc 2011, Aug;74(2):253-61.

[2] Kahi CJ, Hewett DG, Norton DL, Eckert GJ, Rex DK. Prevalence and variable detection of proximal colon serrated polyps during screening colonoscopy. ClinGastroenterolHepatol 2011, Jan;9(1):42-6.

[3] Kahi CJ, Imperiale TF, Juliar BE, Rex DK. Effect of screening colonoscopy on colorectal cancer incidence and mortality. ClinGastroenterolHepatol 2009, Jul;7(7):770-5; quiz 711.

[4] Singh H, Nugent Z, Demers AA, Bernstein CN. Rate and predictors of early/missed colorectal cancers after colonoscopy in manitoba: A population-based study. Am J Gastroenterol 2010, Dec;105(12):2588-96.

[5] Singh H, Nugent Z, Demers AA, Kliewer EV, Mahmud SM, Bernstein CN. The reduction in colorectal cancer mortality after colonoscopy varies by site of the cancer. Gastroenterology 2010, Oct;139(4):1128-37.

[6] Brenner H, Hoffmeister M, Arndt V, Stegmaier C, Altenhofen L, Haug U. Protection from right- and left-sided colorectal neoplasms after colonoscopy: Population-based study. J Natl Cancer Inst 2010, Jan 1;102(2):89-95.

[7] Pickhardt PJ, Nugent PA, Mysliwiec PA, Choi JR, Schindler WR. Location of adenomas missed by optical colonoscopy. Ann Intern Med 2004, Sep 9;141(5):352-9.

[8] Hewett DG, Rex DK. Miss rate of right-sided colon examination during colonoscopy defined by retroflexion: An observational study. GastrointestEndosc 2011, Aug;74(2): 246-52.

[9] Waye JD, Heigh RI, Fleischer DE, Leighton JA, Gurudu S, Aldrich LB, et al. A retrograde-viewing device improves detection of adenomas in the colon: A prospective efficacy evaluation (with videos). GastrointestEndosc 2010, Mar;71(3):551-6.

[10] DeMarco DC, Odstrcil E, Lara LF, Bass D, Herdman C, Kinney T, et al. Impact of experience with a retrograde-viewing device on adenoma detection rates and withdrawal times during colonoscopy: The third eye retroscope study group. GastrointestEndosc 2010, Mar;71(3):542-50.

[11] Leufkens AM, DeMarco DC, Rastogi A, Akerman PA, Azzouzi K, Rothstein RI, et al. Effect of a retrograde-viewing device on adenoma detection rate during colonoscopy: The TERRACE study. GastrointestEndosc 2011, Mar;73(3):480-9.

[12] Kouklakis GS, Kountouras J, Dokas SM, Molyvas EJ, Vourvoulakis GP, Minopoulos GI. Methylene blue chromoendoscopy for the detection of barrett's esophagus in a greek cohort. Endoscopy 2003, May;35(5):383-7.

[13] Kiesslich R, Fritsch J, Holtmann M, Koehler HH, Stolte M, Kanzler S, et al. Methylene blue-aided chromoendoscopy for the detection of intraepithelial neoplasia and colon cancer in ulcerative colitis. Gastroenterology 2003, Apr;124(4):880-8.

[14] Pohl J, Schneider A, Vogell H, Mayer G, Kaiser G, Ell C. Pancolonicchromoendoscopy with indigo carmine versus standard colonoscopy for detection of neoplastic lesions: A randomised two-centre trial. Gut 2011, Apr;60(4):485-90.

[15] Kwan V. Advances in gastrointestinal endoscopy. Intern Med J 2012, Feb;42(2): 116-26.

[16] East JE, Suzuki N, Bassett P, Stavrinidis M, Thomas HJ, Guenther T, et al. Narrow band imaging with magnification for the characterization of small and diminutive colonic polyps: Pit pattern and vascular pattern intensity. Endoscopy 2008, Oct; 40(10):811-7.

[17] Esaki M, Kubokura N, Kudo T, Matsumoto T. Endoscopic findings under narrow band imaging colonoscopy in ulcerative colitis. Dig Endosc 2011, May;23Suppl 1:140-2.

[18] Zhang J, Guo S-B, Duan Z-J. Application of magnifying narrow-band imaging endoscopy for diagnosis of early gastric cancer and precancerous lesion. BMC Gastroenterol 2011;11:135.

[19] Mannath J, Subramanian V, Hawkey CJ, Ragunath K. Narrow band imaging for characterization of high grade dysplasia and specialized intestinal metaplasia in barrett's esophagus: A meta-analysis. Endoscopy 2010, May;42(5):351-9.

[20] Higashi R, Uraoka T, Kato J, Kuwaki K, Ishikawa S, Saito Y, et al. Diagnostic accuracy of narrow-band imaging and pit pattern analysis significantly improved for less-experienced endoscopists after an expanded training program. GastrointestEndosc 2010, Jul;72(1):127-35.

[21] Sabbagh LC, Reveiz L, Aponte D, de Aguiar S. Narrow-band imaging does not improve detection of colorectal polyps when compared to conventional colonoscopy: A randomized controlled trial and meta-analysis of published studies. BMC Gastroenterol 2011;11:100.

[22] Ikematsu H, Saito Y, Tanaka S, Uraoka T, Sano Y, Horimatsu T, et al. The impact of narrow band imaging for colon polyp detection: A multicenter randomized controlled trial by tandem colonoscopy. J Gastroenterol 2012, Mar 3.

[23] Nagorni A, Bjelakovic G, Petrovic B. Narrow band imaging versus conventional white light colonoscopy for the detection of colorectal polyps. Cochrane Database Syst Rev 2012;1:CD008361.

[24] Pasha SF, Leighton JA, Das A, Harrison ME, Gurudu SR, Ramirez FC, et al. Comparison of the yield and miss rate of narrow band imaging and white light endoscopy in patients undergoing screening or surveillance colonoscopy: A meta-analysis. Am J Gastroenterol 2012, Mar;107(3):363-70; quiz 371.

[25] Soetikno RM, Kaltenbach T, Rouse RV, Park W, Maheshwari A, Sato T, et al. Prevalence of nonpolypoid (flat and depressed) colorectal neoplasms in asymptomatic and symptomatic adults. JAMA 2008, Mar 3;299(9):1027-35.

[26] Hsu W-H, Sun M-S, Lo H-W, Tsai C-Y, Tsai Y-J. Carbon dioxide insufflation during withdrawal of the colonoscope improved postprocedure discomfort: A prospective, randomized, controlled trial. Kaohsiung J Med Sci 2012, May;28(5):265-9.

[27] Geyer M, Guller U, Beglinger C. Carbon dioxide insufflation in routine colonoscopy is safe and more comfortable: Results of a randomized controlled double-blinded trial. DiagnTherEndosc 2011;2011:378906.

[28] Wang WL, Wu ZH, Sun Q, Wei JF, Chen XF, Zhou DK, et al. Meta-analysis: The use of carbon dioxide insufflation vs. Room air insufflation for gastrointestinal endoscopy. Aliment PharmacolTher 2012, May;35(10):1145-54.

[29] McGregor SE, Hilsden RJ, Li FX, Bryant HE, Murray A. Low uptake of colorectal cancer screening 3 yr after release of national recommendations for screening. Am J Gastroenterol 2007, Aug;102(8):1727-35.

[30] Hoffman-Goetz L, Thomson MD, Donelle L. Reasons for declining colorectal cancer screening by older canadians: A pilot study. J Cancer Educ 2008;23(1):32-6.

[31] Gupta S, Saunders BP, Fraser C, Kennedy RH, Ignjatovic A, Sala S, et al. The first 3 years of national bowel cancer screening at a single UK tertiary centre. Colorectal Dis 2012, Feb;14(2):166-73.

[32] Marshall DA, Johnson FR, Kulin NA, Ozdemir S, Walsh JME, Marshall JK, et al. How do physician assessments of patient preferences for colorectal cancer screening tests differ from actual preferences? A comparison in canada and the united states using a stated-choice survey. Health Econ 2009, Dec;18(12):1420-39.

[33] Hock D, Ouhadi R, Materne R, Mancini I, Nchimi A. Screening for colorectal cancer in asymptomatic average risk patients: Role of imaging. ActaGastroenterolBelg 2011, Mar;74(1):70-6.

[34] Sieg A. Colon capsule endoscopy compared with conventional colonoscopy for the detection of colorectal neoplasms. Expert Rev Med Devices 2011, Mar;8(2):257-61.

[35] Eliakim R, Yassin K, Niv Y, Metzger Y, Lachter J, Gal E, et al. Prospective multicenter performance evaluation of the second-generation colon capsule compared with colonoscopy. Endoscopy 2009, Dec;41(12):1026-31.

[36] Spada C, Hassan C, Ingrosso M, Repici A, Riccioni ME, Pennazio M, et al. A new regimen of bowel preparation for pillcam colon capsule endoscopy: A pilot study. Dig Liver Dis 2011, Apr;43(4):300-4.

[37] Spada C, Hassan C, Galmiche JP, Neuhaus H, Dumonceau JM, Adler S, et al. Colon capsule endoscopy: European society of gastrointestinal endoscopy (ESGE) guideline. Endoscopy 2012, May;44(5):527-36.

[38] Smith EA, Dillman JR, Adler J, Dematos-Maillard VL, Strouse PJ. MR enterography of extraluminal manifestations of inflammatory bowel disease in children and adolescents: Moving beyond the bowel wall. AJR Am J Roentgenol 2012, Jan; 198(1):W38-45.

[39] Herraiz Hidalgo L, Alvarez Moreno E, CarrascosoArranz J, Cano Alonso R, Martínez de Vega Fernández V. [Magnetic resonance enterography: Review of the technique for the study of crohn's disease]. Radiologia 2011;53(5):421-33.

[40] Tennyson CA, Semrad CE. Advances in small bowel imaging. CurrGastroenterol Rep 2011, Oct;13(5):408-17.

[41] Yamamoto H, Sekine Y, Sato Y, Higashizawa T, Miyata T, Iino S, et al. Total enteroscopy with a nonsurgical steerable double-balloon method. GastrointestEndosc 2001, Feb;53(2):216-20.

[42] Kawamura T, Yasuda K, Tanaka K, Uno K, Ueda M, Sanada K, Nakajima M. Clinical evaluation of a newly developed single-balloon enteroscope. GastrointestEndosc 2008, Dec;68(6):1112-6.

[43] Tsujikawa T, Saitoh Y, Andoh A, Imaeda H, Hata K, Minematsu H, et al. Novel single-balloon enteroscopy for diagnosis and treatment of the small intestine: Preliminary experiences. Endoscopy 2008, Jan;40(1):11-5.

[44] Akerman PA, Cantero D. Spiral enteroscopy and push enteroscopy. GastrointestEndoscClin N Am 2009, Jul;19(3):357-69.

[45] Frieling T, Heise J, Sassenrath W, Hülsdonk A, Kreysel C. Prospective comparison between double-balloon enteroscopy and spiral enteroscopy. Endoscopy 2010, Nov; 42(11):885-8.

[46] Lennon AM, Chandrasekhara V, Shin EJ, Okolo PI. Spiral-enteroscopy-assisted enteral stent placement for palliation of malignant small-bowel obstruction (with video). GastrointestEndosc 2010, Feb;71(2):422-5.

[47] Du Y-Q, Li Z-S, Jin Z-D. Endoscope-assisted brachytherapy for pancreatic cancer: From tumor killing to pain relief and drainage. J IntervGastroenterol 2011;1(1):23-7.

[48] Kim TH, Kim SH, Oh HJ, Sohn YW, Lee SO. Endoscopic ultrasound-guided biliary drainage with placement of a fully covered metal stent for malignant biliary obstruction. World J Gastroenterol 2012, May 5;18(20):2526-32.

[49] Park DH, Koo JE, Oh J, Lee YH, Moon S-H, Lee SS, et al. EUS-guided biliary drainage with one-step placement of a fully covered metal stent for malignant biliary obstruction: A prospective feasibility study. Am J Gastroenterol 2009, Sep;104(9):2168-74.

[50] Will U, Meyer F. [Endoscopic ultrasonography (EUS)-guided transluminalcholangiodrainage (EUCD) - a novel option of interventional endoscopy in the interdiciplinary management of obstructive jaundice]. ZentralblChir 2012, Feb;137(1):20-31.

[51] Cho CM, Dewitt J, Al-Haddad M. Echo-endoscopy: New therapeutic frontiers. Minerva GastroenterolDietol 2011, Jun;57(2):139-58.

[52] Ponnudurai R, Sachithanandan S, George A. Endoscopic ultrasound-guided injection therapy for hepatobiliary disease. J HepatobiliaryPancreatSci 2011, May;18(3):311-8.

[53] Trevino JM, Varadarajulu S. Endoscopic ultrasonography-guided ablation therapy. J HepatobiliaryPancreatSci 2011, May;18(3):304-10.

[54] Kiesslich R, Goetz M, Neurath MF. Confocal laser endomicroscopy for gastrointestinal diseases. GastrointestEndoscClin N Am 2008, Jul;18(3):451-66, viii.

[55] Matloff JL, Abidi W, Richards-Kortum R, Sauk J, Anandasabapathy S. High-resolution and optical molecular imaging for the early detection of colonic neoplasia. GastrointestEndosc 2011, Jun;73(6):1263-73.

[56] Wallace MB, Fockens P. Probe-based confocal laser endomicroscopy. Gastroenterology 2009, May;136(5):1509-13.

[57] Canto MI. Endomicroscopy of barrett's esophagus. GastroenterolClin North Am 2010, Dec;39(4):759-69.

[58] Wallace MB, Sharma P, Lightdale C, Wolfsen H, Coron E, Buchner A, et al. Preliminary accuracy and interobserver agreement for the detection of intraepithelial neoplasia in barrett's esophagus with probe-based confocal laser endomicroscopy. GastrointestEndosc 2010, Jul;72(1):19-24.

[59] Dunbar KB, Okolo P, Montgomery E, Canto MI. Confocal laser endomicroscopy in barrett's esophagus and endoscopicallyinapparentbarrett'sneoplasia: A prospective, randomized, double-blind, controlled, crossover trial. GastrointestEndosc 2009, Oct; 70(4):645-54.

[60] Guo Y-T, Li Y-Q, Yu T, Zhang T-G, Zhang J-N, Liu H, et al. Diagnosis of gastric intestinal metaplasia with confocal laser endomicroscopy in vivo: A prospective study. Endoscopy 2008, Jul;40(7):547-53.

[61] Li C-Q, Li Y-Q. Endomicroscopy of intestinal metaplasia and gastric cancer. GastroenterolClin North Am 2010, Dec;39(4):785-96.

[62] Lim LG, Yeoh KG, Salto-Tellez M, Khor CJL, Teh M, Chan YH, et al. Experienced versus inexperienced confocal endoscopists in the diagnosis of gastric adenocarcinoma and intestinal metaplasia on confocal images. GastrointestEndosc 2011, Jun;73(6): 1141-7.

[63] Sanduleanu S, Driessen A, Gomez-Garcia E, Hameeteman W, de Bruïne A, Masclee A. In vivo diagnosis and classification of colorectal neoplasia by chromoendoscopy-guided confocal laser endomicroscopy. ClinGastroenterolHepatol 2010, Apr;8(4): 371-8.

[64] Kiesslich R, Goetz M, Lammersdorf K, Schneider C, Burg J, Stolte M, et al. Chromoscopy-guided endomicroscopy increases the diagnostic yield of intraepithelial neoplasia in ulcerative colitis. Gastroenterology 2007, Mar;132(3):874-82.

[65] Goetz M, Ziebart A, Foersch S, Vieth M, Waldner MJ, Delaney P, et al. In vivo molecular imaging of colorectal cancer with confocal endomicroscopy by targeting epidermal growth factor receptor. Gastroenterology 2010, Feb;138(2):435-46.

[66] Hsiung P-L, Hsiung P-L, Hardy J, Friedland S, Soetikno R, Du CB, et al. Detection of colonic dysplasia in vivo using a targeted heptapeptide and confocal microendoscopy. Nat Med 2008, Apr;14(4):454-8.

[67] Hurlstone DP, Sanders DS. Recent advances in chromoscopic colonoscopy and endomicroscopy. CurrGastroenterol Rep 2006, Oct;8(5):409-15.

[68] Minami H, Inoue H, Yokoyama A, Ikeda H, Satodate H, Hamatani S, et al. Recent advancement of observing living cells in the esophagus using CM double staining: Endocytoscopicatypia classification. Dis Esophagus 2011, Sep 9.

[69] Anderson MA, Ben-Menachem T, Gan SI, Appalaneni V, Banerjee S, Cash BD, et al. Management of antithrombotic agents for endoscopic procedures. GastrointestEndosc 2009, Dec;70(6):1060-70.

[70] Hagel A, Boxberger F, Dauth W, Kessler H, Neurath M, Raithel M. Colonoscopy-associated perforation: A 7-year survey of in-hospital frequency, treatment and outcome in a german university hospital. Colorectal Dis 2011, Nov 11.

[71] Moss A, Bourke MJ, Williams SJ, Hourigan LF, Brown G, Tam W, et al. Endoscopic mucosal resection outcomes and prediction of submucosal cancer from advanced colonic mucosal neoplasia. Gastroenterology 2011, Jun;140(7):1909-18.

[72] Schurr MO, Hartmann C, Ho C-N, Fleisch C, Kirschniak A. An over-the-scope clip (OTSC) system for closure of iatrogenic colon perforations: Results of an experimental survival study in pigs. Endoscopy 2008, Jul;40(7):584-8.

[73] Voermans RP, Vergouwe F, Breedveld P, Fockens P, van Berge Henegouwen MI. Comparison of endoscopic closure modalities for standardized colonic perforations in a porcine colon model. Endoscopy 2011, Mar;43(3):217-22.

[74] Seebach L, Bauerfeind P, Gubler C. "Sparing the surgeon": Clinical experience with over-the-scope clips for gastrointestinal perforation. Endoscopy 2010, Dec;42(12): 1108-11.

[75] Parodi A, Repici A, Pedroni A, Blanchi S, Conio M. Endoscopic management of GI perforations with a new over-the-scope clip device (with videos). GastrointestEndosc 2010, Oct;72(4):881-6.

[76] Grossmann J, Diening C, Althoff C. [Endoscopic closure of a chronic colonic fistula using the over-the-scope clip (OTSC)]. Dtsch Med Wochenschr 2011, Nov;136(44): 2245-8.

[77] Manta R, Manno M, Bertani H, Barbera C, Pigò F, Mirante V, et al. Endoscopic treatment of gastrointestinal fistulas using an over-the-scope clip (OTSC) device: Case series from a tertiary referral center. Endoscopy 2011, Jun;43(6):545-8.

[78] von Renteln D, Denzer UW, Schachschal G, Anders M, Groth S, Rösch T. Endoscopic closure of GI fistulae by using an over-the-scope clip (with videos). GastrointestEndosc 2010, Dec;72(6):1289-96.

[79] Bini R, Coppola F, Recchia S, Fusca M, Gaia S, Leli R. Endoscopic treatment of post-gastrectomy duodenal fistula with an over-the-scope clip. SurgInnov 2011, Mar;18(1): 102-4.

[80] Naegel A, Bolz J, Zopf Y, Matthes K, Mueller B, Kraus F, et al. Hemodynamic efficacy of the over-the-scope clip in an established porcine cadaveric model for spurting bleeding. GastrointestEndosc 2012, Jan;75(1):152-9.

[81] Hearnshaw SA, Logan RFA, Lowe D, Travis SPL, Murphy MF, Palmer KR. Acute upper gastrointestinal bleeding in the UK: Patient characteristics, diagnoses and outcomes in the 2007 UK audit. Gut 2011, Oct;60(10):1327-35.

[82] Akasaka T, Nishida T, Tsutsui S, Michida T, Yamada T, Ogiyama H, et al. Short-term outcomes of endoscopic submucosal dissection (ESD) for early gastric neoplasm: Multicenter survey by osaka university ESD study group. Dig Endosc 2011, Jan;23(1): 73-7.

[83] Kim ES, Cho KB, Park KS, Lee KI, Jang BK, Chung WJ, Hwang JS. Factors predictive of perforation during endoscopic submucosal dissection for the treatment of colorectal tumors. Endoscopy 2011, Jul;43(7):573-8.

[84] Schurr MO, Baur F, Ho C-N, Anhoeck G, Kratt T, Gottwald T. Endoluminal full-thickness resection of GI lesions: A new device and technique. Minim Invasive Ther Allied Technol 2011, May;20(3):189-92.

[85] Voermans RP, van Berge Henegouwen MI, Bemelman WA, Fockens P. Novel over-the-scope-clip system for gastrotomy closure in natural orifice transluminal endoscopic surgery (NOTES): An ex vivo comparison study. Endoscopy 2009, Dec;41(12): 1052-5.

[86] Giday SA, Kim Y, Krishnamurty DM, Ducharme R, Liang DB, Shin EJ, et al. Long-term randomized controlled trial of a novel nanopowder hemostatic agent (TC-325) for control of severe arterial upper gastrointestinal bleeding in a porcine model. Endoscopy 2011, Apr;43(4):296-9.

[87] Sung JJY, Luo D, Wu JCY, Ching JYL, Chan FKL, Lau JYW, et al. Early clinical experience of the safety and effectiveness of hemospray in achieving hemostasis in patients with acute peptic ulcer bleeding. Endoscopy 2011, Apr;43(4):291-5.

Chapter 16

The Use of Endoscopic Ultrasound-Guided Fine Needle Aspiration (EUS-FNA) in Cytopathology Diagnosis

Lee-Ching Zhu, Qinghua Feng and Verena S. Grieco

Additional information is available at the end of the chapter

1. Introduction

Since the introduction of endoscopic ultrasound (EUS) in the 1980s, EUS-guided fine needle aspiration (EUS-FNA) has become increasingly popular for the diagnosis and staging of gastrointestinal diseases, and peri-gastrointestinal lesions, especially in the areas of pancreatic or peri-pancreatic mass-like lesions. The application of FNA has dramatically expanded the clinical utility of EUS[1-10].

The aims of this chapter are to review:

1. The advantage of EUS-FNA in cytopathology diagnosis over other diagnostic modalities.
2. The impact of on-site cytological interpretation on the diagnostic yield of EUS-FNA.
3. The difference of application of ancillary techniques in cytological as compared to surgical specimens. What are the drawbacks but also the advantages of applying immunocytochemistry (ICC) in EUS-FNA obtained specimens.
4. Why EUS-FNA material can be an ideal source of material for molecular studies.
5. In summary, the full value of EUS-FNA can only be achieved with an integrated approach. We will illustrate this approach by one of our interesting EUS-FNA case studies.

2. Aim 1: The advantage of EUS-FNA in cytopathology diagnosis over other diagnostic modalities

In the absence of EUS-FNA, there are many alternatives for obtaining biopsy specimens of mass lesions in the chest and abdomen [11]. This is done most frequently by transcutaneous ultrasound (TUS), or CT-guided biopsy. Pathology specimens of obstructing lung masses and/or large paratracheal lymph nodes often are obtained at bronchoscopy with forceps or by transbronchial needle aspiration. Pathology specimens of pancreatic masses, especially those causing obstructive jaundice are still commonly obtained at the time of diagnostic or therapeutic ERCP (endoscopic retrograde cholangiopancreatography) with brushing, needle aspiration, or intraductal biopsy forceps. When lesions cannot be accessed by the above techniques, more invasive methods, such as mediastinoscopy or operative biopsy (laparoscopic or open) are used. The primary limitations of TUS and CT-guided aspiration include difficulty in accurately targeting small lesions and finding a safe-skin-to-lesion route, especially for deep-seated retroperitoneal, mediastinal or perirectal lesions. The diagnostic yield of pancreatic malignancies with ERCP biopsy is particularly problematic, with reported sensitivities ranging from 20% to 80%, and most series having yields of a definitive malignant diagnosis of only around 50%. The complication rate for ERCP cytologic brushing is reportedly as high as 11% for the biliary tree and 21% for pancreatic strictures [12-14].

Commercial radial echoendoscopes were introduced by the Olympus Corporation in 1987. Although EUS-FNA was performed successfully with radial echoendoscopes, it was not until 1991, when the linear-array echoendoscopes by Pentax Precision Instruments were introduced, that EUS-FNA has been extensively utilized for a variety of lesions. Fundamentally, EUS-FNA involves passing an 18- to 25-gauge aspiration needle through the biopsy port of an echoendoscope under real-time guidance into a EUS visualized mass lesion, lymph node, lesion within another organ, or fluid collection.

Although EUS is considered superior to MRI or CT with cross-sectional imaging for tumor detection smaller than 2 to 3 cm [15, 16], it is the ability to target and place a needle into suspicious lesions at the closest proximity between the tip of the echoendoscope and the targeted lesion that has made EUS-FNA indispensable in the pre-operative diagnosis, especially in situations where neoadjuvant therapies or non-surgical management might be the clinical choice. Determining the role of EUS-FNA when alternative diagnostic modalities are available is difficult to assess in clinical trials; however, decision analysis models have been used to study the impact of EUS-FNA in lesions of many sites, including non-small-cell lung cancer with mediastinaladenopathy [17, 18], esophageal cancer and pancreatic cancer [19-21]. Commonly employed diagnostic modalities including CT-guided or US-guided FNA, ERCP with brushing, laparoscopic surgical biopsy and EUS-FNA have been analyzed for their costs, failure rate, testing characteristics and complication rate. In each of these analyses, EUS-FNA is the most cost-effective approach as the primary diagnostic modality and the preferred secondary alternative method after a failed initial diagnostic method as the least costly follow-up method.

The overall complication rate of EUS-FNA appears to be about 1-2% [22, 23], comparable to that reported with CT or US-guided FNA or biopsy. However, another significant factor favoring EUS-FNA over transcutaneous biopsy is avoiding the possible risk of needle-tract seeding[24]. During EUS-FNA the aspiration needle travels from the gut lumen to the lesion, a pathway that usually does not involve significant crossing of peritoneal or pleural surfaces. In addition, endosonographers may have multiple options for the most accessible approach to a lesion, such as through esophageal, gastric or duodenal path. In the case of pancreatic neoplasms, because of EUS-FNA imaging advantages, high diagnostic yields and concern over needle-tract seeding with transcutaneous aspiration, the 6th edition of the handbook on cancer staging by the American Joint Committee on Cancer has recommended EUS-FNA as the preferred sampling technique in pancreatic masses if available[25].

Lastly, EUS-FNA has also opened the era of interventional endoscopic ultrasound (IEUS). In the same way as FNA, the close proximity between the needle tip and the targeted organ allows therapeutic procedures, such as injection therapies, to be performed safely and effectively. This includes EUS-guided celiac plexus neurolysis and block for pain relief, drainage of pancreatic pseudocysts and pelvic fluid collections, and implantation of fiducial markers and radioactive seeds into malignant tumors. Other emerging EUS-guided experimental techniques include antitumor injection, ablation of tumors, and vascular access. IEUS is a very promising technique with many potential applications [26-28].

On a different note, performance quality in endoscopy is becoming an important issue for patient care. Currently there is no universally accepted method for performance quality indicators in EUS, mostly because cancer staging accuracy cannot be verified without surgical resection. In addition, FNA yields of many sites (such as mediastinal lymph nodes) vary greatly based on pretest probabilities. Because most pancreatic masses that undergo EUS-FNA have a very high pretest probability of being malignant and most endosonographers agree that pancreatic neoplasms are among the most difficult lesions on which to perform EUS-FNA, the diagnostic yield of EUS-FNA of solid pancreatic masses has become a benchmark for EUS-FNA quality. Much of the data for performance quality has come from series on pancreatic EUS-FNA, which is also the approach of most of our studies discussed in this chapter. In a multicenter retrospective study of 1075 patients who underwent EUS-guided FNA of solid pancreatic masses, the overall diagnostic rate of malignancy was 71%, the median rate per center was 78% and the median rate per endoscopist was 75% [29], remarkably higher than any other aforementioned diagnostic modalities.

The ideal benchmark for pancreatic EUS-FNA performance, however, would be the actual sensitivity and specificity of diagnosing malignancy and require the criterion standard of either surgical pathology or long-term follow-up, which is the focus of our studies in the next section.

3. Aim 2: Efficacy and utility of immediate cytologic interpretation on the diagnostic yield of EUS-FNA of solid and cystic pancreatic and peri-pancreatic lesions

Intra-procedural on-site immediate interpretation by a cytopathologist is not performed in some clinical settings. Having a cytopathologist on site is time-consuming and diverts the pathologist from other duties, and the cytopathologist time is not compensated at the same rate as routine surgical pathology [30, 31]. In the setting of service time pressure, there is a need for evidence based decisions regarding how to allocate pathologists. The clinical impact of immediate interpretation provided by cytopathologists during the EUS-FNA procedure and the statistical significance of this cytologic service has been well-documented[32-43], although with variable conclusions. Many of the previous studies have included a wide range of disease entities sampled by EUS-FNA procedure. In addition, by including cystic lesions, previous analysis has been complicated by the high likelihood of acellular or pauci-cellular specimens obtained from the cystic lesions, which could be interpreted as inadequate on cytology. Thus, the clarity of outcome measurements from previous studies has been hindered by the complexity of the diseases included, and by inclusion of cystic lesions with an unduly high "inadequacy" rate. In addition, many previous studies have used clinical survival years as a surrogate for final assessment of diagnostic accuracy. Our goal in the hereby presented study is to use EUS-FNA of solid pancreatic masses as the benchmark procedure to compare diagnostic yield and accuracy in a strictly defined clinical setting of EUS-FNA performed in the presence or absence of on-site immediate cytologic interpretation. Histologic examination is used as the gold standard for comparison.

To avoid the confounding sampling issues of cystic lesions, this study was focused on the diagnostic yield of EUS-FNA in non-cystic pancreatic mass-like lesions. A computer inventory search located 215 cases during the years 1999-2007 at University of Washington Medical Center and Harborview Medical Center, both in Seattle, WA, USA. These included 100 cases where immediate cytologic interpretation was available and 115 cases without immediate interpretation. Surgical pathology and clinical follow-up information were evaluated whenever possible. Comparison between the cytologic diagnoses with or without on-site immediate cytologic interpretation was facilitated by well-documented cytology reports. "Positive" specimens were defined as suspicious or malignant cytology. "Inadequate" specimens were defined as "rare atypical cells, non-diagnostic"; "essentially acellular specimen", or "gastrointestinal tract carry-over material". "Negative" specimens were defined as "adequate cellularity with benign or reactive features".

As shown in Table 1, the rate of inadequate specimens was significantly lower for cases with immediate cytologic interpretation (1% versus 21%; p <0. 0001). Although not statistically significant, there was a trend toward the need for fewer repeat procedures with the availability of immediate evaluation (rate 5% versus 10%; p <0. 3).

	N = Positive On Cytology	**N = Negative On Cytology**	**Inadequate Case N (%)**	**Repeat EUS-FNA Procedure N (%)**
Immediate Interpretation (N = 100)	60	39	1 (1%)	5 (5%)
No immediate Interpretation (N = 115)	58	33	24 (21%)	11 (10%)
P Value			< 0. 0001	< 0. 3

Table 1. EUS-FNA of non-cystic pancreatic mass-like lesions with or without immediate interpretation for all cases (N=215)

Of the 215 cases, surgical pathology follow-up was available for 55 cases. As would be expected, the majority of pancreatic mass lesions with surgical pathology comprised chronic pancreatitis (n=14), pancreatic ductal adenocarcinoma (n=29), and pancreatic endocrine neoplasms (n=7) (Table 2).

Case Type	Case Number (N)
Chronic pancreatitis	14
Pancreatic ductal adenocarcinoma	29
Pancreatic endocrine neoplasm	7
Solid pseudopapillary neoplasm of pancreas	2
Lymphoma	2
Fibromatosis	1

Table 2. Cases with histologic diagnoses (total N=55)

With histologic follow-up, we identified one false positive case, both at immediate interpretation and at final cytologic review, for which no neoplasm was identified at the open surgery or at repeat EUS-FNA procedure; this may have been a reactive mass that resolved after resolution of inflammation (with 12 months follow up). Cases with negative cytology results usually do not progress to surgical intervention, and surgical resection is also not performed in cases with unresectable malignancy. Due to the expected small number of cytologically negative cases with histologic follow-up, the single false positive case would have weighed un-proportionally in the calculation of specificity and positive predictive value. False negative cases represented well-differentiated pancreatic adenocarcinomas and cases of unrepresentative sampling, including one case of fibromatosis of pancreas. The number of cases with diagnostic discrepancy between cytologic and histologic diagnoses, and the corresponding statistical values, are summarized in Table 3 and Table 4. When comparing cases with on-site cytopathology immediate interpretation to those without, there was a trend toward greater sensitivity (83% versus 65%, p=0.19) with similar specificity (86% versus 100%, p=0.29). There was also a trend toward lower cytologic-histologic discordance rate in cases with availability of immediate interpretation by cytopathologists (16% versus 27%, p=0.34). Positive predictive value was comparable for cases where cytopathologists were present on-site compared with cases where no cytopathologists were present (94% versus 100%, p=0. 32), but the availability of immediate interpretation resulted in a higher negative predictive value (67% versus 47%, p=0.34).

	N=Positive cytology, neoplastic histology (TP)	N= Positive cytology, benign histology (FP)	N=Benign cytology, benign histology (TN)	N=Benign cytology, neoplastic histology (FN)	N= Total histologic follow-up available (TP+FP+TN+FN)
On-Site Interpretation	15	1	6	3	25
No On-Site Interpretation	15	0	7	8	30

TP:True positive cytologic diagnosis

FP:False positive cytologic diagnosis

TN:True negative cytologic diagnosis

FN:False negative cytologic diagnosis

Table 3. Discrepancy between cytologic and histologic diagnoses (N=55)

	Histologic follow-up available	Discordance rate	Sensitivity	Specificity	PPV	NPV
On-Site Interpretation	25	16%	83%	86%	94%	67%
No On-Site Interpretation	30	27%	65%	100%	100%	47%

Histological follow-up available: T=TP+FP+TN+FN

Discordance rate:FP+FN/T

Sensitivity:TP/TP+FN

Specificity:TN/TN+FP

Positive predictive value on cytology (PPV):TP/TP+FP

Negative predictive value on cytology (NPV):TN/TN+FN

Table 4. Performance characteristics according to the availability of on-site cytopathology (N=55 cases)

In this study, the drop of the inadequacy rate from 21% without on-site immediate interpretation to 1% with on-site immediate interpretation is highly statistically significant (p value < 0.0001). The repeat procedure rate dropped correspondingly from 10% to 5%. It has been shown that EUS-FNA would lose its advantage over the other diagnostic options if its failure rate were over 20% [44]. The EUS-FNA procedure in various body sites (thyroid, breast, lung, etc.) generally has a comparable reported failure rate when performed without immediate interpretation, with an average failure rate of 20% and a maximum of reported failure rate of 32% [32, 33, 45-47]. In our current study, without immediate interpretation, our inadequacy rate was 21%, a rate at which the procedure may not be cost effective over other diagnostic options. On-site immediate cytology interpretation of EUS-FNA of solid pancreatic lesions thus results in cost savings, reduced intervals between diagnosis and therapeutic intervention, and enhanced patient care.

An important task at the EUS-FNA procedure is representative sampling of the lesion. With on-site immediate microscopic evaluation of part of the sample, an experienced cytologist should be able to assess the cellularity of the sampling and to differentiate gastrointestinal tract carryover material from moderately to poorly differentiated malignant cells. The presence of dense numbers of inflammatory cells, necrotic debris, and fibrous stromal elements provides good evidence that the endosonographer is actually sampling the targeted lesion. In our experience, on-site communication with immediate feedback is invaluable in guiding the next needle pass. Another indispensable value is that immediate evaluation gives the pathologists the best opportunity to triage the sampled material for its optimal use, including sending fresh specimen for flow cytometry analysis for possible lymphoproliferative disease, sending cyst contents for microbiology tests, or chemical analysis for tumor markers, such as amylase, CEA, CA19-9, etc. All those commonly available laboratory tests cannot be performed once the specimen is fixed.

What is the impact of EUS-FNA on-site evaluation in situations of non-solid pancreatic lesions [48-52]? In our daily practice of cytology, EUS-FNA specimens comprise almost half the volume of our on-site immediate assessment service. There are occasions when the aspirated material has presented with an unusual or unexpected, and yet remarkable gross appearance. On-site availability gives us the advantage of observing the gross appearance of freshly aspirated material. With increased experience, we feel these grossly "unusual" aspirates can actually help to raise our suspicion towards a relatively specific diagnosis and triage the material for certain helpful laboratory tests. In our 2008 publication, we conducted 10-year institutional case review and summarized three different patterns of gross appearance of aspirated material from non-neoplastic pancreatic and peri-pancreatic cystic lesions [53].

3.1. Pattern 1: Grossly yellowish-green pasty material

Case 1: we encountered two patients who presented with almost identical gross and microscopic findings at EUS-FNA. The first patient was a 52-year-old male with a past medical history of acute gallstone pancreatitis 4 years prior, treated by cholecystectomy. He has had no other episodes of pancreatitis after the surgery. During a workup for his nephrolithiasis, CT scan incidentally identified a 3 cm unilocular cyst adjacent to the neck and body of his pancreas. Endoscopic ultrasound was requested in order to evaluate this peri-pancreatic cystic lesion. On site, EUS revealed a 3.4 cm primarily hypoechoic lesion. Aspirated material had an unusual yellowish-green gross appearance with a pasty texture. Microscopically, the smears contain rare squamous cells of gut luminal origin, abundant amorphous material and acellular debris (Figure 1, A). A Hall's stain for bilirubin showed focal staining, suggestive of bile pigment (Figure 1, B). Serum amylase assay was within normal range during this period. In light of the cytological finding and clinical presentation, it was felt that the lesion was most consistent with a small, chronic biloma, which likely developed at the time of his cholecystectomy. Follow up CT scan revealed an unchanged cyst and no further evaluation was recommended.

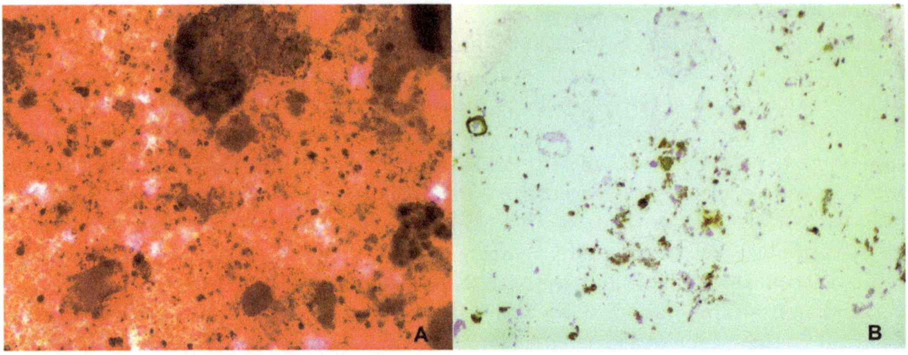

Figure 1. Representative cytologic findings in a case of biloma. Panel A:High-power view showing abundant amorphous material and acellular debris (Papanicolaou stain, 400x). Panel B: A Hall's stain for bilirubin showed focal staining, suggestive of bile pigment (Hall's stain, 400x).

Case 2: the second patient was a 39-year-old male with a history of chronic pancreatitis. During the workup for his intermittent upper abdominal pain, CT scan revealed a 2 cm hypodense mass off the tail of his pancreas. The patient underwent EUS-FNA twice. Each time EUS revealed a 2cm hypoechoic mass off the tail of the pancreas and grossly similar copious yellowish-green material was aspirated and submitted for cytology. Microscopically, both EUS-FNA specimens from this patient revealed almost identical findings as our previous case with abundant bile-stained cyst contents and amorphous debris (Data not shown). No inflammation was present. Concurrent serum CA19-9 assay was within normal limits. Although a specific diagnosis of biloma was not rendered on the original report, findings argue for a benign cystic lesion and a CT follow-up for the stability of the lesion was recommended without further intervention.

3.2. Pattern 2: Grossly tan-white cheesy material

Case 3: this was a 42-year-old male with chronic alcohol use and chronic hepatitis B and HIV co-infection. CT scan found a cystic lesion near the pancreatic tail, which had been stable in size. EUS identified a 2.5 cm complex cystic lesion adjacent to the pancreatic tail with both cystic and solid components. Aspirated material was grossly tan-white in color and semi-solid, cheesy in texture. Most of the material was lost during processing when air-dried or alcohol-fixed slides with Diff-Quik or Papanicolaou staining was attempted. Microscopic examination only revealed abundant amorphous degenerate material (Figure 2, A). Given the suspicion that material was dissolved by alcohol, Oil-Red O stain was performed on air-dried slides and showed variable fat staining (Figure 2, B). Because of the unusual gross appearance, the aspirated material on site was also sent for microbiology (negative findings) and assayed for CEA (164971 ng/ml), and amylase (2357 u/L). The significantly elevated CEA level was concerning for malignancy. The patient subsequently underwent a distal pancreatectomy and splenectomy. Surgical pathology specimen revealed a cyst present in the adipose tissue adjacent to the pancreas filled with tan-white cheesy material. Microscopically, the cyst is lined by mature keratinizing squamous epithelium and lymphoid tissue with germinal centers surrounding the epithelium, consistent with a lymphoepithelial cyst (LEC) of the pancreas (Figure 2, C & D). The possibility of a dermoid cyst was also considered due to the evident sebaceous gland differentiation beneath the squamous epithelium. However, the lack of hair follicles and sweat glands and the presence of dense lymphoid tissue with germinal centers were most consistent with the diagnosis of LEC of the pancreas. We presume that the abundant oily material filling the cyst was partially due to the secretion of the sebaceous glands that accumulated intracytoplasmic lipid droplets and produced oily sebum extracellularly. Mixed in with keratin debris, this material could account for the unusual gross-appearance of that tan-white semi-solid atheromatous material aspirated from this patient on EUS-FNA.

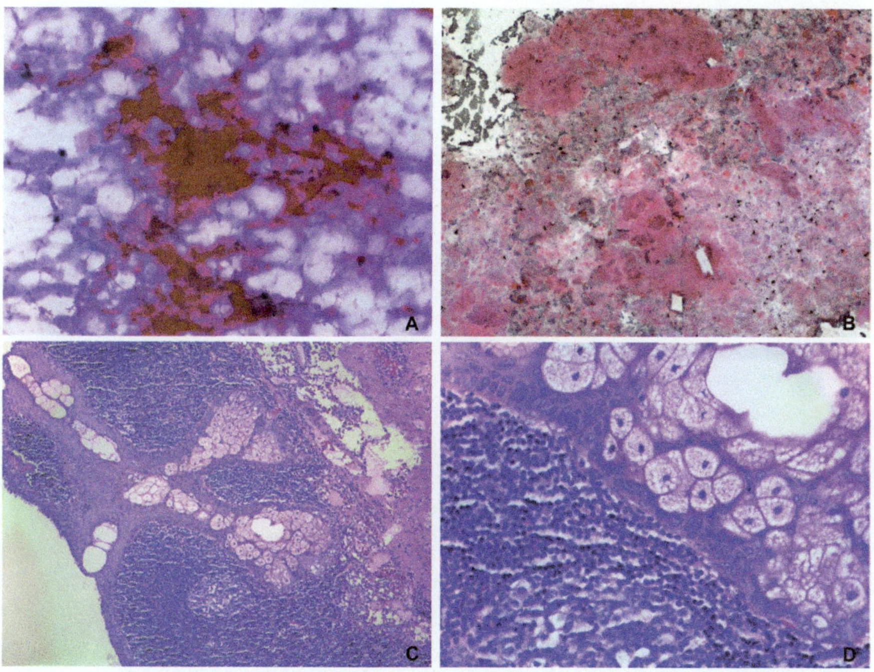

Figure 2. Microscopic findings of a lymphoepithelial cyst of pancreas with sebaceous differentiation. Panel A:High-power view of cytology aspiration revealing abundant amorphous degenerate material (Papanicolaou stain, 400x). Panel B:Oil-Red O stain on air-dried slides showing focally variable fat staining (Oil-Red O 100x). Panel C:Low-power view of the subsequent surgical pathology specimen revealing a pancreatic cystic lesion lined by mature keratinizing squamous epithelium and lymphoid tissue with germinal centers surrounding the epithelium (Hematoxylin and eosin stain, 100x). Panel D:High-power view showing evident sebaceous gland differentiation of the squamous epithelial lining of the cyst (Hematoxylin and eosin stain, 400x).

3.3. Pattern 3: Grossly amber clear fluid, can be darker due to thickness

Cases 4-6: a computer inventory search from year 1997-2007 at University of Washington allowed us to review three additional cases of lymphoepithelial cysts with cytological diagnosis and follow-up surgical resections. The features of these 3 cases are summarized in Table 5. All those surgical-proven lymphoepithelial cysts showed grossly clear fluid on cytology aspiration with color variation described from light yellow to darker-brown. Available laboratory data showed low amylase and CEA level. The follow-up surgical specimens revealed simple lymphoepithelial cysts with no sebaceous gland differentiation.

Cases 7-8: also included in Table 5 are two cases of surgical-proven pancreatic pseudocyst that presented with grossly similar amber clear to brownish fluid on aspiration while concurrent amylase and CEA level were in the normal range.

Case	4	5	6	7	8
Patient	35 yo M	42 yo F	51 yo M	42 yo F	60 yo F
Surgical Diagnosis	LEC	LEC	LEC	Pseudocyst	Pseudocyst
Clinical History	Lower quadrant colic pain for 9 months.	Questionable mild chronic pancreatitis	Choledocolithiasis, s/p cholecystectomy and 3 weeks abdominal pain	Alcohol use; 10yr h/o epigastric pain	Alcohol use; liver cirrhosis and chronic pancreatitis
Imaging Study	4.6 cm cystic lesion at the junction of pancreatic head and body	3.4 cm well-circumscribed radiolucent mass	4. 5 cm heterogeneous microcystic mass adjacent to the uncinate process	3.5 cm circumscribed, heterogenous pancreatic head mass	3.3 cm well demarcated, heterogeneous pancreatic head mass
Gross on EUS-FNA	Clear light yellow fluid	Clear fluid	No fluid obtained	Serosanguinous fluid	Brownish fluid
Cytology Dx	Cystic contents and debris, no epithelium identified	Rare degenerated cells and proteinaceous debris	Degenerative and necrotic adipose tissue	Inflammatory cells, hemosiderin pigment and debris	Inflammatory cells and fragments of fibrous tissue
Lab Data	Amylase: 24-354 U/L; CEA:25.6-34. 5 ng/ml CA19-9:8 U/ml	Amylase:35 U/L; CA19-9:12 U/ml	Amylase:13-53 U/L;	Amylase:18-54 U/L; CEA:3.1 ng/ml CA19-9:4.5-6.1 U/ml	Amylase:12-15 U/L;

** Both lymphoepithelial cyst (LEC) and pancreatic pseudocyst can grossly show amber clear fluid upon fine needle aspiration. Fluid can also be thicker in texture and darker in color due to hemorrhagic changes.*

Table 5. Salient features of 3 cases of LEC and 2 cases of pancreatic pseudocyst.

Our experience tells us that being fully aware of the limitations on cytology diagnosis and the high possibility of non-representative sampling of the lesions, cytologists should be ready to reject or classify the specimens as non-diagnostic in many situations of acellular cytological material and thus avoid misleading the clinical decisions with an erroneous diagnosis. On the other hand, based on the individual institute settings and the availabilities of cytopathologists for on-site immediate assessment, cytology diagnosis tends to ignore the gross appearance of the aspirated material and the background material is also often overlooked microscopically, especially in an acellular cytology specimen. Incorporating those gross material observations can sometimes add valuable information towards a pathological diagnosis.

We presented three entities (8 cases) here in an attempt to highlight the diagnostic value of gross appearance in fine needle aspiration cytology that can provide clues to the nature of a pancreatic or a peripancreatic cystic lesion. These three entities: biloma, pancreatic lymphoepithelial cyst and pancreatic pseudocyst, although considered uncommon and not widely represented in the cytology literature, are actually encountered more commonly now with the rapid advance of our imaging and imaging guided-sampling practices. On cytology specimens, those are the lesions that generally produce acellular or sparsely cellular material (not including carryover material from gastrointestinal luminal origin). However by carefully combining the clinical, radiological, laboratory and cytological findings grossly and microscopically, cytology can help lead to or confirm clinical judgments and aid in patient care.

A biloma is an encapsulated bile collection outside the biliary tree. The underlying causes include iatrogenic, traumatic, and spontaneous injury of the biliary tree causing bile leaks. Its diagnosis can be established upon clinical history, imaging studies, and needle aspiration cytology and chemical analysis of the aspirated fluid. The symptomatic biloma if left untreated may result in significant morbidity and mortality. However, non-surgical intervention is considered the first choice of treatment for biloma, especially in many asymptomatic situations. Alternatively symptomatic biloma may be treated successfully with interventional radiologic techniques instead of open surgery [54, 55]. It was recently reported that endoscopic ultrasound-guided fine-needle aspiration of an infected biloma, together with endoscopic biliary stent placement, resulted in complete resolution of a patient's biloma [56]. Thus, cytological diagnosis of biloma upon EUS-FNA can help a great deal in managing this potentially complex problem.

A wide variety of cystic lesions can arise within or adjacent to the pancreas. They can be generally placed into non-neoplastic and neoplastic categories. The non-neoplastic cystic lesions can be both congenital and acquired. EUS-FNA has emerged as the primary choice for obtaining diagnostic material on pancreatic cystic lesions. Aspirated cystic fluid analysis for pancreatic enzymes, tumor markers, and fluid viscosity can be of great help in the differential diagnosis. Non-neoplastic cysts generally are high on amylase level and low on tumor markers (CEA, CA 19-9) while these tumor markers are generally elevated in malignant cystic neoplasms, but low in non-neoplastic or benign neoplastic cysts. Having said that, exceptions do occur and no standardized values exist among institutions. On cytology specimen, neoplastic cystic lesions usually produce a more cellular aspirate compared to non-neoplastic cysts if appropriately sampled.

The acquired non-neoplastic pancreatic cysts include dermoid cysts, LECs and pseudocysts. Both dermoid cysts and LECs are squamous-lined non-neoplastic cysts. LECs are benign cystic lesions [57] seen predominantly in males, in the fifth to sixth decades of life. They may be unilocular or multilocular. The cyst contents may vary from serous to cheesy/casseous-appearing material depending on the degree of keratin formation. Microscopically, the cysts are lined by well-differentiated stratified squamous epithelium, which may or may not have prominent keratinization. In some areas, the lining may appear more transitional, and in others, flat, cuboidal, or focally denuded. The squamous epithelium is surrounded by a band of dense lymphoid tissue composed of mature T-lymphocytes with intervening germinal centers formed by B cells. The representative aspirate findings are non-specific, showing a mixed population of lymphocytes, histiocytes in a background of keratin debris and proteinaceous debris. Squamous lining cells may be seen. The occurrence of sebaceous glands in LEC of pancreas is well documented [58]. It is unclear whether the florid sebaceous glandular differentiation correlates with the exceedingly elevated CEA and amylase level in our patient. LECs of the pancreas do not appear to be associated with any autoimmune conditions, human immunodeficiency virus infection, lymphoma, or carcinoma. All of these lesions have been documented to occur in their salivary gland counterparts [59]. Dermoid cysts are also rare in the pancreas region. They are reported in younger patients (2nd-3rd decades). The presence of sebaceous glands or hair follicles and absence of closely associated lymphoid tissue is more typical for dermoid cysts and differentiate them from LECs.

Pancreatic pseudocysts account for the vast majority (75-90%) of pancreatic cysts [60]. Pseudocyst lacks an epithelial lining. It develops when a focus of peri-pancreatic fat necrosis is resorbed, producing a debris-filled space rich in pancreatic exocrine enzymes. It is in general composed of an inflammatory fibrous capsule surrounding a region of necrosis. However, the pathologic findings may vary depending on the stage of the process. The cyst contents, originally necrotic fat, transform into a mixture of necrotic cells, enzymes, scavenger cells, cholesterol clefts and sometimes neutrophils. The tissue that surrounds the necrotic material first produces granulation tissue, and eventually becomes a fibrotic pseudocapsule. FNA usually yields clear to dark brown fluid, which often but not always (as in our cases) shows elevated amylase level on fluid analysis. Aspirate smears are again non-specific and composed of granular necrotic debris and mixed inflammatory cells [61]. A clinical history of pancreatitis and confirmatory gross evidence of pancreatitis on imaging should confirm the diagnosis. The diagnosis of pseudocyst on cytology should be considered one of exclusion.

4. Aim 3: Application of immunocytochemistry (ICC) studies in EUS-FNA obtained cytology material

When applying ancillary techniques in cytologic specimens, cytopathologists often encounter the difficulties of limited material, lack of negative or positive controls or lack of internal controls. On the other hand, the presence of internal control material can sometimes add confusion rather than reassurance in ICC-stained material. Nevertheless, by carefully and strategically using the cytology specimen, immunocytochemical studies are often achievable with limited aspiration material. We have used some of the techniques that have been described by others, such as immunostaining over Papanicolaou-stained monolayer slides; applying different antibodies to different areas of one smear slide; or making cell block preparations whenever possible. When unstained material is not available and no cell block is initially prepared, Dr. V. Grieco and her colleagues at Harborview Medical Center, Seattle, Washington, have used a scraped slide technique that transfers smear material on Papanicolaou stained slides into paraffin embedded cell blocks. The cell block can then be used for ICC with appropriate controls. If successful, this may avoid the necessity of obtaining additional tissue. We have routinely used this scraped cell block technique in our daily practice as well as in research projects. We hereby briefly discuss our mucin study project with archival cytology material from 1997-2007 at University of Washington, presented at Digestive Disease Week [62]. Schema of Scraping Technique is illustrated in Figure 3: scraping the material from rehydrated direct smear slides into a cell block preparation.

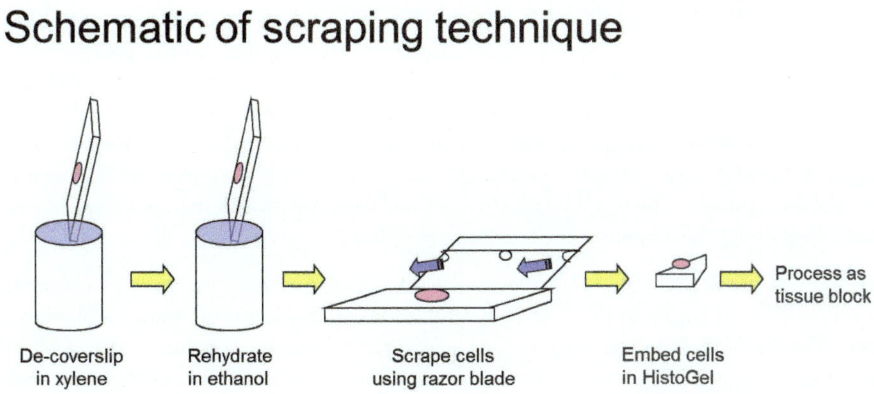

Figure 3. Schema of Scrapped Cell Block Technique:Papanicolaou-stained cellular direct smears are placed in xylene, coverslip removed, and re-hydrated in sequentially graded ethanol to tap water. The cellular material is then scraped from the glass slides using a razor blade, embedded in Histogel and processed with routine cell block preparation.

Cytology diagnosis of mucin-producing pancreatic neoplasms including mucinous non-cystic carcinoma (colloid carcinoma), mucinous cystic neoplasm, and intraductal papillary-mucinous neoplasm (IPMN) is important because of the speculation that disruption of the integrity of these mucinous tumors by an incisional biopsy may cause dissemination of tumor cells with mucin and worsen the prognosis. Mucin-detection is not always an easy task on EUS-FNA specimen. Reactive/inflammatory pancreatitis can cause dilated ducts and-pseudocyst formation with proteinaceous precipitate that can be mistaken as mucinous material. Sheets of carry-over gastric foveolar cells can mimic cells from mucinous neoplasia [63-67]. By applying conventional cytochemistry including PAS (periodic acid-Schiff reaction), PASD (PAS with diastase), alcian blue and mucicarmin, in conjunction withmucin protein (MUC1, MUC2) immunostaining on surgical-proven cytology specimens, this study aims at selecting a practical diagnostic tool to enhance the diagnostic accuracy of detecting mucin-producing pancreatic neoplasms.

Studied material include: 1) Bench FNA specimens performed on autopsy or surgical-obtained normal tissue that are likely to be carried-over during an endoscopic procedure including pancreas, gastric body, pylorus and duodenum; 2) EUS-FNA (with scraped cell block preparation by scraping archival smears into a cell block), along with subsequent surgical specimens on mucinous cystadenoma, borderline mucinous cystic neoplasm, IPMN, colloid carcinoma and ductal adenocarcinma with mucin production; 3) Non-mucin producing lesions including solid pseudopapillary tumor and chronic pancreatitis with dilated duct. Our data demonstrate that mucicarmin is very insensitive in detecting mucin production. We are unable to show reliable mucicarmin staining on both surgical and cytology specimen of IPMN(Figure 4, Panel D-F) as well as mucinous cystic neoplasia cases. MUC1 and MUC 2 immunostains do not consistently pick up mucin production by pancreatic neoplasia on cytology specimens either. In contrast, PAS/PAS-Diastase are a reliable and sensitive marker to stain background mucin material and mucin-producing epithelial cells on cytology, yet specific enough to distinguish proteinaceous precipitate in a pancreatitis case (Figure 4, Panel A-C, precipitate in a dilated duct that was mistaken as possible mucinous material on cytology). The results have directed our daily practice on the use of mucin stains on cytologic diagnosis of pancreatic mucinous neoplasia.

Concomitant use of ICC can greatly enhance the diagnostic accuracy on cytology specimens, especially when it comes to the diagnostic entities invariably requiring immunophenotypic identification, such as in the diagnosis of pancreatic endocrine neoplasia (PENs) [68-72]. However, due to the initial unanticipated nature of the lesion, lack of cytopathologist on site or difficulties of the procedure, sufficient aspirate/biopsy material for cellblock preparation is not always available. By using the scraped cell block technique, a select panel of immunocytochemical studies can be achieved to aid in the diagnosis of PEN. Using the aforementioned scraped cell block technique, figure 5 shows strong expression of the neuroendocrine immuno-marker, chromogranin, by the neoplastic cells. Figure 6 shows neoplastic cells stained positively with the neuroendocrine marker, synaptophysin by directly applying the antibody onto a Papanicolaou-stained charged monolayer slide.

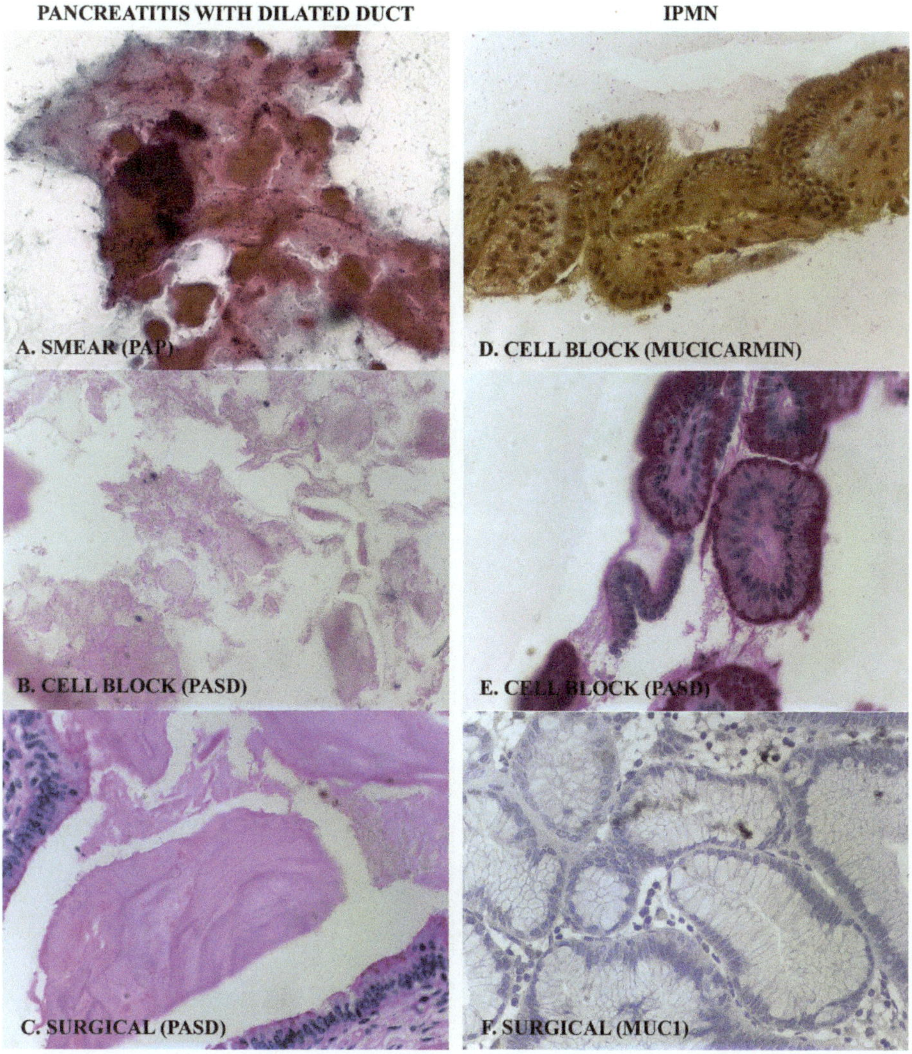

Figure 4. In a case of IPMN, with negative staining for mucicarmine and MUC1, PASD highlighted the mucinous neoplastic cells uniformly (panel D-F). Negative PASD staining in a pancreatitis case with precipitate in a dilated duct that was mistaken as possible mucinous material on cytology initially (panel A-C).

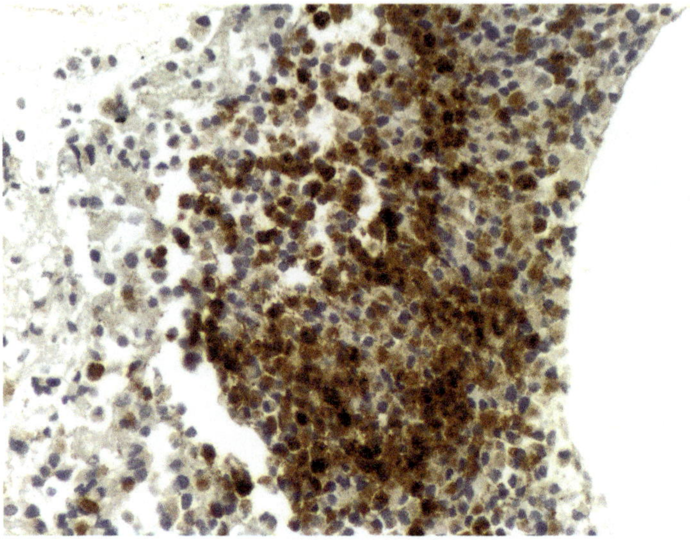

Figure 5. Immunocytochemical stain on a scraped cellblock section displaying strong expression of neuroendocrine marker, Chromogranin by the neoplastic cells (Scraped material for cell block preparation, 400x).

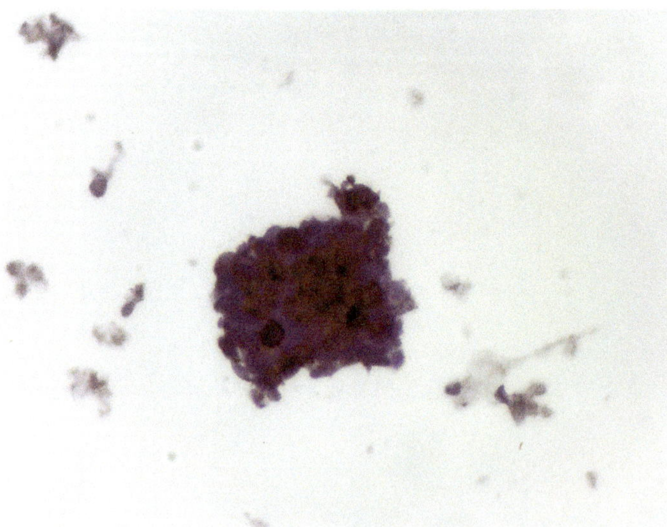

Figure 6. Neoplastic cells on a monolayer slide stained positively with neuroendocrine marker, synaptophysin antibody (400x)

Before leaving this section, it should also be stated that in cytology, as in surgical pathology, the light microscopic appearance of the tumor is more important than a particular staining result and that immunocytochemistry should be used for confirmation of the cytomorphological diagnosis. Be aware of that the staining of cytology specimens is often focal and sometimes difficult to interpret, because of various factors, including limited material, high background staining, and the presence of three-dimensional clusters with non-specific staining and edge artifact. A combined clinical, radiographic and pathologic approach should always be emphasized in rendering each diagnosis.

5. Aim 4: EUS-FNA as a source of material for molecular studies

We are at the beginning of the era of clinical application of molecular probes to assess genetic alterations. Many assays have become clinically available in identifying genetic alterations that serve as prognostic markers and therapeutic targets. EGFR expression in head and neck cancers, non-small cell lung carcinomas, colon cancers, and recently in pancreatic cancers [73-82]; microsatellite instability tests in colon cancer serve as prognostic marker, therapeutic predictive marker and screening test for Lynch syndrome [83-88] are among the most studied areas. Immunodetection of molecular markers on cytology specimen, especially in cancer staging for metastatic disease will be playing a major role as a guide for molecular-targeted therapy. EGFR expression has now been routinely assessed on cell block cytology specimens by many of the commercial or academic laboratories. A prominent example in this regard is FNA diagnosis of thyroid nodules. Given that the cytology reports on thyroid FNA diagnoses are often indeterminate or suspicious, the potential use of diagnostic molecular markers as adjunct methods for cytologic diagnosis appears to be among the most promising area of research [89-98]. Fluorescent (FISH) and chromogenic (CISH) in situ hybridization have recently become part of the diagnostic armamentarium of breast pathologists. HER2 gene amplification testing by FISH and/or CISH has become an integral part of the diagnostic workup for patients with breast cancer [99-105]. FISH or CISH is now used in FNA material with success in many situations, including HER2 assessment in FNA with excellent correlation with the histologic specimens [106-108]. Many other applications, such as N-myc amplication on FNA from neuroblastomas [109, 110] and potential use of multiplex FISH for detection of recurrence of transitional carcinomas on urine specimens [111-114] are also well documented molecular tests using cytology specimens.

Compared to paraffin-embedded tissue, cytology specimens offer the advantage of disaggregated, intact cells, with fewer problems associated with tumor cell homogenization. FISH or CISH probe for diagnosis should be expected to be detected more accurately in cytologic specimen as it contains whole cells and whole nuclei. For the patient, the advantages include low cost, prompt access and the avoidance of surgery.

In carcinogenesis, the majority of molecular alterations occur prior to progressive tumor growth. It has been well documented that resection of small (early) pancreatic tumors and tumors of low histological or cytological grade and stage are correlated with improved survival.

It is, therefore, important to identify these tumors in their early stages. DNA methylation changes are an early event in carcinogenesis and are often present in the precursor lesions of various cancers. Dr. N. Kiviat's lab at Harborview Medical Center, Seattle, Washington, has published extensively in constructing a panel of candidate hypermethylated genes with optimal sensitivity and specificity as a potential screening tool for cervical neoplasia, ovarian carcinoma and lung cancer [115-118]. In collaboration with Dr. N. Kiviat's lab, we performed molecular tests on EUS-FNA of pancreatic lesions in the form of remains in liquid-based preparation, together with bench-performed mock FNA from normal pancreas obtained through Harborview trauma center. We preliminarily tested the hypothesis that a panel of hypermethylated genes with high sensitivity and specificity for pancreatic adenocarcinoma might increase the accuracy of diagnosis of FNA and brush cytology on pancreatic cancer.

Method Excess material from five pancreatic FNAs, three pancreatic duct brushings and nine bile duct brushings from patients who subsequently had histologic evaluation upon surgery were studied. Genomic DNA was isolated from residual cytology brushing sample pellets using QIAamp Blood DNA isolation kit and methylation status of seven genes, was accessed using MethyLight assay after bisulfite conversion [115]. These genes were reported to be frequently methylated in other cancers, including RASSF1A (Ras association domain family 1A gene), UCHL1 (ubiquitin carboxyl-terminal esterase L1), APC (adenomatosis polyposis coli), IGSF4 (also called CADM1, cell adhesion molecule 1), CDH13 (cadherin 13), CCND2 (cyclin D2), and CDKN2A (cyclin-dependent kinase inhibitor 2A, p16). Primers and probes for these genes are listed in Table 6. Sample adequacy after bisulfite conversion was determined by amplification of β-actin gene (ACTB). The percentage of methylated reference (PMR) for each gene was calculated as before [115]. The methylation status of a sample was categorized in two ways: as having any methylation present (PMR>0) and as having high levels of methylation (PMR≥4%), as previously described [115].

Gene	Forward primer (5'-3')	Probe (5'-3')	Reverse primer (5'-3')
ACTB	TGGTGATGGAGGAGGTTTAGTAAGT	6FAM-ACCACCACCCAACACACAATAACAAACACA-TAMRA	AACCAATAAAACCTACTCCTCCCTTAA
APC	TTATATGTCGGTTACGTGCGTTTATAT	6FAM-CCCGTCGAAAACCCGCCGATTA-TAMRA	GAACCAAAACGCTCCCCAT
CCND2	CGTGTTAGGGTCGATCGTGTT	6FAM-ACTACGATAAAATCGCCG-MGB	CTCGCCAAACTTTCTCCCTAAA
CDH13	GATTTTTGGGTTCGGAATGATTT	6FAM-TTTTCGTCGTCGCGATC-MGB	ATCGCCCGACACGAACAA
CDKN2A	TGGAGTTTTCGGTTGATTGGTT	6FAM-ACCCGACCCCGAACCGCG-TAMRA	AACAACGCCCGCACCTCCT
IGSF4	AGGGAGCGAGGTTTTTCGA	6FAM-CGAACCCAACCCGAC-MGB	ACGAAATCCGAACAAACCAATC
RASSF1	TAGGTTTTTATTGCGCGGTTTT	6FAM-CGCGAACCGAACGAA-MGB	TACTTCGCTAACTTTAAACGCTAACAA
UCHL1	TCGCGAAGATGTAGTTTAAGTCGAT	6FAM-ACGCTCACCTCGAAAT-MGB	CGCGCTCTCCGAATAACG

Table 6. Primers and probes for MethyLight assays

Results A total of 17 samples were available for examination. No DNA remained in one bile duct brushing after preparation of smears for microscopic examination. Thus, 16 samples, 12 malignant and 4 benign (by histology) were evaluated. On microscopic examination of the FNA and brush cytologic specimens, 8 of the 12 samples which were later shown to be malignant (on biopsy) were classified as "suspicious" for malignancy while four were called definitively "positive" for malignancy by FNA or brush. The remaining four cases were histologically benign. Two of these cases were called "negative" on microscopic examination of the FNA or brush specimen, one was classified as "atypical" and one as "suspicious for malignancy". The distribution of aberrantly methylated genes of interest among the benign and malignant lesions is presented in Table 7.

Gene	Any Methylation (PMR>0%)				High Methylation (PMR≥4%)			
	Malignant (n=12)		Benign (n=4)		Malignant (n=12)		Benign (n=4)	
UCHL1	9	(75%)	1	(25%)	6	(50%)	0	(0%)
APC	7	(58%)	1	(25%)	3	(25%)	0	(0%)
RASSF1	3	(25%)	0	(0%)	2	(17%)	0	(0%)
IGSF4	3	(25%)	0	(0%)	1	(8%)	0	(0%)
CDH13	8	(67%)	0	(0%)	3	(25%)	0	(0%)
CCND2	10	(83%)	4	(100%)	8	(67%)	2	(50%)
CDKN2A	0	(0%)	0	(0%)	0	(0%)	0	(0%)
CDH13 or RASSF1	(75%)		0%)					
UCHL1, CDH13, or RASSF1					(67%)		(0%)	

Table 7. Promoter Hypermethylation by Histologic Diagnosis

Methylation of three different genes (RASSF1, IGSF4, and CDH13) was present at some level in malignant but not benign samples, and methylation of two other genes (UCHL1 and APC) was present at a higher frequency in the majority of malignant samples but was present in only one of four benign samples. For two genes, methylation was either present in nearly all samples, regardless of histologic diagnosis (CCND2) or was not present in any samples (CDKN2A). For five genes, high levels of methylation (PMR≥4%) were present in malignant cases but were not detected in any of the benign samples. We next identified the combination of genes with the highest sensitivity and specificity for pancreatic cancer.

When any level of methylation was considered as positive, aberrant methylation of CDH13 or RASSF1 provided optimal sensitivity and specificity for cancer, being present in 75% of malignant and 0% of benign specimens (Table 7). Considering high levels of methylation (PMR≥4%), the most sensitive and specific combination of methylated genes was UCHL1, CDH13 and RASSF1 which were positive in 67% of malignant but 0% of benign specimens (Table 7). Next we examined, whether detection of aberrantly methylated genes might increase our ability to accurately classify FNA and brush specimens as "positive" or "negative" for malignancy. Using this approach, FNA and brush specimens were classified as "Positive for malignancy" if *either* cells with malignant morphologic changes *or* any level of methylation of CDH13 or RASSF1 was present (Table 8). Specimens were called "Negative for malignancy" if the cells were morphologically normal *or cells were atypical or suspicious by morphology but* there was no evidence of aberrant methylation of either CDH13 or RASSF1. This algorithm detects 83% of malignant samples while maintaining 100% specificity. We are aware that an independent sample set is necessary to appropriately test this algorithm; however, this pilot data suggests that a panel of hypermethylated tumor suppressor genes might be useful in distinguishing malignancy from benign pancreatic lesions. A similarly sensitive and specific algorithm combining cytologic morphology and a panel of genes methylated at high levels (PMR ≥4% of UCHL1, CDH13 and/or RASSF1 present) was also developed.

Final Diagnosis	Malignant (n=12)	Benign (n=4)
POSITIVE		
morphology consistent with malignancy	4 (33%)	0 (0%)
or aberrant methylation of CDH13	9 (75%)	0 (0%)
or aberrant methylation of RASSF1	10 (83%)	0 (0%)
NEGATIVE		
Negative morphology or		2 (50%)
Atypical or suspicious cell morphology but no aberrant methylation of CDH13 or RASSF1		4 (100%)

Table 8. Cytology or Any Methylation (PMR>0%) vs. Histology

Conclusions. Although the present study was limited by the fact that we were not able to test these algorithms in an independent sample, it appears that FNA and brush cytologic specimens can be more accurately classified as positive or negative for pancreatic cancer by including methylation analysis of tumor suppressor genes.

The variable mixture of tumor cells and normal cells is a major challenge when it comes to the molecular analysis of diagnostic or therapeutic targets in cytologic specimens. Cytologists are needed to play an active role in the adoption and application of molecular techniques, since we are able to interpret the results in the light of cytological morphology. Our pilot data holds promise for further research to conduct a genome wide search for additional aberrantly methylated genes with high sensitivity and specificity for pancreatic cancer and which are not methylated in other tissues (such as colon, liver, stomach, duodenum) which can be frequently or incidentally present as carry-over material in FNA and brush specimens from pancreatic lesions.

6. Aim 5: Achieving the full value of EUS-FNA with an integrated approach: A EUS-FNA case study

A 67-year-old woman was found to have a large retroperitoneal mass of uncertain etiology. The mass appears to invade the inferior vena cava and renal vein. Two prior attempts of CT and ultrasound guided biopsy were non-diagnostic due to the biopsy specimen consisting predominantly of necrotic tissue. Endoscopic ultrasound and enteroscopy were requested to re-evaluate the lesion and re-attempt biopsy.

In the initial effort of EUS-FNA, rare clusters of neoplastic cells having round nuclear contour, mild nuclear crowding and overlapping, vesicular chromatin pattern, and distinct nucleoli are noted in a background of extensive necrosis and blood. Fresh material sent for flow cytometry analysis contained an abnormal CD56- and EpCAM-positive population. Abnormal B or T cell populations were not identified. A cytologic impression was issued as: Positive for neoplasm with features suggestive of neuroendocrine origin. Before implementing chemotherapy as neuroendocrine tumor, our astute clinician ordered indiumIII octreotide scan for clinical correlation and found no evidence of focal radiotracer uptake in the abdominal mass. The diagnosis was subsequently felt not sufficiently conclusive for therapy as neuroendocrine neoplasia. A repeat biopsy was requested. During the second attempt of EUS-FNA, there was extrinsic appearing compression at the second, third, and fourth portions of the duodenum with no evidence of mucosal lesions or ulcerations. A large (greater than 12 cm) heterogeneous hypoechoic mass lesion was identified adjacent to the head and neck of the pancreas. One component of the mass appeared to be cystic (Figure 7, panel A, with needle inside the cystic area), and a more solid component was also identified (Figure 7, panel B). The former was sampled with FNA, the latter with a core biopsy. Nine total FNA passes were obtained with on-site immediate interpretation:

Pass 1 (core biopsy):Blood and necrotic material, non-diagnostic.

Pass 2 (core biopsy):Blood, necrotic material and sheets of bland epithelium. Additional diagnostic material requested.

Pass 3 (needle aspirate):Chiefly blood with atypical cells present.

Pass 4 (needle aspirate):Chiefly blood.

Pass 5 (needle aspirate):Chiefly blood.

Pass 6 (needle aspirate):Placed directly into saline.

Pass 7 (needle aspirate):Atypical cells present, defer to permanents.

Pass 8 (needle aspirate):Atypical cells present, defer to permanents.

Pass 9 (needle aspirate):Placed directly into saline for cell block preparation.

Many clusters of viable cells were obtained during the second attempt of EUS-FNA, displaying cytological features including three dimensional clusters, loose monolayer and individual monotonous cells, microfollicular pattern and nuclear grooves (coffee bean-like nuclei). The tumor cells are uniform and lack nuclear hyperchromasia and pleomorphism (Figure 7, panel C-E). Given the ample material obtained, a cell block was prepared and a more complete panel of antibodies for ICC was able to be performed, with the following results (19 antibody stains performed on cytology specimen, figure 7, panels E, F):

Antibody	Results
AE1/AE3	Positive, focally
CALRETININ	Positive
CD10	Negative
CD34	Negative
CD56	Positive, uniformly
CD68/KP-1	Negative
1A4	Positive, focally
DESMIN	Negative
S100	Negative
CHROMOGRANIN	Negative
SYNAPTOPHYSIN	Negative
C-KIT	Negative
INHIBIN	Positive, uniformly
MELAN A	Negative
CD45 (T200)	Negative
EMA	Negative
NSE	Positive, focally
ER (clone 1D5)	Negative
ER (clone SP1)	Positive

Table 9.

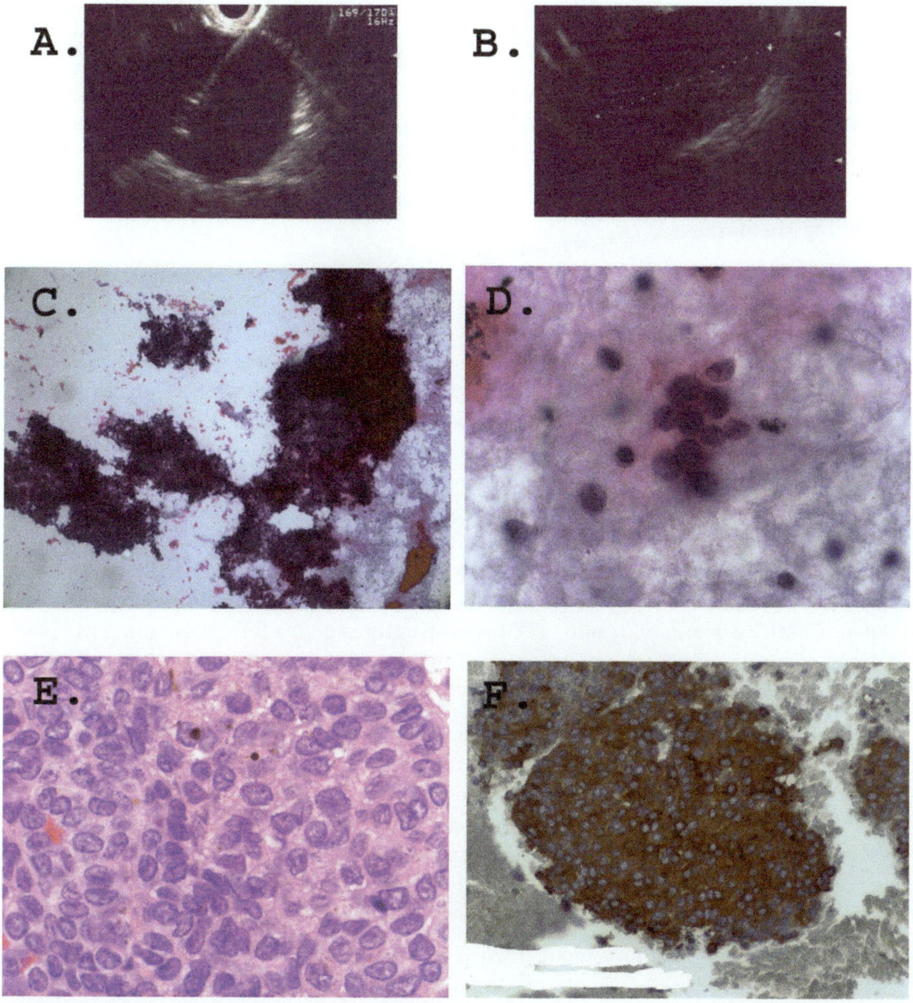

Figure 7. EUS-FNA diagnosis of granulosa cell tumor. A heterogeneous hypoechoic mass lesion identified by EUS. One component of the mass appearsto be cystic (panel A, with needle inside the cystic area); A more solid component (panel B); Ample viable material obtained on repeat EUS-FNA (panel C, Pap smear 100 x); Cytomorphology of neoplastic cells on smear (panel D, oil immersion, 1000 x); Cytomorphology of neoplastic cells on cell block section (panel E, oil immersion, 1000 x); Application of inhibin antibody on cell block section (panel F, 400 x).

The combined cytologic and immunophenotypic profile leads to the following final diagnosis:

Retroperitoneal mass, endoscopic ultrasound-guided FNA: Consistent with metastatic/ recurrent granulosa cell tumor. See comment.

Comment: The cytologic appearance of this tumor, along with the overall immuno-phenotype demonstrated by calretinin and inhibin positivity, supports the diagnosis of granulosa cell tumor. Additional studies performed at PhenoPath Laboratory using the more sensitive anti-ER antibody SP1 document expression of estrogen receptor (in contrast to the negative anti-ER studies using the 1D5 clone), further supporting the diagnosis of granulosa cell tumor.

After the diagnosis, patient recalls that she had a procedure for granulosa cell tumor about 30 years ago in Mexico.

Granulosa cell tumor may pose a diagnostic challenge in cytology preparations. First, there is some similarity between the granulosa tumor cells and reactive mesothelial cells. Indistinct cell borders, high nuclear cytoplasmic ratio and indentation of the nuclear membrane are helpful features in distinguishing granulosa tumor cells from mesothelial cells. Secondly, although nuclear features, especially nuclear grooves, are one of the classic features on granulosa cell tumor, they can also be seen in other ovarian tumors such as Brenner tumor and other sex cord-stromal tumor. Other characteristic histological features for granulosa cell tumor, such as Call-Exner bodies, a second population of elongated theca cells, are rarely evident on cytology specimens. Lastly, as occurred in our case, cells of carcinoid, especially pancreatic neuroendocrine tumors in this anatomic site, share many features of granulosa cells. Judicious use of a panel of immunocytochemistry (with the availability of sufficient sampling material) can be of great help in this scenario. Granulosa cell tumor is positive for inhibin, CD99, calretinin, vimentin, CD56, is generally negative for cytokeratin, EMA, Ber-Ep4, and is negative for neuroendocrine markers synaptophysin and chromogranin. Brenner tumor and other sex cord-stromal tumor usually are positive for cytokeratin and EMA.

As illustrated in this case, clinical-pathologic correlation is essential with octreotide scan preventing a diagnostic pitfall of neuroendocrine neoplasia. The on-site cytology interpretation performed for each of 9 EUS-FNA passes played a pivotal role in obtaining adequate viable diagnostic material, considering the sampling difficulty due to extensive tumor necrosis despite the apparent large size of the tumor by imaging study. A more complete ICC panel was thus able to be performed. The ICC results together with cytomorphology led to a diagnosis consistent with the subsequently retrieved clinical history.

Thus, our final note: the full value of FNA is only achieved with the integrated approach: the integration of clinical information, light microscopic analysis, results of ancillary studies, and even the gross appearance of the aspiration material will inform and lead us to a more accurate pathology diagnosis that can help tremendously in directing patient care.

Acknowledgements

The authors want to express their sincere gratitude to Drs. Nancy B. Kiviat (University of Washington, Seattle, WA), Melissa P. Upton (University of Washington, Seattle, WA) and Stephen J. Rulyak (Evergreen Medical Center, Gastroenterology, Seattle, WA), for their professional guidance, insightful discussions and tremendous technical support.

Author details

Lee-Ching Zhu[1*], Qinghua Feng[2] and Verena S. Grieco[3]

*Address all correspondence to: zhu.c@ghc.org

1 Anatomic Pathology, Group Health Permanente, Seattle, WA, USA

2 Department of Pathology, School of Medicine, University of Washington, Seattle, WA, USA

3 Harborview Medical Center, Anatomic Pathology, Seattle, WA, USA

References

[1] Rosch T, Lightdale CJ, Botet JF, et al:Localization of pancreatic endocrine tumors by endoscopic ultrasonography. N Engl J Med.1992;326(26):1721-26.

[2] Voss M, Hammel P, Molas G, et al:Value of endoscopic ultrasound guided fine needle aspiration biopsy in the diagnosis of solid pancreatic masses. Gut.Feb 2000;46(2): 244-9.

[3] Yoshinaga S, Suzuki H, Oda I, Saito Y:Role of endoscopic ultrasound-guided fine needle aspiration (EUS-FNA) for diagnosis of solid pancreatic masses.Dig Endosc; 2011 May;23Suppl 1:29-33.

[4] Zhang S, Defrias DV, Alasadi R, Nayar R:Endoscopic ultrasound-guided fine needle aspiration (EUS-FNA): experience of an academic centre in the USA. Cytopathology; 2010 Feb;21(1):35-43.

[5] Hwang CY, Lee SS, Song TJ, Moon SH, Lee D, Park do H, Seo DW, Lee SK, Kim MH:Endoscopic ultrasound guided fine needle aspiration biopsy in diagnosis of pancreatic and peripancreatic lesions: a single center experience in Korea. Gut Liver; 2009 Jun;3(2):116-21.

[6] Raddaoui E:Clinical utility and diagnostic accuracy of endoscopic ultrasound-guided fine needle aspiration of pancreatic lesions: Saudi Arabian experience.ActaCytol; 2011;55(1):26-9.

[7] Fisher L, Segarajasingam DS, Stewart C, Deboer WB, Yusoff IF:Endoscopic ultrasound guided fine needle aspiration of solid pancreatic lesions: Performance and outcomes.J GastroenterolHepatol; 2009 Jan;24(1):90-6.

[8] Nakahara O, Yamao K, Bhatia V, Sawaki A, Mizuno N, Takagi T, Shimizu Y, Koshikawa T, Yatabe Y, Baba H:Usefulness of endoscopic ultrasound-guided fine needle

aspiration (EUS-FNA) for undiagnosed intra-abdominal lymphadenopathy.J Gastroenterol; 2009;44(6):562-7.

[9] Moehler M, Voigt J, Kastor M, Heil M, Sengespeick C, Biesterfeld S, Dippold W, Kanzler S, Galle PR:Endoscopic ultrasonography-guided fine-needle aspiration (EUS-FNA) as primary diagnostic tool for unclear lesions in the upper gastrointestinal tract.Dtsch Med Wochenschr; 2011 Feb;136(7):303-8.

[10] Fritscher-Ravens A, Izbicki JR, Sriram PV, et al:Endosonography-guided, fine-needle aspiration cytology extending the indication for organ-preserving pancreatic surgery.Am J Gastroenterol. Sep 2000;95(9):2255-2260.

[11] Erickson, RA: EUS-guided FNA.GastrointestEndosc. 2004 Aug;60(2):267-79.

[12] De Bellis M, Sherman S, et al:Tissue sampling at ERCP in suspected malignant biliary strictures, part 1, GastrointestEndosc2002;56:552-61.

[13] De Bellis M, Sherman S, et al:Tissue sampling at ERCP in suspected malignant biliary strictures, part 2, GastrointestEndosc2002;56:720-30.

[14] Vandervoort J, Soetikno RM, et al:Accuracy and complication rate of brush cytology from bile duct versus pancreatic duct.GastrointestEndosc 1999;49:322-7.

[15] Rösch T, Lorenz R, Braig C et al: Endoscopic ultrasound in small pancreatic tumors. Z Gastroenterol 1991;29:110-5.

[16] Vilmann P, Saftoiu A:Endoscopic ultrasound-guided fine needle aspiration biopsy:equipment and technique.J GastroenterolHepatol.Nov2006;21(11):1646-1655.

[17] AabakkenL, Silvestri GA, Hawes R, et al:Cost-efficacy of endoscopic ultrasonography with fine-needle aspiration vs. mediastinotomy in patients with lung cancer and suspected mediastinaladenopathy.Endoscopy 1999;31:707-11.

[18] Harewood GC, Wiersema MJ, Edell ES, et al: Cost-minimization analysis of alternative diagnostic approaches in a modeled patient with non-small cell lung cancer and subcarinal lymphadenopathy.Mayo ClinProc 2002;77:155-64.

[19] Harewood GC, Wiersema MJ:A cost analysis of endoscopic ultrasound in the evaluation of esophageal cancer.Am J Gastroenterol 2002;97:452-8.

[20] Harewood GC, Wiersema MJ:A cost analysis of endoscopic ultrasound in the evaluation of pancreatic head adenocarcinoma.Am J Gastroeneerol 2001;96:2651-6.

[21] Chen VK, Arguedas MR, Kilgore ML, et al:A cost-minimization of analysis of alternative strategies in diagnosing pancreatic cancer.Am J Gastroenterol 2004;99:2223-34.

[22] O'Toole D, Palazzo L, Arotcarena R et al:Assessment of complications of EUS-guided fine-needle aspiration.GastrointestEndosc 2001;53:470-4.

[23] Chieng DC, JhalaD, Jhala N et al:Endoscopic ultrasound –guided fine-needle aspiration biopsy: a study of 103 cases. Cancer 2002;96:232-9.

[24] Dumonceau JM, Polkowski M, Larghi A, Vilmann P, Giovannini M, Frossard JL, Heresbach D, Pujol B, Fernández-EsparrachG, Vazquez-Sequeiros E, Ginès A:European Society of Gastrointestinal Endoscopy.Indications, results, and clinical impact of endoscopic ultrasound (EUS)-guided sampling in gastroenterology: European Society of Gastrointestinal Endoscopy (ESGE) Clinical Guideline.Endoscopy; 2011 Oct; 43(10):897-912.

[25] Exocrine pancreas.In: Greene FL, Page DL, Fleming ID, et al. editors. AJCC cancer staging handbook. 6thed. New York: Springer-Verlag;2002. p.182.

[26] Klapman JB, Chang KJ:Endoscopic ultrasound-guided fine-needle injection. GastrointestEndoscClin N Am. 2005 Jan;15(1):169-77.

[27] Tarantino I, Barresi, L:Interventional endoscopic ultrasound: Therapeutic capability and potential.World GastrointestEndosc 2009 Oct 15;1(1):39-44.

[28] Cho CM, Dewitt J, Ai-Haddad M:Echo-endoscopy: new therapeutic frontiers. Minerva GastroenterolDietol. 2011 Jun;57(2):139-58.

[29] Savides TJ, Donohue M, Hunt G, et al:EUS-guided FNA diagnostic yield of malignancy in solid pancreatic masses:a benchmark for quality performance measurement.GastrointestEndosc 2007;66:277-82.

[30] Layfield LJ, Bentz JS, and Gopez EV:Immediate on-site interpretation of fine-needle aspiration smears: a cost and compensation analysis.Cancer 2001;93319-322.

[31] Schwartz MR: Endoscopic ultrasound-guided fine-needel aspiration-time, diagnostic challenges and clnical impact. Cancer Cytopathology 2004;102(4):203-205.

[32] Klapman JB, Logrono R, Dye CE, et al:Clinical impact of on-site cytopathology interpretation on endoscopic ultrasound-guided fine needle aspiration.Am J Gastroenterol 2003;98:1289-94.

[33] Alsohaibani F, Girgis S, SandhaGS:Does onsite cytotechnology evaluation improve the accuracy of endoscopic ultrasound-guided fine-needle aspiration biopsy?Can J Gastroenterol. 2009 Jan;23(1):26-30.

[34] Jhala N, Jhala D,Etoum I, Vickers SM, et a:Endoscopic ultrasound-guided fine-needle aspiration biopsy: a powerful tool to obtain samples from small lesions.Cancer 2004;102(4):239-246.

[35] Erickson RA, Sayage-Rable L, Beissner S:Factors predicting the number of EUS-guided fine-needle passes for diagnosis of pancreatic malignancies. Gastrointestinal Endoscopy 2000;51(2):184-190.

[36] Jhala NC, Jhala DN, Chhieng DC, et a:Endoscopic ultrasound-guided fine-needle aspiration-a cytopathologist's perspective.AJCP 2003; 120(3):351-367.

[37] JhalaNC,Eltoum IA, Eloubeidi MA, et al:Providing on-site diagnosis of malignancy on endoscopic-ultrasound-guided fine-needle aspiration: should it be done?Annals DiagPathol 2007;11:176-181.

[38] Dumonceau JM, Koessler T, vanHooft JE, Fockens P:Endoscopic ultrasonography-guided fine needle aspiration: Relatively low sensitivity in the endosonographer population.World J Gastroenterol; 2012 May 21;18(19):2357-63.

[39] Iqbal S, Friedel D, Gupta M, Ogden L, Stavropoulos SN:Endoscopic-ultrasound-guided fine-needle aspiration and the role of the cytopathologist in solid pancreatic lesion diagnosis.Patholog Res Int; 2012;2012:317167.

[40] Cherian PT, Mohan P, Douiri A, Taniere P, Hejmadi RK, Mahon BS:Role of endoscopic ultrasound-guided fine-needle aspiration in the diagnosis of solid pancreatic and peripancreatic lesions: is onsite cytopathology necessary?HPB (Oxford); 2010 Aug;12(6):389-95.

[41] HikichiT, Irisawa A, Bhutani MS, et al:Endoscopic ultrasound-guided fine-needle aspiration of solid pancreatic masses with rapid on-site cytological evaluation by endosonographers without attendance of cytopathologists.J Gastroenterol2009;44(4):322-8.

[42] Nguyen YP, Maple, JT, Zhang, Q, et al:Reliability of gross visual assessment of specimen adequacy during EUS-guided FNA of pancreatic masses.GastrointestEndosc 2009;69(7):1264-70.

[43] Boujaoude J:Role of endoscopic ultrasound in diagnosis and therapy of pancreatic adenocarcinomas. World J Gastro 2007;13(27):3662-3666.

[44] Eltoum IA, Jhala CD, Crowe DR, et al:Cumulative sum procedure in evaluation of EUS-guided FNA cytology: the learning curve and diagnostic performance beyond sensitivity and specificity.Cytopathology 2007;18:143-50.

[45] Nasuti JF, Gupta PK and Baloch ZW:Diagnostic value and cost-effectiveness of on-site evaluation of fine-needle aspiration specimens: review of 5,688 cases.Diagn. Cytopathol. 2002;27:1-4.

[46] Shin HJC, Lahoti S, and Sneige N:Endoscopic ultrasound-guided fine-needle aspiration in 179 cases.Cancer (Cancer Cytopathol) 2002;96:174-80.

[47] Savoy AD, Raimondo M, Woodward TA, et al:Can endosonographers evaluate on-site cytologic adequacy?A comparison with cytotechnologists.GastrointestEndosc 2007;65(7):953-7.

[48] de Jong K, Poley JW, van Hooft JE, Visser M, Bruno MJ, Fockens P:Endoscopic ultrasound-guided fine-needle aspiration of pancreatic cystic lesions provides inadequate material for cytology and laboratory analysis: initial results from a prospective study.Endoscopy; 2011 Jul;43(7):585-90.

[49] Karim Z, Walker B, Lam E:Lymphoepithelial cysts of the pancreas: the use of endoscopic ultrasound-guided fine-needle aspiration in diagnosis.Can J Gastroenterol; 2010 Jun;24(6):348-50.

[50] Barresi L, Tarantino I, Granata A, Curcio G, Traina M:Pancreatic cystic lesions: How endoscopic ultrasound morphology and endoscopic ultrasound fine needle aspiration help unlock the diagnostic puzzle. World J GastrointestEndosc; 2012 Jun 16;4(6): 247-59.

[51] Bhatia V, Rastogi A, Saluja SS, Kumar M, Bihari C, Kalayarasan R, Gupta NL:Cystic pancreatic lymphangioma. The first report of a preoperative pathological diagnosis by endoscopic ultrasound-guided cyst aspiration. JOP; 2011 Sep;12(5):473-6.

[52] Coe AW, Evans J, Conway J:Pancreas cystic lymphangioma diagnosed with EUS-FNA. JOP; 2012 May;13(3):282-4.

[53] ZhuLC and Grieco V:Diagnostic value of unusual gross appearance of aspirated material from endoscopic ultrasound-guided fine needle aspiration of pancreatic and peripancreatic cystic lesions.ActaCytol. 2008 Sep-Oct;52(5):535-40.

[54] Dev V, Shah D, Gaw F, Lefor AT:Gastric outlet obstruction secondary to post cholecystectomy biloma:case report and review of the literature. JSLS. 1998;2(2):185-8.

[55] Chang ML, Lin DY:Symptomless cyst formation at the location of a biloma resolved with a single aspiration:case report. Chang Gung Med J. 2000;23(12):794-8.

[56] Ponnudurai, R:Endoscopic ultrasound-guided drainage of a biloma: A novel approach. Endoscopy 2006;38:199.

[57] Policarpio-Nicolas,ML, Shami VM, Kahaleh M, Adams RB, Mallery S, Stanley MW, Bardales RH, Stelow EB:Fine-needle aspiration cytology of pancreatic lymphoepithelial cysts. Cancer (Cancer Cytopathol) 2006;108:501-6.

[58] Fujiwara H, Kohno N, Nakaya S, Ishikawa Y:Lymphoepithelial cyst of the pancreas with sebaceous differentiation. J Gastroenterol 2000;35:396-401.

[59] Adsay NV:Cystic lesions of the pancreas.Modern Pathology, 2007;20:S71-S93.

[60] Solcia EN, Capella C, Kloppel G:Tumors of the pancreas. Fascicle 20 in Atlas of Tumor Pathology, 3rd series. Armed Forces Institute of Pathology, Washington DC:1997, 215-223.

[61] Weinstein LJ: Pancreas, in Cytology, Diagnostic principles and clinical correlates. Cibas ES and Ducatman BS, Saunders, Philadelphia 2003, 367-382.

[62] Zhu L and GriecoV:Identifying mucin on cytology specimens from EUS-FNA procedures.Digestive Disease Week, Washington, DC, 2007.

[63] Ringel J, Löhr M:The MUC gene family: their role in diagnosis and early detection of pancreatic cancer.Mol Cancer. 2003 Jan 7;2:9

[64] Hruban RH, Maitra A, Kern SE, Goggins M:Precursors to pancreatic cancer.GastroenterolClin North Am. 2007 Dec;36(4):831-49.

[65] Albores-Saavedra J, Simpson K, Dancer YJ, Hruban :.Intestinal type adenocarcinoma: a previously unrecognized histologic variant of ductal carcinoma of the pancreas.Ann DiagnPathol. 2007 Feb;11(1):3-9.

[66] Furukawa T, Klöppel G, VolkanAdsay N, et al:Classification of types of intraductal papillary-mucinous neoplasm of the pancreas: a consensus study.Virchows Arch. 2005 Nov;447(5):794-9. Epub2005 Aug 9.

[67] Giorgadze TA, Peterman H, Baloch ZW, Furth EE, Pasha T, Shiina N, Zhang PJ, Gupta PK:Diagnostic utility of mucin profile in fine-needle aspiration specimens of the pancreas: an immunohistochemical study with surgical pathology correlation.2006 Jun 25;108(3):186-97.

[68] Zhu L and Peck A: Endoscopic ultrasound guided fine needle aspiration of pancreatic endocrine neoplasms:Diagnostic challenges and the role of immunocytochemistry.Check Sample, ASCP, 2008.

[69] Eloubeidi MA, Tamhane AR, Buxbaum J:Unusual, metastatic, or neuroendocrine tumor of the pancreas:a diagnosis with endoscopic ultrasound-guided fine-needle aspiration and immunohistochemistry.Saudi J Gastroenterol;2012 Mar-Apr;18(2):99-105.

[70] Chang F, Vu C, Chandra A, Meenan J, Herbert A:Endoscopic ultrasound-guided fine needle aspiration cytology of pancreatic neuroendocrine tumours: cytomorphological and immunocytochemical evaluation. Cytopathology. Feb 2006;17(1):10-17.

[71] NotoharaK,Hamazaki S, Tsukayama C, et al:Solid-pseudopapillary tumor of the pancreas: immunohistochemical localization of neuroendocrine markers and CD10. Am J SurgPathol. Oct 2000;24(10):1361-1371.

[72] Portela-Gomes GM, Hacker GW, Weitgasser R:Neuroendocrine cell markers for pancreatic islets and tumors.ApplImmunohistochemMolMorphol. 2004 Sep;12(3):183-92.

[73] Carlsson J:Potential for clinical radionuclide-based imaging and therapy of common cancers expressing EGFR-family receptors.Tumour Biol. 2012 Jun;33(3):653-9. Epub 2012 Jan 7.

[74] Matthaios D, Zarogoulidis P, Balgouranidou I, Chatzaki E, Kakolyris S:Molecular pathogenesis of pancreatic cancer and clinical perspectives.Oncology. 2011;81(3-4): 259-72. Epub 2011 Nov 23.

[75] Stella GM, Luisetti M, Inghilleri S, CemmiF,Scabini R, Zorzetto M, Pozzi E:Targeting EGFR in non-small-cell lung cancer: lessons, experiences, strategies.Respir Med. 2012 Feb;106(2):173-83. Epub 2011 Nov 21

[76] Bohanes P, LaBonte MJ, Winder T, Lenz HJ:Predictive molecular classifiers in colorectal cancer.SeminOncol. 2011 Aug;38(4):576-87.

[77] Cervera P, Fléjou JF:Changing pathology with changing drugs: tumors of the gastrointestinal tract.Pathobiology.2011;78(2):76-89. doi: 10.1159/000315535. Epub 2011 Jun 15.

[78] Saijo N:Critical comments for roles of biomarkers in the diagnosis and treatment of cancer.Cancer Treat Rev. 2012 Feb;38(1):63-7. Epub 2011 Jun 8.

[79] William WN Jr:Oral premalignant lesions: any progress with systemic therapies?CurrOpinOncol. 2012 May;24(3):205-10.

[80] Smith RA, Tang J, Tudur-Smith C, Neoptolemos JP, Ghaneh P:Meta-analysis of immunohistochemical prognostic markers in resected pancreatic cancer.Br J Cancer. 2011 Apr 26;104(9):1440-51. Epub 2011 Mar 29. Review.

[81] Larsen AK, Ouaret D, El Ouadrani K, Petitprez A:Targeting EGFR and VEGF(R) pathway cross-talk in tumor survival and angiogenesis.PharmacolTher. 2011 Jul; 131(1):80-90. Epub 2011 Mar 23.

[82] Murphy M, Stordal B:Erlotinib or gefitinib for the treatment of relapsed platinum pretreated non-small cell lung cancer and ovarian cancer: a systematic review.Drug Resist Updat. 2011 Jun;14(3):177-90. Epub 2011 Mar 24.

[83] Iacopetta B, Grieu F, Amanuel B:Microsatellite instability in colorectalcancer.Asia Pac J ClinOncol. 2010 Dec;6(4):260-9. doi: 10.1111/j.1743-7563.2010.01335.x. Epub 2010 Oct 26.

[84] Imai K, Yamamoto H:Carcinogenesis and microsatellite instability: the interrelationship between genetics and epigenetics.Carcinogenesis. 2008 Apr;29(4):673-80. Epub 2007 Oct 17.

[85] Lawes DA, SenGupta S, BoulosPB:The clinical importance and prognostic implications of microsatellite instability in sporadic cancer.Eur J SurgOncol. 2003 Apr;29(3): 201-12.

[86] Chapusot C, Martin L, Puig PL, Ponnelle T, Cheynel N, Bouvier AM, Rageot D, Roignot P, Rat P, Faivre J, Piard F:What is the best way to assess microsatellite instability status in colorectal cancer? Study on a population base of 462 colorectalcancers.Am J SurgPathol. 2004 Dec;28(12):1553-9.

[87] Shia J, Ellis NA, Paty PB, Nash GM, Qin J, Offit K, Zhang XM, Markowitz AJ, Nafa K, Guillem JG, Wong WD, Gerald WL, KlimstraDS:Value of histopathology in predicting microsatellite instability in hereditarynonpolyposiscolorectal cancer and sporadic colorectalcancer.Am J SurgPathol. 2003 Nov;27(11):1407-17.

[88] Edmonston TB, Cuesta KH, Burkholder S, Barusevicius A, Rose D, Kovatich AJ, Boman B, Fry R, Fishel R, Palazzo JP:Colorectal carcinomas with high microsatellite instability: defining a distinct immunologic and molecular entity with respect to prognosticmarkers.Hum Pathol. 2000 Dec;31(12):1506-14.

[89] Kouniavsky G, Zeiger MA:The quest for diagnostic molecular markers for thyroid nodules with indeterminate or suspicious cytology.J SurgOncol. 2012 Apr 1;105(5): 438-43.

[90] Bartolazzi A, Bellotti C, Sciacchitano S:Methodology and technical requirements of the galectin-3 test for the preoperative characterization of thyroidnodules.ApplImmunohistochemMolMorphol. 2012 Jan;20(1):2-7. Review.

[91] Freitas BC, Cerutti J:.Genetic markers differentiating follicular thyroid carcinoma from benign lesions.Mol Cell Endocrinol. 2010 May 28;321(1):77-85. Epub 2009 Nov 20.

[92] Nikiforova MN, NikiforovYE:Molecular diagnostics and predictors in thyroid cancer.Thyroid. 2009 Dec;19(12):1351-61.

[93] Arora N, Scognamiglio T, Zhu B, Fahey TJ 3rd:Do benign thyroid nodules have malignant potential? An evidence-based review.World J Surg. 2008 Jul;32(7):1237-46.

[94] Carpi A, Nicolini A, Marchetti C, Iervasi G, Antonelli A, Carpi F:Percutaneous large-needle aspiration biopsy histology of palpable thyroid nodules: technical and diagnostic performance.Histopathology. 2007 Aug;51(2):249-57.

[95] Kapur U, WojcikEM:Follicular neoplasm of the thyroid--vanishing cytologicdiagnosis?DiagnCytopathol. 2007 Aug;35(8):525-8.

[96] Ogilvie JB, Piatigorsky EJ, Clark OH:Current status of fine needle aspiration for thyroidnodules.Adv Surg. 2006;40:223-38.

[97] Carpi A, Mechanick JI, Nicolini A, Rubello D, Iervasi G, Bonazzi V, Giardino :Thyroid nodule evaluation: what have we really learned from recent clinical guidelines? BiomedPharmacother. 2006 Sep;60(8):393-5. Epub 2006 Aug 4.

[98] Mechanick JI, Carpi A:Progress in the preoperative diagnosis of thyroid nodules: managing uncertainties and the ultimate role for molecularinvestigation.Biomed-Pharmacother. 2006 Sep;60(8):396-404. Epub 2006 Aug 1

[99] Lambros MB, Natrajan R, Reis-FilhoJS:Chromogenic and fluorescent in situ hybridization in breast cancer.HumPathol. 2007 Aug;38(8):1105-22.

[100] Lee JA, Shaheen M, Walke T, Daly M:Clinical and health economic outcomes of alternative HER2 test strategies for guiding adjuvant trastuzumabtherapy.Expert Rev Pharmacoecon Outcomes Res. 2011 Jun;11(3):325-41.

[101] Ross JS:Update on HER2 testing for breast and upper gastrointestinal tract cancers.Biomark Med. 2011 Jun;5(3):307-18.

[102] Penault-Llorca F, Bilous M, Dowsett M, Hanna W, OsamuraRY, Rüschoff J, van de Vijver M:Emerging technologies for assessing HER2amplification.Am J ClinPathol. 2009 Oct;132(4):539-48.

[103] Ross JS:Breast cancer biomarkers and HER2 testing after 10 years of anti-HER2therapy.Drug News Perspect. 2009 Mar;22(2):93-106.

[104] Sauter G, Lee J, Bartlett JM, Slamon DJ, Press MF:Guidelines for human epidermal growth factor receptor 2 testing: biologic and methodologicconsiderations.JClinOncol. 2009 Mar 10;27(8):1323-33. Epub 2009 Feb 9.

[105] Cuadros M, Villegas R:Systematicreview of HER2breast cancer testing.ApplImmunohistochemMolMorphol. 2009 Jan;17(1):1-7.

[106] Bayani J, Squire JA:Fluorescence in situ Hybridization (FISH).CurrProtocCell Biol. 2004 Sep;Chapter 22:Unit 22.4.

[107] Shabaik A, Lin G, Peterson M, HastehF, Tipps A, Datnow B, Weidner N:Reliability of Her2/neu, estrogen receptor, and progesterone receptor testing by immunohistochemistry on cell block of FNA and serous effusions from patients with primary and metastatic breast carcinoma.DiagnCytopathol. 2011 May;39(5):328-32.

[108] Hanley KZ, Birdsong GG, Cohen C, SiddiquiMT:Immunohistochemical detection of estrogen receptor, progesterone receptor, and human epidermal growth factor receptor 2 expression in breast carcinomas: comparison on cell block, needle-core, and tissue block preparations.Cancer. 2009 Aug 25;117(4):279-88.

[109] Barroca H, Carvalho JL, da Costa MJ,Cirnes L, Seruca R, Schmitt FC:Detection of N-myc amplification in neuroblastomas using Southern blotting on fine needle aspirates.ActaCytol. 2001 Mar-Apr;45(2):169-72.

[110] Fröstad B, Martinsson T, Tani E, Falkmer U, Darnfors C, Skoog L, Kogner P:The use of fine-needle aspiration cytology in the molecular characterization of neuroblastoma in children.Cancer. 1999 Apr 25;87(2):60-8.

[111] Constantinou M, Binka-Kowalska A, Borkowska E, Zajac E, Jałmuzna P, Matych J, Nawrocka A, Kałuzewski B:Application of multiplexFISH, CGH and MSSCP techniques for cytogenetic and molecular analysis of transitional cell carcinoma (TCC) cells in voided urine specimens.J Appl Genet. 2006;47(3):273-5.

[112] Halling KC, KippBR:Bladder cancer detection using FISH (UroVysion assay).AdvAnatPathol. 2008 Sep;15(5):279-86.

[113] vanRhijn BW, van der Poel HG, van der KwastTH:Urine markers for bladder cancer surveillance: a systematic review.Eur Urol. 2005 Jun;47(6):736-48. Epub 2005 Mar 23.

[114] Dey P:Urinary markers of bladder carcinoma.ClinChimActa. 2004 Feb;340(1-2):57-65.

[115] Feng Q, Balasubramanian, A, Hawes SE et al:Detection of hypermethylated genes in women with and without cervical neoplasia.J Natl Cancer Inst 2005;97:273-82.

[116] Hawes SE, Stern JE, Feng Q, Wiens LW, Rasey JS, Lu H, Kiviat NB, Vesselle H:DNA-hypermethylation of tumors from non-small cell lung cancer (NSCLC) patients is as-

sociated with gender and histologic type.Lung Cancer. 2010 Aug;69(2):172-9. Epub 2009 Nov 28.

[117] Feng Q, Deftereos G, Hawes SE, Stern JE, Willner JB, Swisher EM, Xi L, Drescher C, Urban N, Kiviat NB:DNA hypermethylation, Her-2/neu overexpression and p53 mutations in ovarian carcinoma.GynecolOncol. 2008 Nov;111(2):320-9. Epub 2008 Aug 30.

[118] Feng Q, Hawes SE, Stern JE, Dem A, Sow PS, Dembele B, Toure P, Sova P, Laird PW, Kiviat NB:Promoter hypermethylation of tumor suppressor genes in urine from patients with cervical neoplasia.CancerEpidemiol Biomarkers Prev. 2007 Jun;16(6):1178-84.

Permissions

The contributors of this book come from diverse backgrounds, making this book a truly international effort. This book will bring forth new frontiers with its revolutionizing research information and detailed analysis of the nascent developments around the world.

We would like to thank Assoc. Prof. Somchai Amornyotin MD, FRCAT, for lending his expertise to make the book truly unique. He has played a crucial role in the development of this book. Without his invaluable contribution this book wouldn't have been possible. He has made vital efforts to compile up to date information on the varied aspects of this subject to make this book a valuable addition to the collection of many professionals and students.

This book was conceptualized with the vision of imparting up-to-date information and advanced data in this field. To ensure the same, a matchless editorial board was set up. Every individual on the board went through rigorous rounds of assessment to prove their worth. After which they invested a large part of their time researching and compiling the most relevant data for our readers. Conferences and sessions were held from time to time between the editorial board and the contributing authors to present the data in the most comprehensible form. The editorial team has worked tirelessly to provide valuable and valid information to help people across the globe.

Every chapter published in this book has been scrutinized by our experts. Their significance has been extensively debated. The topics covered herein carry significant findings which will fuel the growth of the discipline. They may even be implemented as practical applications or may be referred to as a beginning point for another development. Chapters in this book were first published by InTech; hereby published with permission under the Creative Commons Attribution License or equivalent.

The editorial board has been involved in producing this book since its inception. They have spent rigorous hours researching and exploring the diverse topics which have resulted in the successful publishing of this book. They have passed on their knowledge of decades through this book. To expedite this challenging task, the publisher supported the team at every step. A small team of assistant editors was also appointed to further simplify the editing procedure and attain best results for the readers.

Our editorial team has been hand-picked from every corner of the world. Their multi-ethnicity adds dynamic inputs to the discussions which result in innovative outcomes. These outcomes are then further discussed with the researchers and contributors who give their valuable feedback and opinion regarding the same. The feedback is then collaborated with the researches and they are edited in a comprehensive manner to aid the understanding of the subject.

Apart from the editorial board, the designing team has also invested a significant amount of their time in understanding the subject and creating the most relevant covers. They scrutinized every image to scout for the most suitable representation of the subject and create an appropriate cover for the book.

The publishing team has been involved in this book since its early stages. They were actively engaged in every process, be it collecting the data, connecting with the contributors or procuring relevant information. The team has been an ardent support to the editorial, designing and production team. Their endless efforts to recruit the best for this project, has resulted in the accomplishment of this book. They are a veteran in the field of academics and their pool of knowledge is as vast as their experience in printing. Their expertise and guidance has proved useful at every step. Their uncompromising quality standards have made this book an exceptional effort. Their encouragement from time to time has been an inspiration for everyone.

The publisher and the editorial board hope that this book will prove to be a valuable piece of knowledge for researchers, students, practitioners and scholars across the globe.

List of Contributors

Karel Geboes
Department of Pathology, University of Leuven KUL, Leuven, Belgium

Anne Jouret-Mourin
Department of Pathology, Saint Luc Hospital, UCL, Brussels, Belgium

Karen Geboes
Department of Gastroenterology, Digestive Oncology, University of Gent, Gent, Belgium

George Pados, Anastasios Makedos and Basil Tarlatzis
1st Dept. of OB-GYN, School of Medicine, Aristotle University of Thessaloniki, General Hospital, N. Efkarpia, Greece

Somchai Amornyotin
Department of Anesthesiology and Siriraj GI Endoscopy Center, Faculty of Medicine, Siriraj Hospital, Mahidol University, Bangkok, Thailand

Petr Lukes, Michal Zabrodsky, Jaroslav Betka, Eva Foltynova and Jan Betka
Department of Otorhinolaryngology, Head and Neck Surgery, First Faculty of Medicine, Charles University in Prague and University Hospital Motol, Czech Republic

Jan Plzak and Martin Chovanec
Department of Otorhinolaryngology, Head and Neck Surgery, First Faculty of Medicine, Charles University in Prague and University Hospital Motol, Czech Republic
Institute of Anatomy, First Faculty of Medicine, Charles University in Prague, Czech Republic

Pongsakorn Tantilipikorn
Division of Rhinology & Allergy, Faculty of Medicine Siriraj Hospital, Mahidol University, Bangkok, Thailand

Charles A. Elmaraghy and Kris R. Jatana
Department of Pediatric Otolaryngology-Head and Neck Surgery, Nationwide Children's Hospital, Columbus, Ohio, USA
Department of Otolaryngology-Head and Neck Surgery, Wexner Medical Center at The Ohio State University, Columbus, Ohio, USA

Timothy P. McEvoy
Department of Pediatric Otolaryngology-Head and Neck Surgery, Nationwide Children's Hospital, Columbus, Ohio, USA

Rickul Varshney, Faisal Zawawi, Marc A Tewfik and Saul Frenkiel
McGill University, Jewish General Hospital, 3755 Chemin de la Cote-Sainte-Catherine, Montreal, Quebec, Canada

Mihai Olteanu, Costin Teodor Streba, Bogdan Oprea, Raluca Marinas, Mimi Floarea Nitu and Tudorel Ciurea
University of Medicine and Pharmacy of Craiova, Romania

Emilia Crisan
University of Medicine and Pharmacy of Craiova, Romania
"Marius Nasta" Pulmonology Institute, Bucharest, Romania

Alexander Aloy
Department of Anaesthesia and General Intensive Care Medicine, Vienna, Austria

Matthaeus Grasl
Department of Otorhinolaryngology, Head & Neck Surgery, Vienna, Austria

R. Peric, M. de Mol, N. van Walree and J.G. Aerts
Department of Pulmonary Diseases Erasmus MC Rotterdam and Amphia Hospital Breda, The Netherlands

Nurten Akyurek Savas
Baskent University, Department of Gastroenterology, Istanbul Hospital, Turkey

Paul Mitrut and Liliana Streba
Department of Internal Medicine, University of Medicine and Pharmacy of Craiova, Romania

Anca Oana Docea and Cornelia - Daniela Calina
Department of Pharmacology, University of Medicine and Pharmacy of Craiova, Romania

Puru Naidu, Jessica Packer, Maheshi Samaraweera and John G. Calleary
Department of Urology, Morth Manchester General Hospital, UK

D. Sorrentino
Department of Gastroenterology, Nambour General Hospital, University of Queensland, Australia
Sunshine Coast Clinical School, Australia
University of Udine Medical School, Udine, Italy

J. Van Den Bogaerde
Department of Gastroenterology, Nambour General Hospital, University of Queensland, Australia
Sunshine Coast Clinical School, Australia

Lee-Ching Zhu
Anatomic Pathology, Group Health Permanente, Seattle, WA, USA

Qinghua Feng
Department of Pathology, School of Medicine, University of Washington, Seattle, WA, USA

Verena S. Grieco
Harborview Medical Center, Anatomic Pathology, Seattle, WA, USA